BRAIN MAPPING RESEARCH PROGRESS

BRAIN MAPPING RESEARCH PROGRESS

INES C. GIRARD
AND
JADE S. ANDRE
EDITORS

Nova Biomedical Books
New York

For permission to use material from this book please contact us:
Telephone 631-231-7269; Fax 631-231-8175
Web Site: http://www.novapublishers.com

Library of Congress Cataloging-in-Publication Data

Brain mapping research progress / [edited by]
Ines C. Girard and Jade S. Andre.
p. ; cm.
Includes bibliographical references and index.
ISBN 978-1-60456-784-7 (hardcover)
1. Brain mapping. I. Girard, Ines C. II. Andre, Jade S.
[DNLM: 1. Brain Mapping. 2. Brain--physiology. WL 335 B81429 2009]
RC386.6.B7B633 2009
616.8'0475--dc22

2008050991

Published by Nova Science Publishers, Inc. ✢ New York

Contents

Preface		**vii**
Chapter I	**Neural Signal Estimation through Time-Resolved Functional Imaging** *C.W. Tyler and L.T. Likova*	**1**
Chapter II	**DNA Damage Response and Apoptosis of Postmitotic Neurons** *Inna I. Kruman and Elena I. Schwartz*	**33**
Chapter III	**Hallmarks of Apoptotic-Like Cell Death in Response to Hypoxic Injury in Various Developmental Models Are Closely Related to Brain Immaturity** *Jean-Luc Daval and Christiane Charriaut-Marlangue*	**57**
Chapter IV	**The Use of Neural Stem Cells in Treating Traumatic Brain Injury in Rats** *Shu-Yuan Yang and Hui Liu*	**75**
Chapter V	**Subdural Interictal EEG Analysis for Extracting Discriminating Features towards Electrode Classification Using Artificial Neural Networks** *Mercedes Cabrerizo, Malek Adjouadi, Melvin Ayala and Prasanna Jayakar*	**87**
Chapter VI	**Laboratory Memory Tasks and Autobiographical Recollection: Cognitive and Neurofunctional Evidence for Differential Forms of Episodic Memory** *Martina Piefke*	**109**
Chapter VII	**Brain Electric Source Imaging by an Iterative Correlation Matrix Based Multiple Signal Classification Approach** *Dezhong Yao*	**137**
Chapter VIII	**Mapping of Brain Operational Architectonics** *Andrew A. Fingelkurts and Alexander A. Fingelkurts*	**157**

Chapter IX **Neural Mechanisms in Anxiety and Panic** **199**
Marcus Lira Brandão and Julia Maria dos Santos

Chapter X **Phase Synchronization at Different Frequency Bands Induced by the Emotional Film Stimuli of Happiness, Sadness and Fear** **219**
Tommaso Costa, Elena Rognoni, Dario Galati and Manuella Crini

Index **247**

Preface

Brain mapping is a set of neuroscience techniques predicated on the mapping of (biological) quantities or properties onto spatial representations of the (human or non-human) brain resulting in maps. All neuroimaging can be considered to be a part of brain mapping. Brain mapping techniques are constantly evolving, and rely on the development and refinement of image acquisition, representation, analysis, visualization and interpretation techniques. Functional and structural neuroimaging are at the core of the mapping aspect of brain mapping. This book presents the latest research in the field.

An algorithm dedicated at discriminating between electrodes that lead to a seizure onset as opposed to those electrodes that do not, are examined in this book by using interictal subdural EEG data.

The most effective method for localizing the effects of neural activation throughout the human brain is Functional Magnetic Resonance Imaging (fMRI). This book provides a new level of specificity in the basis of advanced approaches of using fMRI to study brain function as deep as at the level of the neural processing.

Programmed cell death or apoptosis is a relevant process in the physiology and pathology of the nervous system. DNA damage response in postmitotic neurons is discussed and the elucidation of these mechanisms, which promise to provide multiple points of therapeutic intervention in neurodegenerative diseases, are examined as well.

This book explains the temporal features of brain injury in three different developmental models of oxygen deprivation, capable of inducing apoptotic cell death. The hallmarks of hypoxia-induced apoptosis that may vary according to brain maturity, are also looked at. In addition, the neuroprotective effect of transplants of Neural Stem Cells (NSCs) after experimental traumatic brain injury were investigated and are discussed in this book.

Chapter I – The most effective method for localizing the effects of neural activation throughout the human brain is Functional Magnetic Resonance Imaging (fMRI). However, there is currently no method able to derive from the fMRI signal the particular neural signals underlying the measured BOLD waveforms. The goal of the present analysis is therefore to achieve time-resolved estimation of the neural signals determining the temporal waveforms in event-related fMRI. This analysis provides a new level of specificity in the basis of advanced approaches of using fMRI to study brain function as deep as at the level of the neural processing. In particular, we can resolve details of neural response dynamics down to the millisecond level for the analysis of visual processing and its temporal deficits.

For this purpose, the authors develop a nonlinear dynamic forward model of the metabolic demand arising from the transmitter release in the minimal set of component neural populations that account for each fMRI waveform. This model allows derivation of the neural signals underlying the wide variety fMRI waveforms evoked from even the most elementary brief stimuli. Estimation of signal delays between cortical regions is enhanced by an autonormalization procedure to provide maximum temporal precision in mapping the causal interactions among functional subunits across the cortex by means of the pattern of simultaneous covariation in the fMRI responses. This technique is also robust to feedback processes, allowing the mapping of recursive feedback signal between cortical regions at different levels in the response hierarchy.

Chapter II – Programmed cell death or apoptosis is a relevant process in the physiology and pathology of the nervous system. Apoptosis is an organized form of cell death which is triggered by different factors including DNA damage. A growing body of evidence suggests that DNA damage and genomic instability are involved in neuronal abnormalities and may play a central role in neurodegeneration. DNA strand breaks and DNA lesions have been reported in Parkinson's and Alzheimer's diseases and as an early event after reperfusion of ischemic brain. DNA damage has been found to activate a cell death program in terminally differentiated postmitotic neurons. Since the genome is continuously damaged by a variety of endogenous and exogenous agents and the majority of DNA damage is produced by oxyradicals, generated by normal aerobic metabolism, neurons are particularly susceptible to DNA damage due to the high rate of oxidative metabolism. To maintain genomic integrity, cells are equipped with special defense mechanism, DNA damage response, to remove DNA damage by DNA repair pathways or eliminate damaged cells via apoptosis. Generally, differentiated cells, like neurons, are deficient in DNA repair and more vulnerable to DNA damage-initiated apoptosis. For example, neurons are more vulnerable than astrocytes to DNA-damaging conditions such as ionizing radiation. Breast cancer patients receiving hemotherapy commonly experience long-lasting cognitive impairment. It is known that radiotherapy may cause CNS toxicity. DNA damaging agents including γ-irradiation induce neuronal apoptosis *in vitro*, suggesting the direct adverse effect of these DNA damaging agents on neurons. The importance of DNA repair for neuronal survival is illustrated by disorders observed in patients with hereditary DNA repair abnormalities. These disorders combine the predisposition to cancer with progressive neurodegeneration. Although indirect evidence suggests that DNA damage and repair mechanisms play critical roles in neuronal survival, the pathways involved are poorly understood. Recently, the authors found that cell cycle activation is essential for DNA damage-induced neuronal apoptosis which suggests that the cell cycle machinery is a critical element of the DNA damage response not only in cycling but also in quiescent cells. Here, the authors discuss the DNA damage response in postmitotic neurons and possible mechanisms by which neurons are forced to apoptosis versus DNA repair thereby controlling cell fate. Elucidation of these mechanisms promises to provide multiple points of therapeutic intervention in neurodegenerative diseases.

Chapter III – With regard to the specificity of the developing brain, a better understanding of cellular mechanisms involved in perinatal hypoxic-ischemic injury would help to prevent neurological impairments. The authors therefore examined temporal features of brain injury in three different developmental models of oxygen deprivation capable of inducing apoptotic cell death. Nuclear staining by DAPI (4,6-diamidino-2-phenylindole) was used to identify healthy, apoptotic and necrotic nuclei as well as for cell counting in cultures and brain sections. DNA fragmentation was monitored by in situ terminal dUTP nick end labeling (TUNEL) and electrophoresis on agarose gels. Also, the expression profile of apoptosis-related proteins Bax and Bcl-2 was studied by immunohistochemistry. In all cases, oxygen deprivation induced significant delayed cell death with morphological features of apoptosis and a progressive increase in the Bax/Bcl-2 protein ratio, except in the penumbra of the ischemic infarct where Bcl-2 remained predominant. As in the control newborn brain that still exhibited physiological death, hypoxia-associated DNA breakdown led to small fragments of ~200 bp in the cortex of hypoxic rat pups. Ladder pattern and TUNEL-positive cells exhibiting apoptotic bodies were only present in the penumbra of 7 day-old ischemic rats. These data indicate that hallmarks of hypoxia-induced apoptosis may vary according to brain maturity, possibly through specific nuclease activities. While retaining a part of the developmental death program, the newborn brain seems to be prone to an apoptotic-like response that resembles physiological programmed death.

Chapter IV – Objective

In this study the authors investigated the neuroprotective effect of transplants of Neural Stem Cells (NSCs) after experimental traumatic brain injury.

Methods

NSCs were derived from human fetal hippocampi. The cells were injected into the cerebral cortex of rats subjected to experimental traumatic brain injury. The effect on the motor function scores of the rats was assessed. The techniques of immunohistochemistry and TUNEL were applied to define the NSCs' differentiation and neuroprotection.

Results

Brain injured animals that received transplants of NSCs had marked and significantly improved motor scores compared with control groups. Animals that received NSCs transplants had significantly more surviving neurons compared with the vehicle treated brain injured rats.

In situ TUNEL assay demonstrated fewer apoptotic cells in animals that received NSCs transplants than those of the control group.

Conclusions

These results demonstrate the neuroprotective and functional efficacy of NSC transplants after experimental traumatic brain injury.

Chapter V – This study introduces an algorithm dedicated at discriminating between electrodes that lead to a seizure onset from those electrodes that do not, using interictal subdural EEG data. The significance of this study is in classifying among all of these channels, all containing interictal spikes that are asynchronous and independent of location, which are selected randomly, those channels that lead to seizure from those that do not with the purpose of focusing the attention on those electrodes during epileptogenic focus localization. The main epileptogenic focus is supposed to evolve from the tissue located at the channels that present interictal activity, but sometimes this is no the case. The purpose is to gain a better understanding of the dynamics of subdural EEG, while characterizing the common behaviors of interictal EEG channels prior to an ictal activity. The merits of this algorithm are: (a) its fast computational time and (b) its integrated signal processing design that identifies based on different parameters, electrodes leading or not to seizure. EEG signals were transformed into quantitative measures to account for those morphological characteristics of interictal signals deemed important in the classification process of channels leading or not to a seizure.

Chapter VI – The classic model of episodic memory refers to both laboratory tasks requiring the conscious recall or recognition of experimental materials and autobiographical recollection of one's personal past experiences. Recent research in cognitive neuroscience, however, showed evidence that laboratory and autobiographical memory may share aspects of conscious retrieval and reference to the temporal and spatial context at the time of encoding of information, but are different from each other in some important respects. The autobiographical memory domain is characterized by self-referential information processing, subjective emotional evaluation of memories, and the accompanying autonoetic conscious awareness. In contrast, laboratory episodic memory requires the effortful search for impersonal target information and the intentional use of retrieval strategies. Subregions of the prefrontal, medial temporal, and retrosplenial cortices appear to be differentially involved in the neural processing of each type of episodic memory, thus suggesting that they are supported by anatomically and functionally overlapping, but also segregated neural circuits. The empirical data reviewed here support the view that laboratory and autobiographical episodic memory can at least in part be distinguished on the cognitive-behavioral and the neurofunctional levels. Accordingly, the review proposes an integrated view of laboratory and autobiographical forms of episodic memory which accounts for an overlap, but also emphasizes the unique features distinguishing the two memory types.

Chapter VII – How to localize the neural electric activities effectively and precisely from the scalp EEG recordings is a critical issue for clinical neurology and cognitive neuroscience. In the 1980s and 1990s, suggested approaches included the dipole localization, cortical imaging, scalp Laplacian and 3D tomography. The 3D tomography may be realized by a direct linear inversion, or an indirect algorithm such as the subspace projection scanning method named MUltiple SIgnal Classification (MUSIC). However, the classical MUSIC algorithm is limited for its assumption of random noise. In this work, the authors propose to use a delay-correlation matrix instead of the previous zero-delay-correlation matrix in the signal-subspace estimate of the MUSIC algorithm to get a better performance over a spatial coherent but temporal random noisy disturbance. Then an Iterative application of the Delay-correlation MUSIC (IDM) is emphasized to derive a reasonable reconstruction of the multi-sources. The present simulation and empirical data experiment show that final promising results are obtained.

Chapter VIII – Recent neuroscience is lacking of consistent theory and methods for understanding the mechanisms through which the brain orchestrate the symphony of perceptions, thoughts and actions. The aim of this Chapter is to contribute to a better understanding of such mechanisms by establishing methodological foundations of the Operational Architectonics framework of brain and mind functioning. The theory the authors offer provides a framework for mapping and understanding important aspects of the brain mechanisms that constitute perception, cognition, and eventually consciousness.

Chapter IX – Depending on the nature of the aversive stimuli or threatening conditions different types of fear responses are elaborated in the brain. Conditioning procedures using light, tones and contexts used as conditioned stimuli associated to unconditioned stimuli of moderate intensity causes orientated and active forms of defense reaction. Organized and oriented defense reactions seem to be linked to anxiety. On the other hand, intense fear conditioning or past experience with stressful situations originate active but disorganized forms of defensive responses that ensures emotional states of different nature. The faulty performance of these animals in the fear-potentiated startle and contextual fear procedure show similarities with panic attacks in man. A sequential pattern of defense reaction made up of arousal, immobility, escape and an incapacitating immobility is also seen when the prey are exposed to potential, distal and proximal signals emitted by the approaching predator. Efforts have been made to characterize the neural circuits recruited in the organization of the defensive reactions during these conditions. The prefrontal cortex, hippocampus and ventral periaqueductal gray are mainly involved in the integration of anxiety-like responses whereas the dorsal periaqueductal gray constitutes the main neural substrates for the integration of aversive states related to panic. In this chapter the authors summarize the evidence linking the brain's defense systems to the concept of anxiety-panic. The neural substrates of aversion in the hypothalamus seem to be in the middle of these processes. As a working hypothesis, it is advanced that past experience with stressors may lead to an emotional shift from the neural circuits responsible for the production of the usual defensive responses to environmental stressful events in higher brain structures towards disturbed or maladaptive defense responses related to panic attacks in brainstem structures. Therefore, prior experience with stressor events may shift orientated, active and organized motor patterns of appropriate defensive behaviors in response to contextual aversive stimuli towards non-oriented, fragmentary and uncoordinated motor acts. With great probabilities the switch mechanisms for these processes are part of the neural substrates of defense located at the level of the amygdala and the hypothalamus.

Chapter X – The neural large-scale dynamics and the connectivity pathways among spatially separated neural groups are conceived as a fundamental brain mechanism to integrate and process information.

The new measures of nonlinear interdependencies applied to EEG recordings, such as phase synchronization, have been recently shown to be highly sensitive to detect the dynamical change underlying the brain functions.

In the present chapter, the patterns of interdependency among different brain regions were investigated extracting the Synchronization Index (SI) from EEG response to different emotional and non-emotional film stimuli. The three basic emotions of happiness, fear and sadness were induced with the goal to investigate the synchronization patterns at different frequencies bands specifically associated with the valence dimension (positive vs. negative) and with the distinct basic emotional systems.

The comparisons among the experimental conditions showed several significant SI changes. The results demonstrated an overall decrease of SI during emotional stimulation compared to neutral, indicating an increase of complexity in the cortical dynamics. Further differences were found among the specific emotions, involving a distinct couple of electrodes with topographical effects at the frequencies bands examined. During happiness, the authors found a large pattern of synchronization in the left frontal hemisphere, especially in delta and theta waves, while fear, compared to neutral stimuli, showed a higher right synchronization, especially in beta waves. Largely different SI patterns emerged in the comparisons between the two negative emotions of fear and sadness, suggesting that the basic emotions are mediated by specific synchronized activity. The observed emotion-related SI change supports the view that coupling-decoupling patterns among the neural networks may be a relevant neural mechanism for the emotional processing and that SI nonlinear analysis may contribute to describe how the brain generates the emotion.

In: Brain Mapping Research Progress
Editors: Ines C. Girard and Jade S. Andre

ISBN: 978-1-60456-784-7

Chapter I

Neural Signal Estimation through Time-Resolved Functional Imaging

C.W. Tyler and L.T. Likova
Smith-Kettlewell Eye Research Institute
San Francisco

Abstract

The most effective method for localizing the effects of neural activation throughout the human brain is Functional Magnetic Resonance Imaging (fMRI). However, there is currently no method able to derive from the fMRI signal the particular neural signals underlying the measured BOLD waveforms. The goal of the present analysis is therefore to achieve time-resolved estimation of the neural signals determining the temporal waveforms in event-related fMRI. This analysis provides a new level of specificity in the basis of advanced approaches of using fMRI to study brain function as deep as at the level of the neural processing. In particular, we can resolve details of neural response dynamics down to the millisecond level for the analysis of visual processing and its temporal deficits.

For this purpose, we develop a nonlinear dynamic forward model of the metabolic demand arising from the transmitter release in the minimal set of component neural populations that account for each fMRI waveform. This model allows derivation of the neural signals underlying the wide variety fMRI waveforms evoked from even the most elementary brief stimuli. Estimation of signal delays between cortical regions is enhanced by an autonormalization procedure to provide maximum temporal precision in mapping the causal interactions among functional subunits across the cortex by means of the pattern of simultaneous covariation in the fMRI responses. This technique is also robust to feedback processes, allowing the mapping of recursive feedback signal between cortical regions at different levels in the response hierarchy.

Overview

The basic capability of functional Magnetic Resonance Imaging (fMRI) is mapping the spatial organization of the cortical and subcortical responses throughout the brain to a variety of stimulus and behavioral paradigms. It is often considered to have high spatial resolution (0. 25 – 1 million voxels), but low temporal resolution (0.5 – 5 *s*) relative to other methods for mapping human brain function (such as high-density EEG analysis). Of course, even the spatial resolution is low relative to single-unit neurophysiological recoding, but this is largely attributable to the signal/noise ratio. Inplane spatial resolution as high as 150 μ has been reported at 9.4 Tesla in cat cortex (Harel et al., 2006) and less than 1 mm^3 voxels in human (Barth and Norris, 2007). As improved technologies come on line, these spatial limitations are expected to be continually decreased.

The temporal limit is not so tractable. The inherent time constants of the BOLD signal are about 5 *s*, several orders of magnitude slower than the neural signal that is driving it. This slow time course incurs a severe limitation on the use of fMRI for application to deficits in temporal processing and diseases such as multiple sclerosis, where the conductions delays are of the order of tens of *ms* (Regan, Milner and Heron, 1976; Neima & Regan, 1984; Stefano et al., 1991; Werring et al., 2000; Russ et al., 2002; Levin et al., 2006). For a reasonable recording time and voxel size (*e. g.*, 3 x 3 x 3 mm) the signal/noise ratio for the most effective stimuli rarely exceeds 10:1. At such signal/noise ratios, deconvolution of the BOLD response can improve its temporal resolution by about a factor of 5 (Glover, 1999; Logothetis, 2003). However, that for the underlying neural signal can only be improved to about 1 sec, which is far short of what is required to measure typical neural delays. Single-parameter estimation, such as response delay, can improve the temporal resolution to 100 *ms* or better for narrowly targeted brain regions (Menon, Luknowsky and Gati, 1998; Henson et al., 2002), but this requires the assumption that the BOLD signal has a unitary waveform, which is often not the case. Even minor deviations from a stable waveform violate the assumptions of such single-parameter analysis and invalidate the delay measure.

Indeed, most commonly used fMRI analysis techniques, such as the SPM analysis package, make the assumptions of a unitary BOLD waveform kernel for an instantaneous stimulus, which, together with the assumption of superposition linearity, allows the prediction of the BOLD response waveform for any stimulus type or duration in any brain area. In fact, however, major deviations from a standard BOLD waveform may be found, even in the same cortical regions, for variations in stimulus conditions. D'Avossa, Shulman and Corbetta (2003) reported strong differences in waveform for attention modulation of response to the motion or color of a cue/stimulus pairing with about 5 *s* duration. Likova and Tyler (2007) showed striking differences within each of many cortical regions for manipulation of the perceptual organization in result of instantaneous changes in random-noise field. A similar variety of BOLD waveforms for a set of visual stimuli within given cortical regions are reported in a later section of the present paper. Such local waveform differences must derive from differences in the *neural* signals driving the BOLD activation, since the metabolism and hemodynamics should be invariant within a given cortical region. These results imply that the fMRI signal contains much more information than commonly appreciated. It is therefore important to develop a coherent analysis of the neural-to-BOLD processing sequence in order to derive a clear understanding of the neural signal variation revealed by the BOLD variations.

There is at present no method of transcending the BOLD temporal limitations in order to estimate the neural signals underlying the measured fMRI waveforms. The present analysis is therefore designed to provide *time-resolved estimation* of the *neural signals* underlying the particular characteristics of the temporal BOLD waveforms for a particular stimulus processed by a particular cortical region. We propose a *Nonlinear Forward Modeling* approach to provide a compact account of the measured waveform with the minimal number of neural predictors. This approach utilizes prior knowledge of the expected temporal properties of neural signals and of their consequent metabolic demand. This approach is reminiscent of the spectral analysis of the composition of stars, in which each element has a characteristic pattern of emission lines and the net spectrum is the sum of an unknown mixture of these predetermined patterns. The result is a specification of prevalence of each element in the star. In the case of the neural signals, the result is the amplitude and delay of each of the neural components that, when summed, account for the measured waveform for a particular stimulation condition and cortical region. The predictors are non-linear because there is a nonlinear relationship between the neural response and the metabolic demand that it generates, but we can assume that the component metabolic demands sum linearly together.

The next step in neuroscience, beyond spatial and temporal mapping, is the establishment of the causal relations among the network of activated cortical and subcortical locations. We introduce an autonormalization procedure to provide maximum temporal precision in mapping the functional subunits across the cortex by means of pattern of simultaneous covariation. The causal mapping of such delays can then be tracked through responsive cortical and subcortical regions to determine the causal networks with unprecedented accuracy. The technique is also robust to feedback processes, allowing the mapping of recursive feedback signal between regions lower and higher in the response hierarchy (when the delay is sufficiently long to disambiguate the feedback signals from the feedforward projections).

The Chain of Processing

In general terms, the stimulus S(t) impinging on the subject generates a sequence of neural responses starting with the transduction into a neural signal within the sensory receptors, which then propagates to the brain and activates various populations of neurons within the voxels being analyzed by the fMRI technique. For instance, the signals arriving from the retina generate synaptic activation of the populations of cortical cells, which generates an energetic demand for the restoration of the neurotransmitter molecules carrying the activation signals. The chain of cortical processing, illustrated in the block diagram of figure 1, progresses from the neural events through the metabolic demand mediated by the neighboring astrocyte glial cells to the processes of oxygen delivery by the adjacent capillaries that is detected by the imaging methodology.

We will treat the *neural responses* within each voxel as generated by sets of homogeneous populations with similar signal waveforms $N_i(t)$ within each population. Each neural response then generates a *local metabolic demand $M_i(t)$* that may have a nonlinear relationship to the neural signal waveform. The *integrated metabolic demands G(t)* are met primarily by the astrocytes, which integrate the required energy consumption over time and space and make a *complementary oxygen demand G(t)* on the adjacent vasculature. The *hemodynamic processes H(t)* provide the requisite oxygen exchange to replenish the energy depletion in the astrocytes. The fMRI BOLD analysis provides an estimate *Y(t)* of the ratio of oxygenated to deoxygenated hemoglobin in the blood complement of a given voxel. The *post-neural* processing stages are often modeled as a *linear hemodynamic response kernel* convolved with the presumed neural signal. However, this approach overlooks the key role of the *pre-hemodynamic* processes of the *glial* intermediaries. To incorporate the contributions of these processes, we will term it a *'metabolic response kernel'* (MRK) incorporating *both* the glial and hemodynamic components of the metabolic recovery processes. The MRK will be convolved with a non-linear transform of the presumed neural signal to provide an estimate of the neural metabolic demand that is being met by the combined glial and hemodynamic metabolic response. The fMRI analysis also has a finite dynamic response time, but it will be treated as negligible and linear with respect to the MRK of the glial/hemodynamic response.

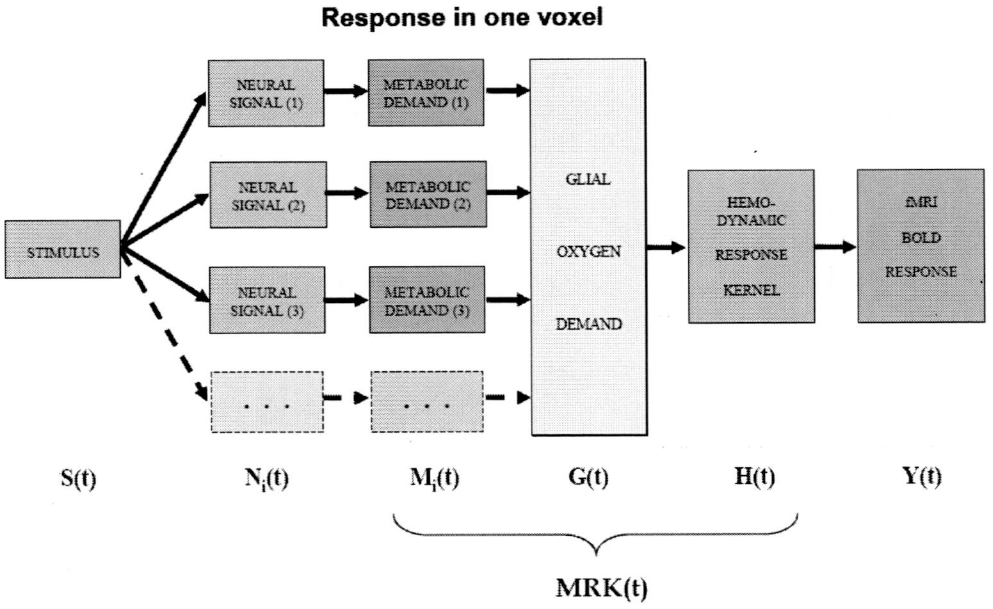

Figure 1. Block diagram of the main processing stages that lead up to the BOLD signal. The subscript i indicates that the stage incorporates multiple components within the voxel.

Table 1. Mathematical model of the operations involved in the generation of the BOLD signal from the input stimulus, S(t)

Output	Generation logic	Features
Neural signal	$N_i(t) = f[S(t) \otimes n_i(t)]$	Nonlinear transducer
Neural metabolic demand	$M_i(t) = f[N_i(t) \otimes m(t)]$	Nonlinear transducer
Glial oxygen demand	$G(t) = \sum M_i(t) \otimes g(t)$	Multiple linear integrator
Hemodynamic response	$H(t) = G(t) \otimes h(t)$	Linear (slow)
Paramagnetic response	$BOLD(t) = H(t) \otimes p(t)$	Linear (fast)
	$\approx \sum M_i(t) \otimes MRK(t)$	Combines four linear stages

The terms in figure 1 are related by a series of mathematical operations specified in table 1. The three operators are: (i) linear convolution ($\otimes$), a nonlinear, zero-memory transducer ($f[\,]$) and a linear integrator ($\sum$). In this model, which is considerably elaborated from the conventional analyses, we make the simplification that each stage consists of the linear convolution of the output signal from the previous stage with a temporal response kernel (which is designated by lower case initial for the name of that stage). Where necessary to model the physiological processes, the linear convolution kernel is elaborated with one of the nonlinear operators.

To pursue the analysis of neural responses underlying BOLD signals, we consider the responses to rapid stimulus events in an event-related paradigm. The measured event-related BOLD response *Y(t)* for this paradigm will be termed the *Peri-Event Response Function* (PERF), to distinguish it from *h(t)*, the underlying *hemodynamic response function* (HRF), or *kernel.* (The HRF is the kernel specific to the dynamics of blood oxygenation and is based on the assumption that its input is an invariant Dirac pulse.) The PERF is thus defined as the averaged BOLD activity synchronized with any repeated stimulus event. It incorporates the full sequence of linear or nonlinear neural, metabolic/hemodynamic response properties that follow the stimulus event of whatever form. Unlike the HRF, the PERF concept does not make any assumptions about the stimulus or the mechanism, location or linearity of the measured responses.

Time-Resolved fMRI

Although the time resolution of FMRI is low relative to the full time resolution of single unit activity, it must be recognized that many single-unit studies are noise-limited and use response integration up to 500 *ms* or so, and that many interesting perceptual processes have durations and delays this long and longer. Thus, resolving fMRI delays in the range below 1 sec can deliver important information, as demonstrated by Menon et al. (1998). These authors were able to resolve reaction-time delays of the order of 100 *ms*, and Henson et al. (2002) used the basis function of the HRF derivative to determine the sign of the advance or delay of the BOLD response (although the latter approach assumes a unitary HRF in all response regions, which may confound delays with other waveforms differences (Bellgowan, Saad and Bandettini, 2003). Similarly, Sun et al. (2005), working with a frequency domain technique, used the slope of the phase of the fMRI spectrum as an index of relative neural delay between brain areas. This method allowed the mapping of causal influences from a chosen brain areas to the rest of the brain with a typical accuracy of about 500 *ms*.

The present analysis is focused on the *time* domain, with the goal of extracting the maximum possible information about the neural signals underlying particular BOLD activation profiles. It is important to realize that there are many situations in which the neural response properties are reflected in the BOLD signals, even if the time-resolution is insufficient to reproduce the exact neural signal. Examples of such 'transparency' of response properties are particularly clear in the case that the full metabolic response kernel is monophasic.

This seems to be a fair approximation in the case of fMRI because the canonical response kernel (commonly known as the HRF) provided in the SPM-5 software package, although biphasic, has a negative lobe of less than 10% of the amplitude of the positive lobe. It is therefore only a minor approximation of this standardized kernel to assume that it has no negative lobe, which is the assumption made for the following analysis. (As will be explained below, the residual biphasic component can be readily attributed to neural rebound signals.) Armed with this assumption, we show how several properties of the neural signal are reflected in the recorded PERF waveform. (For the purpose of this demonstration, we are assuming a linear relationship between the neural response and the PERF in order to make its properties clear before introducing the nonlinear aspects discussed in the previous section.)

Polarity. The PERF polarity will be an accurate reflection of the polarity of the neural response for any monophasic neural response.

Latency. Any delay in the neural response will also be reflected in the consequent PERF. Of course, the metabolic processing sequence may introduce additional delays, but neural delays such as response reaction times or perceptual ambiguity delays should be accurately reflected in the PERF once the inherent delays of the MRK are taken into account.

Transience. It is an established property of the BOLD response that it is largely sustained for an appropriately sustained neural response (Birn, Saad and Bandettini, 2001; Boynton et al., 1996; Glover, 1999; Logothetis, 2002, 2003; Shmuel et al., 2006). Hence, transience of the PERF for a sustained stimulus implies a transience of the underlying neural response. For example, the onset of a sustained light is known to generate transient neural responses in most cortical neurons responding to it. Such stimulation will generate a transient PERF even though the stimulation and photoreceptor response are sustained.

Number of phases. For a monophasic MRK (HRF), the PERF will have the same number of phases as the input stimulus, if the neural input is balanced for positive and negative lobes. Thus, the fact that the measured PERF is typically biphasic does not imply that the MRK is necessarily biphasic. The negative lobe may derive from a biphasic neural response to a stimulus rather than to blood dynamics.

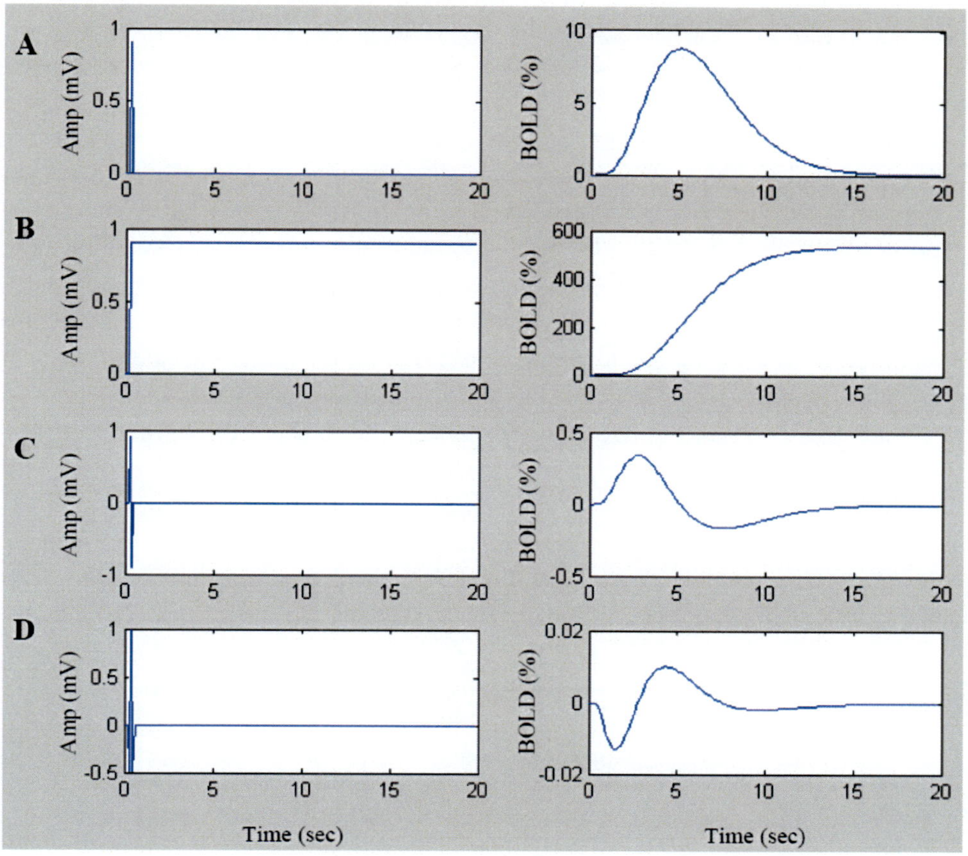

Figure 2. Left panels: (*A*) neural impulse response, (*B*) step response, (*C*) balanced doublet and (*D*) balanced triplet response. Right panels present convolution of each of these responses with the MRK shown in *A* (right). Note that differences in neural response characteristics (left panels) at the time scale of 100 *ms* generate profound changes in the simulated PERF waveforms (right panels) on a much longer timescale, which in turn are diagnostic of the differences in the neural signals.

These properties of the PERF are illustrated in the simulation of figure 2, for which the MRK (HRF) is assumed to be the gamma function shown in figure 2A, right. (We use the term "gamma function" as shorthand for the gamma probability density function that is the theoretical limit of the Gamma Distribution, which is the sum of k exponentially-distributed random variables). Gamma probability density functions have the form $a.\ t^{k-1}.\ e^{-t/\tau}$ (where t is the time dimension, a is a scaling parameter and k and τ are shape constants). Each left-hand panel shows a different neural waveform with a time-course typical of those seen in neurophysiological recordings. Convolution with the MRK of figure 2A (right) generates the predicted BOLD waveforms of the right-hand column of figure 2. The important point made by this simulation is that most typical features of measured PERF waveforms could arise from convolution of a simple gamma-function MRK with a variety of neural signals modulated within less than 100 *ms*.

Conversely, under the assumption of a uniform MRK, the neural signal properties can be inferred from the form of the PERF. Thus, if the PERF rises to a sustained plateau (figure 2B, right), we may infer that the neural signal was sustained (figure 2B, left). If the PERF is biphasic (figure 2C, right), we may infer that the neural signal was biphasic (figure 2C, left). If the PERF is triphasic (figure 2D, right), we may infer that the neural signal was correspondingly triphasic (figure 2D, left). Figure 2 illustrates that, under appropriate assumptions the form of the BOLD response can act as a kind of "temporal microscope" for the form of the underlying neural response. Although it cannot resolve the precise temporal parameters (*e. g.*, whether the response lobes have durations of 1, 10 or 100 *ms*), many of the aspects of the waveform structure are reflected in the BOLD waveform. The interpretation is particularly straightforward if the BOLD metabolic/hemodynamic kernel is monophasic, and we are emphasizing that previous suggestions that it is biphasic are contaminated by the likelihood that the underlying neural signal is itself biphasic. Under the logic of the analysis in figure 2, this property would generate the biphasic form of empirical hemodynamic kernel that is commonly observed, but it seems that no previous analysis of BOLD properties has take this possibility into account. Based on this analysis, we propose that (i) it is more plausible to assume that the true metabolic kernel has a monophasic form, and that (ii) the biphasic property that is often empirically observed (but is quite variable over brains and cortical regions; Bellgowan, Saad & Bandettini, 2003; Handwerker et al., 2003), is a function of the neural processing that precedes the metabolic demand, as illustrated in figure 2.

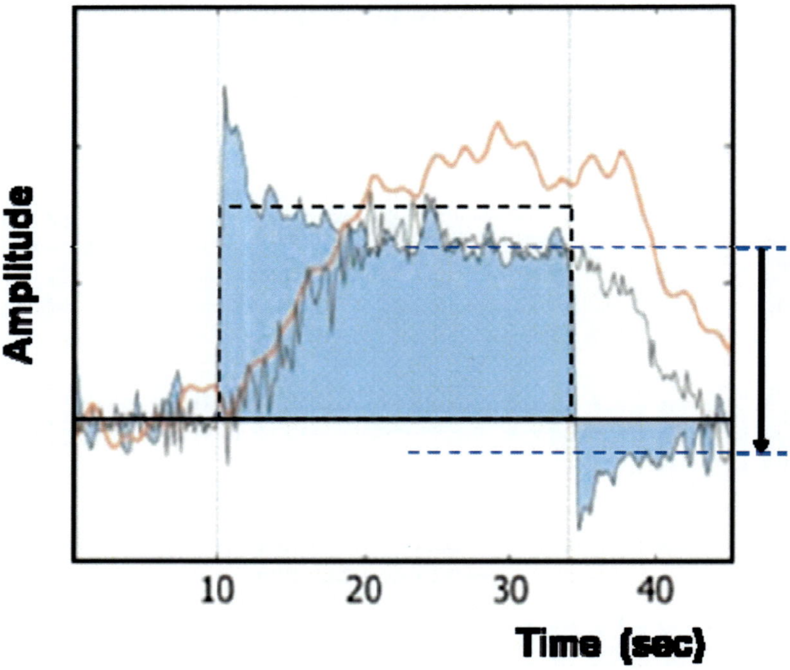

Figure 3. Time course of the local field potentials (blue trace), BOLD (red trace) and predicted BOLD (black trace) to a continuous dynamic stimulus (black dotted rectangle) of 24 s duration. From Logothetis (2003). Blue dashed lines show the inhibitory rebound level predicted from the average level of the second half of the BOLD response.

The Neural Signal

Logothetis and colleagues (Logothetis, 2002, 2003; Logothetis & Wandell, 2004; Shmuel et al., 2006) have made the case that the most likely basis of the metabolic demand driving the BOLD signal is the energetic load deriving from the total conductance changes in the postsynaptic membrane generated by a range of processes consequent on transmitter release at the synaptic inputs to each neuron. The summed metabolic demand in the nexus of active cortical neurons adjacent to a capillary forms the drive for the metabolic response in that region of cortex. These authors argue that the transmitter release is tightly coupled to the activation of the post-synaptic receptors on the recipient cell membrane and consequently to the energetic demands of the membrane receptor activation and to a lesser extent to the subsequent recycling of the transmitter molecules. The majority of these energetic demands are met by glycolysis of glutamate to glutamine in the neighboring astrocytes (Shank and Aprison, 1979; Wang and Floor, 1994). The glutamine is then taken up by the neurons for reconversion to glutamate for use as a transmitter, releasing energy within the neuron in the process. Since cells are predominantly linear summators of the excitatory and inhibitory transmitter release across their synaptic population, it seems to follow that the energetic demand driving the BOLD signal is most closely coupled to the net transmitter signal impinging on the cells, and hence to intracellular potential in the cells.

A comprehensive model of the BOLD therefore requires an accurate model of the intracellular potential dynamics coupled to sensory stimulation. As is highlighted by the data of Logothetis (2003), there are adaptive effects in the neural response that become evident for long-duration activation by continuous dynamic stimuli (figure 3). The LFP recordings (blue curve) from monkey V1 reveal that the adaptation has a complex time course that can be approximated by two exponentials with time constants of about 1 sec and 60 sec, respectively. These are remarkably prolonged neural processes that are on the time scale of BOLD activation, and will therefore affect the form of the recorded BOLD signal from the same general region of cortex (figure 3, black trace). The importance of this adaptation effect is emphasized by the fact that the recorded LFP signal does not fully match the BOLD activation predicted (red curve, figure 3) on the basis of General Linear Model (GLM) of convolution of a hemodynamic response kernel with the stimulus time course, and therefore a more comprehensive model is required, going beyond the standard GLM model. (This analysis applies when the stimulus is continuously refreshed to support the assumption that the neural signal would be well approximated by the stimulus waveform).

Notice that the negative LFP signal following the stimulus *offset* in figure 3 has a similar (but inverted) time course relative to that following the stimulus *onset*. This inversion implies that the adaptation effect is a subtractive *inhibition* (rebound prediction shown by the blue dashed lines) rather than solely a multiplicative form of fatigue (which would have no negative rebound). If it were a multiplicative gain control, the amplitude of signal change at offset would be substantially less than that at onset, whereas the two amplitudes are similar within about 10%.

The mechanism of this subtractive inhibition appears to be the tonic intracellular hyperpolarization induced by pattern adaptation, as described by Carandini and Ferster (1997, 2000). However, the stimulus driving this response was a *dynamic* contrast modulation, and hence this gives us a solid basis to treat the sustained LFP signal as deriving from a full-wave rectified transform of the intracellular potential. This leads to a model of the LFP from any nearby neuron as the integrated response of instantaneous signal of the rectified intracellular potential, convolved with an exponential decay function. However, in its simple form, such a model will have a single exponential decay, whereas the data in figure 3 clearly show a short decay to a stable response level followed by a slow decay of about 10% over the 30 sec of the full stimulus epoch.

An implementation of the *parallel-process model* we have proposed on that basis is shown in figure 4 for a qualitative fit to the data of figure 3. It is based on two decaying exponential components with time constants of 1 and 60 *s* (figure 4a). These components were convolved with a neural signal derived from the convolution of the rectangular form (box-car) of the continuous stimulus for 3 and 12 s (cf., Logothetis, 2003), the latter corresponding to the rectangle in figure 3. This model captures the qualitative features of the data (figure 3) with the sum of the two component response (dashed curves in figure 4c). These components represent the average responses of two separate neural populations contributing to the recorded LFP. Note that it is difficult to obtain the integrated response, i.e., the combination of the two component slopes of figure 4c with any kind of serial model, because this would imply a convolution of the two exponentials that would necessarily result in a function dominated by the slower process rather than allowing both processes full expression.

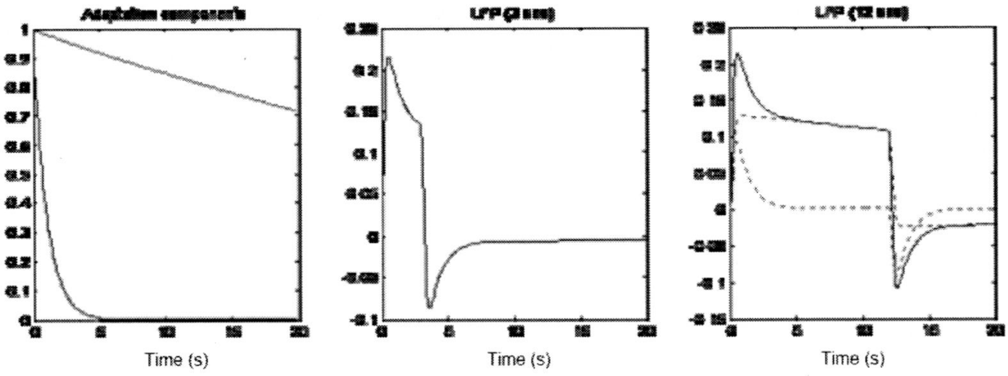

a *b* *c*

Figure 4. a) Two exponential decay processes used to account for the adaptation effects in figure 3. *b*) The sum of the two components in 4*a* each convolved with a 3 sec stimulus time course. c) *Dashed curves*: the two components in 4*a* each convolved with a 12 sec stimulus time course; *full curve*: the sum of the two convolved responses.

Temporal Properties of Human Vision

To place the temporal analysis of human visual processing on a firm footing, it is critical to have a secure understanding of the linearity of the signals passing from the retina to the cortex that form the basis of visual perception. This knowledge is achieved by psychophysical measurements of the temporal integration function (Bloch, 1885; Barlow,

1958). An example of such measurements for three base intensities of red (660 nm) light is depicted in figure 5, which shows three properties of relevance. One is that, below 10 *ms* duration, detection thresholds have an accurately reciprocal relation to pulse duration down to durations as low a 10 μs (at the higher mean intensities) at the 35° eccentricity. This behavior implies that temporal summation is accurately linear over this extreme range. The number of quantal absorptions per cone implied by the reciprocal relationship is indicated next to each curve. If, on the other hand, the cone or subsequent neural responses had an amplitude saturation, for example at a level of 1 million quanta (6 log quanta) per cone per second, the required energy above this point would be disproportionately large and the curves above this point would show an increasing slope. However, they remain accurately proportional, implying full linearity.

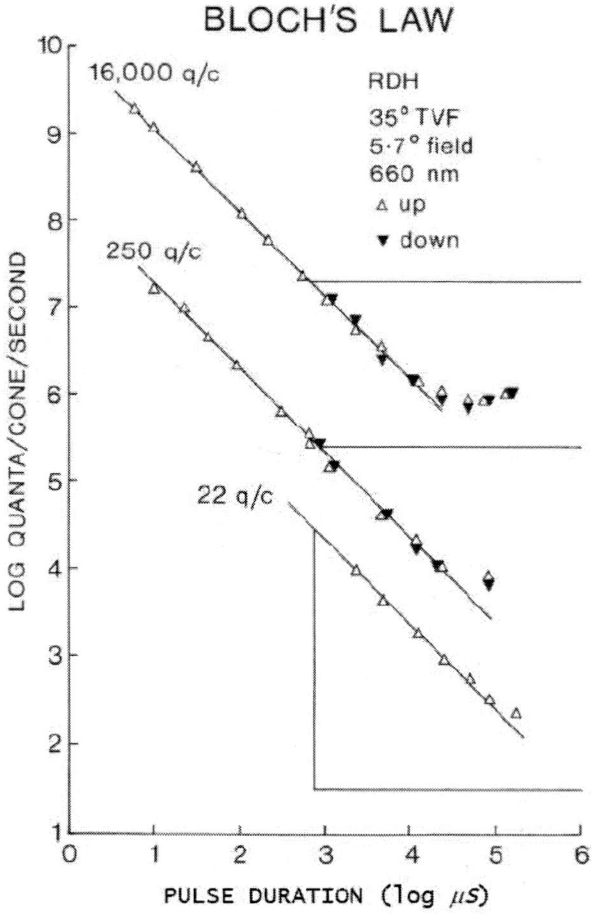

Figure 5. Bloch's Law linearity and the temporal integration limit across the intensity range. Psychophysical thresholds were measured with an optimized staircase method for high-intensity 660 nm light-emitting diodes projecting to a 5.7° field at 35° eccentricity on the horizontal temporal meridian. The stimuli had base luminances of 0.7, 4.7 and 6.7 log cd/m^2 (intensities of 1. 4, 5.4 and 7.4 log quanta/cone/s at this retinal location) with a 180° white surround of matching intensity.

The second linearity test is to compare detection thresholds for *pulse increments* and *pulse decrements* (open and filled symbols, respectively, in figure 5). This comparison is possible only for threshold amplitude less than the base luminance level because the luminance decrement can not exceed its base level. Where the comparison could be made, there was no significant difference between the increment and decrement thresholds, implying that the temporal response of the human visual processing is linear with respect to the sign of the internal response.

The final issue addressed by these psychophysical data is that temporal integration fails beyond the range of the neural impulse response, and the detection threshold conforms to a horizontal line (Regan and Tyler, 1970; Gorea and Tyler, 1986; Sekiguchi, Williams and Brainard, 1993). This slope transition occurs at about 15, 20 and 100 *ms* for the three stimulus intensities (22q/c, 220q/c and 16000q/c respectively), which are typical values for this eccentricity. Since the highest intensity is close to the limit that is comfortable for the human viewer, and the lowest is close to the cone detection threshold (a 6 log unit range), this range of transition durations corresponds to the range of neural integration times expected for human vision. Thus, these psychophysical measurements provide an important constraint on the range of integration times operative in the underlying neural signals. These in turn constrain the neural response time constants allowable for the "temporal microscope" analysis of the neural response properties driving human BOLD signals.

In this connection, it should be noted that the temporal properties of the human psychophysics are compatible with the known properties of the responses recorded at the outer segments of human cones. Recordings from monkey cone outer segments (Schneeweis and Schnapf, 1995, 1999) show voltage response with roughly the right properties to account for human psychophysics, showing early response peaks with time constants of the order to 20 *ms*. The recordings in Schneeweis and Schnapf, (1995) match those from human cones (Kraft, Schneeweis and Schnapf, 1993), implying that voltage responses for human and monkey cones would also be similar. The difference between that 20 *ms* estimate and the 12 *ms* of figure 5 can easily be accounted for by the difficulty of recording up to the highest intensities, and the use of filter cutoffs no higher than 100 Hz in the physiological recordings.

Stepwise Incremental Estimation of the Neural Dynamics

One useful approach to the issue of the neural dynamics underlying the BOLD response has been published by Bandettini and Ungerleider (2001), on the basis of a temporal summation experiment reported in Birn, Saad and Bandettini (2001). The stimuli consisted of counterphasing checkerboard patches with durations increasing in factors of 2 from 0. 25 to 2 *s* (together with a 20 *s* duration). The key result was that the BOLD responses did not increase proportionately with stimulus duration, as would be expected for linear summation of a neural response of constant amplitude through convolution with the BOLD impulse response kernel. Instead, the amplitude showed little increase from the short durations (figure 6a), implying either a nonlinear summation process or a disproportionate strength of neural signals for short duration stimuli.

Bandettini and Ungerleider (2001) proposed an analysis for the derivation of the implied neural signal under the assumption that the integration process underlying the generation of the BOLD response was indeed equivalent to a linear convolution operation. To derive the neural signal estimate, they took the difference between BOLD response areas for each successive pair of stimulus durations as an estimate of the amplitude of the neural signal for the time interval defined by the difference in stimulus durations. The result is reproduced in figure 6b. It implies that the neural signal has a pronounced early transient followed by a sustained phase of stable amplitude out to 20 s (red box function).

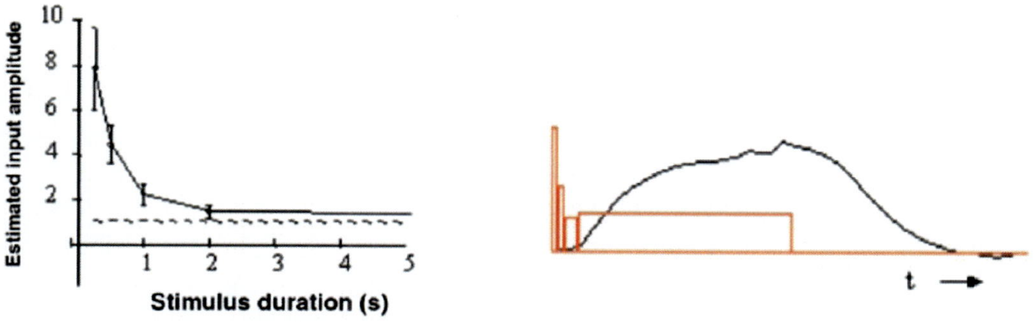

a b

Figure 6. *a*) Response amplitudes as a function of the duration of a counterphase checkerboard stimulus. *b*) Convolution model (black line) of the amplitude of the presumed neural response (red rectangles) that would have generated the data in *a*. Reproduced from Bandettini and Ungerlieder (2001).

As revealing as this analysis was, however, it does not seem to have been followed up by further estimates of the neural signals underlying the BOLD response to other stimulus types or in other cortical regions. Perhaps the reason is that the analysis requires an extended series of stimulus conditions. It should be clarified that the 250 *ms* neural transient estimated from the Bandettini and Ungerleider (2001) analysis is resolved only to the duration specified by that stimulus condition. The true underlying neural transient could have been much shorter. For example, the analysis could not distinguish between a neural transient of 250 *ms* and one of the 40 *ms* duration typical of neural responses. Only if the stimulus series had the requisite temporal sampling could the actual duration of the neural transient be determined (under the linearity assumptions of the analysis). Birn, Saad and Bandettini (2001) studied 5 durations, but a series of 12 or more would be required to cover the required range expected for neural signals (even under their assumption that the signal fluctuations would be likely to be proportionately slower as duration increased, permitting the temporal sampling to be logarithmically spaced). Thus, the neural integration time is of the order of 10 *ms* (figure 5), so stimulus durations of, say, 8, 16, 32, 64, 125, 250, 500 *ms*, and 1, 2, 4, 8, and 16 *s*, would adequately cover the required range with log-spaced sampling. If there were reason to suspect transient but delayed neural signals to be included in the response of a particular cortical area, however, a finer sampling density would be required. BOLD responses for stimuli of very short duration have recently been reported by Uludag, Yesilyurt and Ugurbil (2006), so this approach to neural signal estimation should be practicable, even though intensive stimulation conditions would be required to obtain adequate sampling resolution.

Dynamic forward Modeling

The analysis of figure 6 is a rudimentary kind of modeling, in the sense that it begins with an assumed form for the underlying neural signal. This form is a boxcar, based on the (unstated) assumption that the neural response is fast enough to follow the stimulus exactly, within the resolution visible in the plotted functions. The neural response is then convolved with a metabolic response kernel (*MRK*(t) in figure 1) to generate a model BOLD response that is fitted to the data with the amplitude as one free parameter. This parameter then, according to the linearity assumption, determines the inferred amplitude of the neural signal (red box function in figure 6b) that must have given rise to the measured BOLD response. This logic was applied by Bandettini and Ungerlieder (2001) in incremental fashion to each new temporal segment of the stimulus.

We can expand the forward modeling approach to reveal some remarkable properties of the neural response to extremely brief stimuli such as those reported by Uludag, Yesilyurt and Ugurbil (2006). By the use of high luminance LED stimulators, this group have been able to record BOLD responses to stimuli as brief as 1 *ms* (figure 7a). This achievement does not imply, of course that the underlying neural response is as brief as this, but their data provides the opportunity to apply the forward modeling concept to a model neural signal that has full temporal resolution. We will show that the *forward modeling* approach is able to reveal precise details of the neural response at it native time resolution. Based on an appropriate model of the temporal summation experiment, there is essentially no limit to the temporal resolution to which the underlying neural response can be determined.

The starting point for this analysis is the model neural response function we have developed to fit the LFP data of figure 3. This function was convolved first with the stimulus time-course and then with a unitary MRK to generate a predicted cortical BOLD summation function (figure 7b, blue dashed curve). The form of the predicted response was then optimized for best fit to the actual BOLD responses of figure 7a by varying the parameters of the model neural response (which operates like a hidden layer in a neural network model). The integrated areas for the optimized BOLD fits are plotted in figure 7b for comparison with the empirical area data. The resultant estimate of the neural signals are shown at two time scales in figure 7c,d. This analysis again implies that there is a neural transient followed by an extended sustained plateau, but now reveals the precise temporal properties of the neural response. The transient peaks at about 20 *ms* and that the plateau has an adaptive decay with a time constant of about 800 *ms*. Thus, the *forward modeling* approach in combination with the temporal integration paradigm can overcome the inherent limitations of the slow BOLD signal to quantify details of neural processing at the millisecond time scale.

Note that a single exponential attention term can account well for the integrated response growth beyond 500 *ms*. However, below this duration, no adjustment of the relative weightings could improve the fit to the temporal integration data. Running the optimization with the two-component function of figure 4c results in the neural response function (red curves in figure 7c,d). The fit is improved by a factor of three (which is a significant improvement on the chi-square test at $p < 0.\ 01$). Note that resulting neural transient implied by this optimization to the BOLD signals is so brief that the time axis had to be scaled to 60 *ms* to show its features (figure 7d).

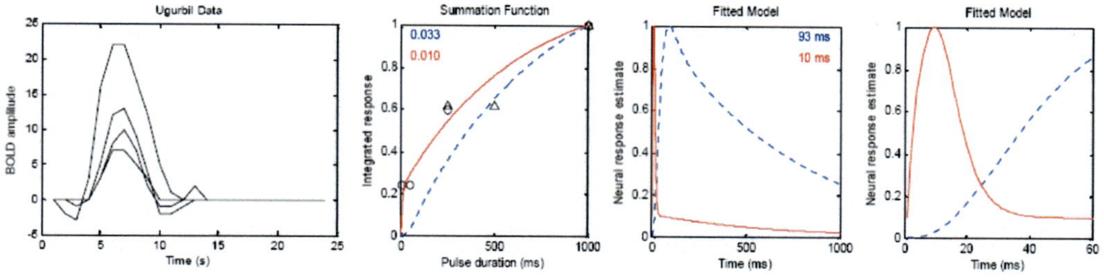

Figure 7. a. BOLD responses to high-luminance flashes from for stimulus durations of 1, 3, 5, and 1000 *ms* duration (curves of increasing amplitude), replotted from Uludag et al. (2006). *b*. Integrated BOLD response data from *a* (open circles), together with further areal integration data from Birn et al (2001, open triangles), for stimulus durations of 5, 50, 250 and 1000 *ms*. Dashed blue curve shows the initial predictions of the neural-response model prior to optimization. The full red curve shows the *optimization* of this model to the BOLD data depicted. Blue and red numbers represent the residual errors for the two cases. *c*. Non-optimized (blue) and best-fitting (red) neural response estimates on a long time-scale. Blue and red numbers represent the peak latencies for the two cases. *d*. The early phase of the non-optimized and best-fitting neural responses on a short time-scale. This result illustrates that forward modeling of temporal summation data can resolve details of the underlying neural response in human cortex on a millisecond time scale.

This characterization of the *neural* response characteristics in the human brain makes it clear that the *dynamic forward analysis* is capable of resolving differences in neural response time constants of the order of a few milliseconds. Previous studies have established that fMRI can resolve neural time delays of the order of 100 *ms* or less (Menon, Luknowsky and Gati, 1998). However, this range still falls short of resolving temporal properties in the typical range of neural transients. The present analysis shows that, with the right paradigm, the finest details at the level of neural temporal processing are accessible from analysis of the fMRI signal. We emphasize, of course, that this analysis is applicable to every voxel of fMRI recording, and thus the responses of local neural populations can be resolved to the millisecond level at a spatial resolution of the order single hypercolumns anywhere in the cerebral cortex.

Nonlinear Dynamic forward Modeling

In this section, we propose a more biophysically-based development of the *forward modeling* approach that we term *Nonlinear Dynamic Forward modeling* (NDF modeling). Rather than simply characterizing the nonlinearities in the behavior of the BOLD waveform (Birn, Saad and Bandettini, 2001; Bandettini et al., 2002) or attempting to infer the potentially complex properties of the underlying neural mechanisms from the form of the BOLD response (Glover, 1999; Logothetis, 2002, 2003a,b; Logothetis and Wandell, 2004), the concept of forward modeling is to start *from the 'cause'* – the neural signal, instead from the 'consequence" – the BOLD signal. Thus we incorporate into the model as much knowledge as possible about the likely neural substrate and then optimize the details to best fit the BOLD waveform. This knowledge includes known nonlinearities both of the population of neural responses to the stimulus but also of the metabolic requirements of the neural processing that lead to the measurable BOLD response.

The *dynamic forward modeling* discussed in the previous section is *linear* in the sense that it assumes no nonlinearity in the model linking the neural response to the BOLD response (or indeed in linking the stimulus waveform to the BOLD response) [1]. It merely estimates the *gain* of the neural response for each stimulus duration, which can vary by a linear process. For example, the transient neural response to a contrast onset would have such a characteristic, as detailed in the previous section.

A more general form of forward modeling is to incorporate a range of possible nonlinearities into the structure of the model, which we term *nonlinear dynamic forward* (NDF) modeling. The range of possible nonlinearities at each stage of the model is vast, so the approach is not feasible unless one incorporates Bayesian constraints in the modeling, based on the known biophysics of the neuronal responses likely to underlie the BOLD activation. The groundwork for such constraints has been provided by Logothetis and Wandell (2004). Thus, the starting point for the NDF modeling will be the neural signal, whose first effect in terms of the chain of BOLD dynamics is to create a metabolic demand *G(t),* in the neighboring glial cells *(*see figure 1).

Since little is known about the glial dynamics of transmitter recovery, we will pursue two options as to their effects. One is that the *metabolic demand* derives from the transmitter recovery cycle following the release of transmitter consequent to an axonal spike. Since axonal spikes represent only the positive aspect of the intracellular voltage and since 90% of cortical synapses are excitatory (Shank and Aprison, 1979; Wang and Floor, 1994), one option is to treat the signal transmitted from one cortical stage to the next as a half-wave rectified version of the dynamic neural signal. This prediction is shown as the blue curves in figure 8Aa, which is an overlay of the model estimates of the neural responses to stimulus pulses that double in duration from 8 *ms* to 16 s (eight doublings). For this example, the neural response has balanced excitation and inhibition, so there is only an initial transient response even to the prolonged pulses, with the negative lobe at offset being thresholded out by the rectification. (Note that the local metabolic demand, M_i(t), per se, has the same time course in this model as the transmitter recovery from which it derives. The energetic processes required for the recovery of the initial state, however, form an oxygen-based chain of glial metabolic response, *G*(t), that may have substantially slower time course at one or more stages.)

The other option is to consider the instantaneous metabolic demand of both polarities relative to the mean background level (i.e., the demand of both excitatory and inhibitory cells, or both 'on' and 'off' cells), implying that the signal generating the metabolic demand is a full-wave rectified version of the intracellular voltage. This option is shown in figure 8Aa, as the red curve, whose spikes represent the instantaneous metabolic demand for the

[1] Strictly speaking, many GLM models contain an implied nonlinearity, in that a flickering counterphase stimulus should generate both positive and negative activations in a typical neural array, tending to cancel to a null signal. It is only if there is a rectifying nonlinearity in the neural response that they should sum to a waveform approximating the integrated amplitude of the stimulus waveform. However, we are adopting the common convention here that a neural signal matching the net stimulus contrast over time is considered to be linear.

offset transient for each of the pulse duration doublings (which were thresholded out by in the blue curve).

We may now pursue the response to these two options for metabolic demand through the biophysical chain to the measured BOLD signal. The first element in this chain is the astrocytes, which provide glucose to the neuron and replenish its supply by ATP metabolism fueled by oxygen from a neighboring blood vessels. It is important to emphasize that the astrocyte metabolic processes are as slow relative to the intracellular signal dynamics, as are the processes of hemodynamic oxygen supply. The time constants of the astrocyte responses is known to be of the order of several seconds (Kelly and van Essen, 1974; Filosa, Bonev and Nelson, 2004; Metea and Newman, 2006), and it is clear that there must be a substantial pre-hemodynamic component from these slow responses. However, at present too little is known of their dynamics and/or nonlinearities to securely assign precise time constants to the astrocyte related component relative to the hemodynamic component. We will therefore treat the entire chain from the metabolic demand to the magnetic resonance signal in the traditional fashion, as a unitary linear kernel. This kernel is often termed the hemodynamic response function (HRF), but in view of its likely substantial astrocyte contribution, we will give it the more general term of the metabolic response kernel (MRK).[2] Our main goal is to estimate the properties of the neural signal properties, and it will be seen that there is sufficient information to provide a rich analysis of these properties, and to account for the empirical nonlinearities of the BOLD signal, as long as the metabolic supply chain conforms to the linearity assumption.

The way in which NDF modeling captures the underlying neural properties is laid out in figure 8 (indexed in row/column notation). This figure shows the consequences of the assumption that the neural impulse response has balanced positive and negative lobes, and of various degrees of imbalance of the negative lobe. It also compares two forms of nonlinearity of the metabolic demand. (The figure does not show the neural responses themselves, but takes the metabolic demand as the starting point for the analysis.) The point of the figure is to illustrate that subtle properties of the neural response and its metabolic effects have dramatic effects on the measured BOLD waveform, and that therefore the BOLD waveform characteristics in well-controlled experiments can be diagnostic of the fine details of the neural and metabolic processes in the brain regions from which the BOLD signals derive.

The first row of figure 8 shows the development of the BOLD response waveform through the pulse duration series for which the metabolic demand derives from a balanced neural signal. Half- and full-rectified versions of the metabolic demand are shown in figure 8Aa (blue and red curves). The resultant BOLD waveforms are computed under the assumption of a gamma function model of the MRK (HRF), as developed in figure 2. Because the balanced neural signal generates only a spike in the half-rectified version (column *b*) of the neural metabolic demand, the predicted BOLD waveform approximates the form of the MRK for all durations, varying only in amplitude as the neural signals integrate the energy in the pulse stimuli. After the first two durations the BOLD amplitude asymptotes to a stable value.

---

[2] The term "kernel" is preferred because it is conceptualized as the theoretical response to an imaginary stimulus of infinitely short duration and unit area, termed a "Dirac pulse".

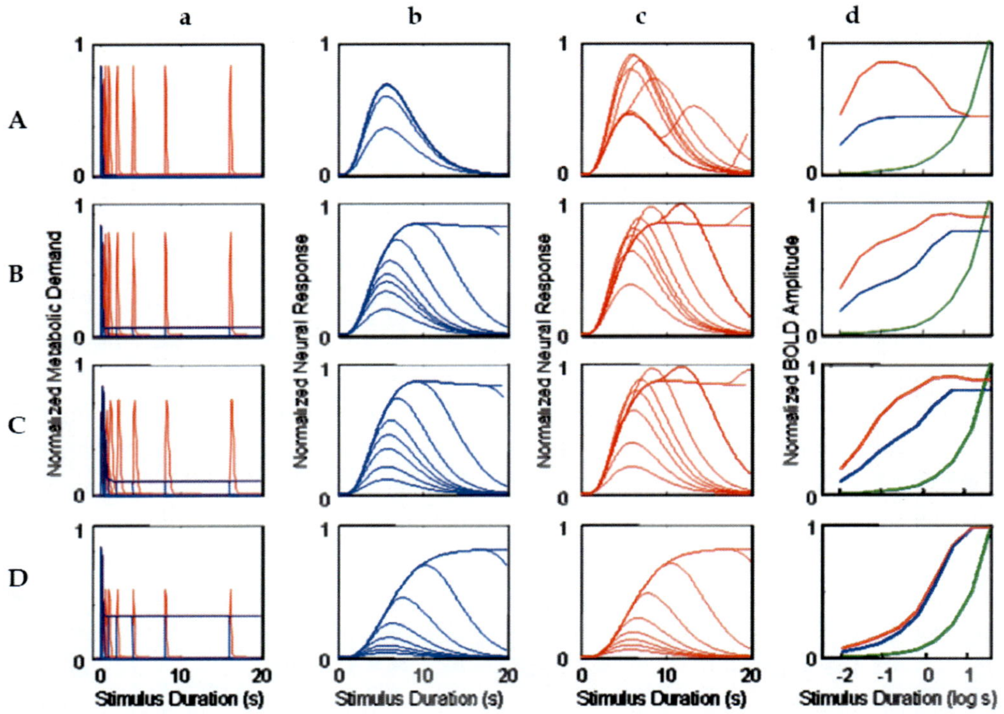

Figure 8. Simulations of four different types of BOLD response for monophasic metabolic demand signals (and a monophasic Metabolic Response Kernel). The rows represent the results for A: metabolic demands with a purely transient time course, B-D: responses with a mixed transient and sustained time course, in which the sustained component is respectively 12%, 18% and 50% of the amplitude of the transient component (based on different ratios of neural excitation/inhibition). For each type, column (*a*) shows the assumed metabolic demand, column (*b*) plots the BOLD responses over duration for the half-wave-rectified model of metabolic demand, column (*c*) plots the BOLD responses over duration for a full-wave-rectified model, and column (*d*) plots the duration summation curves for peak amplitude (blue curve: half-wave-rectified model, red curve: full-wave-rectified model, green curve: full linear summation). Note the use of the logarithmic abscissa to focus on the brief duration regime. The progression of the model BOLD responses and the form of the summation curves are diagnostic of both the relative weighting between the sustained and transient components of the neural signal and the form of rectification feeding the metabolic demand.

The development of the peak amplitude in the BOLD temporal summation series is shown as the blue curve in figure 8Ad. The critical point of this plot is that the asymptotic corner of this summation curve occurs at 40 *ms*, which is the value of the time constant assumed for the neural signal. Thus, the form of the BOLD amplitude summation series (figure 8, column *d*) is diagnostic of the time constant of neural integration down to the millisecond range. There is no limit in principle to the temporal resolution that can be achieved by this methodology since it is estimated from the amplitude variation of the BOLD signal as a function of stimulus duration, not from the its temporal aspects .

The reduction in peak amplitude is captured in the red temporal summation curve of figure 8Ad, showing a reduction by a factor of two for long durations. (The green curve in figure 8Ad represents the values expected for fully proportional summation of the energy in the stimulus pulse; it is an accelerating curve due to the logarithmic abscissa.)

It is evident that the temporal summation properties of this first model of the nonlinear dynamics is not close to those observed in typical fMRI studies (such as those reproduced in figure 7), but it is presented to illustrate the power of NDF modeling to evaluate particular properties of the neural signal dynamics. In this case, the main culprit is the exact balance of excitation and inhibition in the model, bringing the response for long-duration stimuli back to baseline after about 15 sec (when typical data show a much slower decline over time). However, notice that relaxing the assumption of such a balanced response by even a small amount is enough to obtain much more plausible predictions.

The case of the full-rectification model of the metabolic demand is shown in figure 8Ac. Here the second neural response peak (i.e., that from the stimulus offset) plays key a role in varying the BOLD waveform, which first extends in time and then shows a two-peaked structure with reduced amplitude for long-duration stimuli.

Figure 8Ba shows the *half-* and *fully-rectified* version of the metabolic demand to the same pulse duration series, where the neural inhibition is now assumed to be reduced in energy by 1.5% relative to the excitation. This small imbalance is magnified by the convolution with the sustained stimulus, and thus it results in a sustained component that is 12% of the amplitude of the initial transient (blue curve in figure 8Ba) and then into an almost fully sustained set of BOLD response functions (figure 8Bb, compare to *Ab*). Thus, the *form* of the BOLD response functions can be strongly *diagnostic* of even slight variations in the properties of brief *neural* signals. Again, the nature of the metabolic demand function (half- or fully-rectified) has a big impact on the form of the BOLD response, determining whether an offset peak is evident at the tail of the responses even when they are sustained (figure 8 Bc). Such a peak has been reported in some studies but is not always evident. Thus it remains an empirical question to what extent it is representative of BOLD waveforms. Intermediate forms of the rectification model are required to capture the empirical properties in detail.

Note that the amplitude series in figure 8Bb and c show bands of denser packing, where the amplitude changes were not proportional to the doublings of stimulus duration. This property has often been called a "nonlinearity" of the BOLD response, but it is generated here by a linear convolution process, so for clarity we will refer to it as a "non-proportionality" (see Section 3). Viewed in terms of the peak amplitude summation plots of figure 8Bd the regions of dense packing form an intermediate "shelf" or asymptote. It is again evident that the onset of this intermediate 'shelf' in the summation curve corresponds to the integration time of the underlying neural signal, while the second asymptote corresponds to the 5 sec integration time of the MRK (HRF). Careful measurement of this summation function can therefore provide estimates of both the neural and the metabolic time constants in the neural > BOLD signal chain.

This point is emphasized by the response set in row *C* of figure 8. The key difference from the parameters used in row B of figure 8, is that the neural time constant was doubled from 50 *ms* to 100 *ms* (and the excitation/inhibition imbalance was also increased to 7% to maintain the same form of offset peak). It is evident that (i) the summation curve (figure 8Cd) takes a measurably different form, and that (ii) the accuracy of estimation of the neural time constant is limited not by the BOLD time constant but only by the variability of the BOLD amplitude measures. For example, this analysis shows that the neural time constant can be estimable to an accuracy of about 0. 1 log units if the BOLD response functions can be measured to an achievable accuracy of about 10%. Note that the values of 50 and 100 *ms* were chosen here for illustrative convenience, and the estimation of a time constant of, say, 10 *ms* should be equally good.

The final case (figure 8Dd) shows the NDF predictions of increasing the excitation/inhibition imbalance of the neural response to 50% in order to model a system that is predominantly sustained in nature. Under these conditions, the impact of the initial transient becomes essentially negligible, and the summation curves (figure 8Dd) become indistinguishable from proportional summation (i.e., they run parallel to the green curve). This manipulation illustrates that the power of the NDF analysis depends on the neural processing being predominantly transient, and that the properties of the underlying neural mechanisms would not be accessible to this form of analysis in predominantly sustained systems. Luckily, however, the well-established deviation from proportionality for short-duration stimuli implies that the neural system is, in practice, predominantly transient and is therefore amenable to this form of analysis.

In summary, NDF modeling of the full-range duration summation series provides a powerful tool for the analysis of detailed properties of the underlying *neural* signals, including their *time constants*, their *excitation/inhihibition ratio* and the form of *nonlinearity* coupling them to the metabolic recovery processes.

Multicomponent Optimization of the NDF Model to BOLD Responses for a Family of Luminance-Based Stimuli

Background

We have empirically evaluated the NDF model on the basis of BOLD fMRI data that we have recorded in visual stimulation experiments in human. Critically, we have estimated the neural signals underlying the BOLD responses generated by different stimuli *in one and the same* ROI. The rational beyond it is the fact that BOLD waveforms within one and the same cortical region may vary dramatically as a function of the stimulus type, in spite that the metabolic/hemodynamic response functions (MRK) must remain invariant in the region (Likova and Tyler, 2007; d'Avossa, Schulman and Corbetta, 2003). Consequently, differences in the BOLD response waveform must be interpreted as due to differences in the neural response waveforms to the different stimuli.

Task-related differences in BOLD waveform between different brains and between different areas in the one and same brain have been previously reported in long-duration cognitive tasks. These differences could readily be resolved on the typical BOLD time scale, and can be *equivalently* explained by vascular differences between brains and between brain areas as well as by neural differences. However, the preferred interpretation is that differences in BOLD waveform is more likely to be due to differences in hemodynamics (e.g., Handwerker, Ollinger and D'Esposito, 2004) rather than in neural signal dynamics. We now make the crucial point that if there are significant waveform deviations *within the same* cortical areas ensure that they reflect neural processing differences specific for each of the visual stimuli. The stimulus paradigm that we have previously developed following this logic generates distinct percepts of spatial structures from different but very brief, practically instantaneous, temporal changes (Likova and Tyler, 2007). The BOLD response to any instantaneous stimuli (impulses) is traditionally considered to have a constant shape and is used as the HRF estimate in the most popular methods and software packages (*e. g.*, SPM, etc.). However, measuring the waveform for a whole set of different 'impulse' stimuli revealed significant waveform deviations within *the same* cortical areas, thus ensuring that they reflect neural processing differences specific for each of the visual stimuli.

Experimental Paradigm

For the purposes of the empirical evaluation of NDF modeling, we wanted to have very basic stimuli with well known psychophysical and electrophysiological characteristics and to determine the variety of responses *within each* of defined cortical regions, so that any difference would have to be attributed to differences in the neural processing for the four stimulus types as opposed to differences in metabolic/hemodynamic response properties. We have developed a stimulus paradigm including a set of four basic types of luminance transients. They were based either on a uniform field or a checkerboard of 6 arcmin squares, designed to target mechanisms with either low or high spatial-frequency tunings. The uniform gray field was switched to either zero or double the gray luminance for a pulse of 400 *ms* duration. The checkerboard stimuli had 100% luminance contrast and were presented from a uniform gray pre-stimulus state for either 100 *ms* or 400 *ms*.

Results

An example of the variety of cortical responses obtained in retinotopic areas V1 combined for both hemispheres (blue curves) is shown in figure 9, row ***A***, together with the monophasic MRK (green curves) estimated for the same subject. For the checkerboard stimuli (upper panels), the response was almost monophasic for the 100 *ms* duration but was strongly biphasic for the 400 *ms* duration. For the dark pulse, the response was again approximately monophasic, while the response to the bright luminance pulse shows a striking increase in the BOLD signal many seconds after the primary peak.

A similar variety of BOLD response types was seen in the response from cortical area hV4 (figure 9, row *B*), although here the pattern was different from that for the early visual areas. The responses to the checkerboard stimuli were similar to those for V1 except that the early peak for the 400 *ms* duration was substantially reduced. However, the response for the dark pulse was now predominantly a later negativity, while that for the bright pulse had both early and late peaks of entirely positive response. Thus, for both cortical regions, the variety of response waveforms implied a large variation in the neural signals for the four brief stimulus types (whose duration was short enough that they would each be expected to generate the same PERF under the standard GLM analysis.)

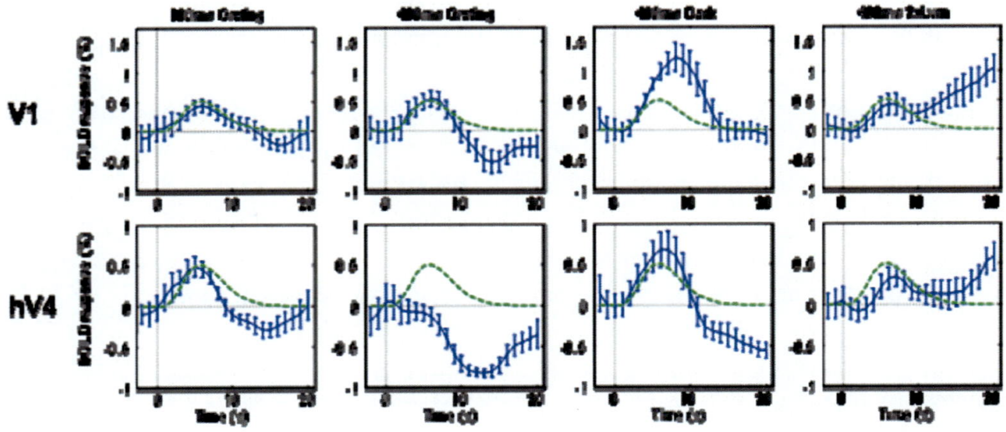

Figure 9. Variety of BOLD response waveforms obtained in retinotopic areas V1 and hV4 for the set of brief grating stimuli of 100 *ms* and 400 *ms* duration, and uniform-field increment and decrement stimuli of 400 *ms*. Note that many of these responses differ substantially from the form of the typical MRK (dashed green lines). The BOLD waveforms differ within each retinotopic area, although the similarity of characteristics between the two areas indicates that the differences are stable and repeatable.

Analysis

Our analysis utilizes the *Nonlinear Dynamic Forward* (NDF) modeling approach based on the assumptions of figure 1, that the neural signals from the neural populations within a small region of cortex generate local metabolic demands that may be nonlinearly related to the neural signals but which sum linearly to form the net activation signal. The linear convolution of the net activation signal with a metabolic response kernel (MRK) thus generates an adequate prediction of the recorded BOLD signal. The nonlinearity lies in the presence of multiple summed components, each derived by linear convolution of the component metabolic demands with the unitary MRK. It may also incorporate the rectification process illustrated in figure 8 (red curves), but such a rectification was not needed for the present analysis.

To analyze the BOLD response waveforms, we assume a blend of two types of gamma functions, based on common features of responses recorded from neurons in early visual areas. The parameters are chosen to typify the shapes encoded by gamma functions, namely with exponent values of k = 1 and 5. These values generate, respectively, a brief and prolonged form of delayed gamma function. These two components are designed to constitute a minimum set of the neural signal properties required to account for the varieties of BOLD responses that are encountered in figure 9. The components were optimized to the waveform for each stimulus type simultaneously with the optimization of a unitary HRF (figure 10A) for the transmutation of the metabolic demand into a predicted BOLD waveform. Note that the HRF used for this analysis is itself assumed to be from the family of (monophasic) gamma functions, on the grounds that many BOLD waveforms are found to be monophasic. The monophasic form of many empirical BOLD waveforms tends to exclude the possibility that the HRF is, in general, multiphasic because it is highly implausible that the neural signal underlying a monophasic BOLD response would happen to have the right form to cancel the multiple phases if the HRF was, in fact, multiphasic.

The novel analysis we propose consists of (i) the simultaneous optimization of the a set of neural components (ii) convolved with the unitary HRF separately for all four stimulus types together with (iii) the rise and fall parameters of HRF. The results of the analysis for the V1 dataset for the battery of four stimulus types we have run with fMRI, is that two components were sufficient to account for >95% of the BOLD variance in each case. Although the average responses exhibit a wide variety of waveforms, the unitary HRF (figure 10A) has the typical form known from previous studies, peaking at about 6 s and returning to baseline by about 18 s. The center row (figure 10C) shows the optimized pair of neural signals in each case, with their parameters optimized to provide the fits shown in the top row (figure 10B). The contribution of each component to the BOLD signal is shown in figure 10D. Note that, although the delay parameter was free to vary, the delays remained close to zero for each primary positive component. The second component was negative (inhibitory) in two cases, with either long delays or a very slow time course, illustrating the unexpected properties of the components required to account for the full variety of BOLD waveforms.

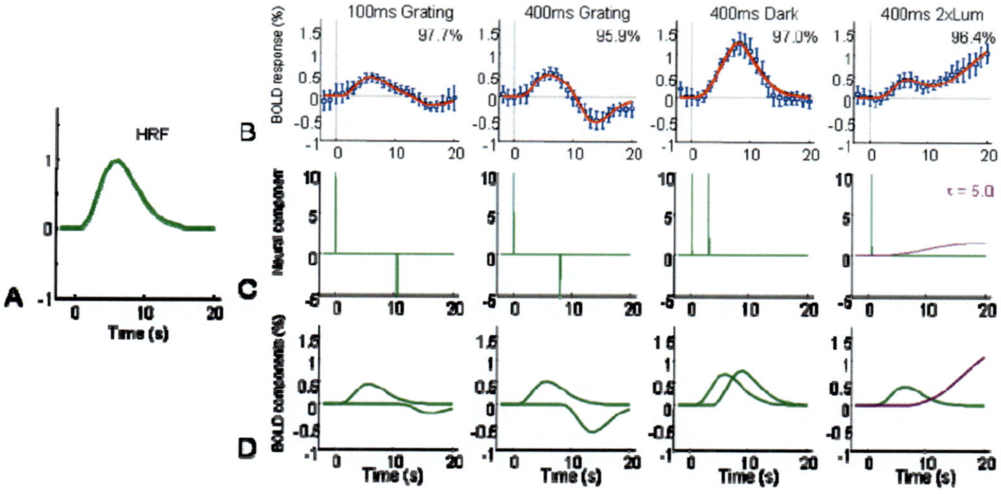

Figure 10. Dynamic forward modeling optimization of neural components to the BOLD responses for cortical area V1, with simultaneous optimization of the unitary HRF to convert the neural signals into the BOLD waveform predictions. *A*. Optimized monophasic HRF. From left to right, the data in the columns correspond to (i) 100 *ms* grating, (ii) 100 *ms* grating, (iii) 400 *ms* dark pulse (decrement), (iv) 400 *ms* bright pulse (increment). *B*. Measured BOLD waveforms for each stimulus type (blue) with best-fitting waveforms (red) and percent variance accounted for. *C*. Optimized neural components for the two-component case. *D*. Individual BOLD waveforms for the separate components making up the summed BOLD waveforms in *B*. Two-component optimizations gave satisfactory fits to all waveforms with minimal delay in the first neural components. Different temporal properties are selected by the optimization to account for the variety of different waveforms.

Of course, any such estimation of the parameters of a set of components underlying a noisy empirical function will have some error variance. A standard approach to the estimation of the parameter variance is the jackknife statistic (Pitman, 1937; Miller, 1964). In general this procedure consists of the removal of each measured point of a function and successive refitting of the parameter estimation to the remaining data for each "*k*th deleted" dataset. The variance of the fits to the loss of each measured point can then be used to infer the overall variance. This approach provides a means of determining the sensitivity of each parameter to the noise contaminating the measured responses. Thus, the jackknife approach provides a means of setting the confidence interval on any of the measured parameters. This capability will be particularly relevant in the next section of the application to the measurement of the causal dynamics of information flow through the cortex.

Causal Cortical Dynamics

The effective connectivity approach (Friston, 1994; Friston et al., 1993a) was proposed to resolve the direction-of-influence ambiguity by defining explicit statistical models of directed neuronal interactions, and it was further advanced by covariance structural equation modeling (Buchel and Friston, 1997; McIntosh and Gonzalez-Lima, 1994), nonlinear system identification techniques (Friston and Buchel, 2000), such as Bayesian estimation of deterministic state-space models (Friston et al., 2003). However, the classic 'effective connectivity' methods have the problem that they rely on a priori specification of a model that contains pre-selected regions and prior knowledge about the existence and direction of influence connections between them. Thus, a conceptual advance toward effective connectivity mapping without pre-selection was the use of "Granger causality" (Granger, 1969; Sims, 1980), to determine both the existence and the direction of interactions from empirical data. Granger causality analysis has been applied to electrophysiological animal data (Baccala and Sameshima, 2001; Bernasconi and Konig, 1999; Bernasconi et al., 2000; Brovelli et al., 2004; Freiwald et al., 1999) and EEG data (Hesse et al., 2003; Kaminski et al., 2001) and to fMRI data (Goebel et al., 2003, 2004). Consequently, various methods for modeling of fMRI time series in the context of Granger causality have been proposed, such as a vector autoregressiion (VAR) (Roebroeck et al., 2005) and wavelet-dynamic vector autoregression (Sato et al., 2006), among others. However, a key problem for the successful application of Granger causality to fMRI signals is its low temporal resolution, due to the fact that the BOLD signal is only an indirect measure of the neuronal responses and thus the neuronal responses are temporally blurred by the metabolic delays of this signal.

The NDF analysis of the underlying neural components sheds further light on the Granger causality. Granger (1969) argued that the flow of time is a natural property incorporated into our concept of causality, and that only associations with a finite lag should be considered to be causal. In its usual implementation, Granger causality is based on a cumulation of significant regression coefficients between two signals across time lags between the two signals. Only the regression coefficients with a time lag are incorporated in the Granger coefficient of causation to the lagged variable. Subsequently, Goebel et al. (2003) and Roebroeck et al. (2005) have proposed the use of Granger Causality approach (as vector autoregressive models) and shown their utility in the analysis of fMRI experiments.

Thus, Granger causality is somewhat problematic when considered in terms of typical neural event sequences, where 'events' consist of signals with extended time courses. If one signal has a short time course and another has a long time course, for example, it is natural to think of their peaks as specifying the timings in their designation as events. If the signal with a short time course goes into a system with a long time constant it will 'cause' a prolonged 'event' peaking at a later time, conforming to the Granger concept. If, on the other hand, the signal with the long time constant has the nonlinear effect of triggering the signal with a short time constant at an early point in the rising phase (of the long-time constant signal), it could happen that the *caused* event peaks earlier than the causal event, reversing the order of inference in the Granger analysis. Thus, particular kinds of nonlinearity, such as trigger events, can violate the assumptions required by Granger, so its inferences should be regarded as probabilistic rather than definitive.

As stated, the Granger causality calculation has the implicit problem that it lacks temporal specificity because takes the *autoregressive spread* of information in each analyzed signal into account by cumulating over *all* delay intervals. The result is purely the causal direction and strength of the connection between any pair of signal sources. We propose an alternative approach based on *temporal cross-correlation* that provides *fine-grain temporal information* about the signal delays between the sources. When there is delayed signal transmission from one signal 'channel' to another, the cross-correlation function between the two signals will exhibit an asymmetry with a peak at the lag corresponding to the transmission delay (Knapp and Carter, 1976). Cross-correlation captures the second-order moments of the full autoregression statistics of the Granger causality formalism. However, Granger causality loses the information about specific delays by summing the lagged mutual information over all lags. The *cross-correlation* approach allows the identification of the specific lag by the *autonormalization* of the two signals being compared in the cross-correlation to remove the effect of their temporal autocorrelations.

An example of a single lag between two signals is shown in figure 11. The broad spread of positive and negative lags of the original autocorrelation is converted to a narrow spike that clearly specifies the *unitary delay* characterizing the connection between the two sources. This compensation may be achieved simply by dividing the Fourier Transform of the cross-correlation signal by its Fourier Amplitude Spectrum, then transforming back to the time domain. This *autoregressive normalization* should account for the temporal spread of all signals feeding into each of the measured activation areas. The essence of the autoregressive] normalization is to collapse the spread of delays due to the build-up and decay in the responsive system to a single characteristic time-shift representing the transmission delay between the two signals, which will be termed the *autonormalized delay*. From this perspective, each autonormalized delay represents a *specific causal link* between the two components. (As in all non-manipulative inferences of causality, there is always the possibility that an apparent causal link of A > B actually represents separate links of C > A and C > B, the latter having extra delay. Such possibilities can be excluded by direct manipulation of the signal at A. In the absence of such manipulation, the inference of causality can only be treated as the parsimonious hypothesis.)

If there is more than one autonormalized delay spike, it implies separate causal links between these systems. The usual implementation of Granger causality throws away this differential information by cumulating the (lagged) delays into a single index, but in the autonormalization approach each lag represents a specific causal link, allowing them to be considered separately rather than being cumulated together. Thus, our novel approach to causality treats each autonormalized delay as a separate causal link between pairs of signals in a network of interconnected cortical regions, with the ability to account for parallel causal links.

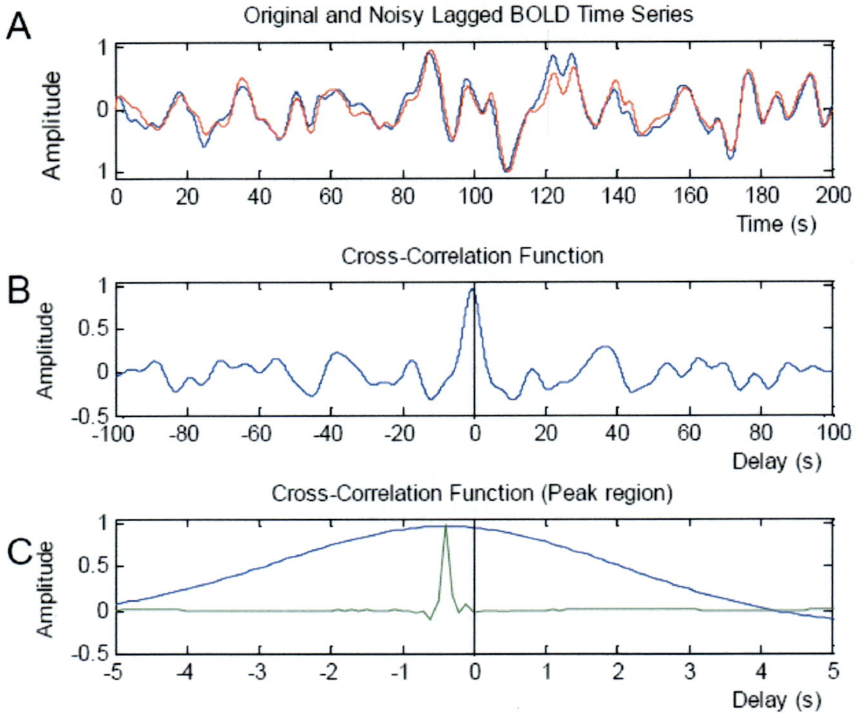

Figure 11. Autonormalization of the cross-correlation for time-resolved delays. *A*). A random time series convolved with a physiologically plausible MRK giving it substantial self-correlations (blue) and a delayed noisy copy of the same signal (red). *B*). Cross-correlation between the original and delayed time series. *C*). Expanded central region of *B*(blue) with autonormalized version of the same function (green). Note that, for this case of a single delay, the autonormalization compresses the causal signal essentially to a single time sample, thus greatly increasing the temporal resolution of the method.

The proposed autonormalization approach is also able of revealing an inhibitory influence between cortical regions, and indeed *separate excitatory and inhibitory* influences between the regions. A simulation of this capability is shown in figure 12. The simulated BOLD waveform was generated again as an MRK-filtered noise model signal that was delayed relative to its input signal and then fed back to the input with a negative weight. As a result, the autonormalized cross-correlation function between input and output (green trace) has *both* a positive and a negative correlation peak indicating delays of 7 s for the feedforward and 4 s for the feedback. These delays are derived from the simulation based on realistic temporal properties of the BOLD signal, indicating that there is a far greater ability to resolve specific temporal interactions through the BOLD signal than previously appreciated.

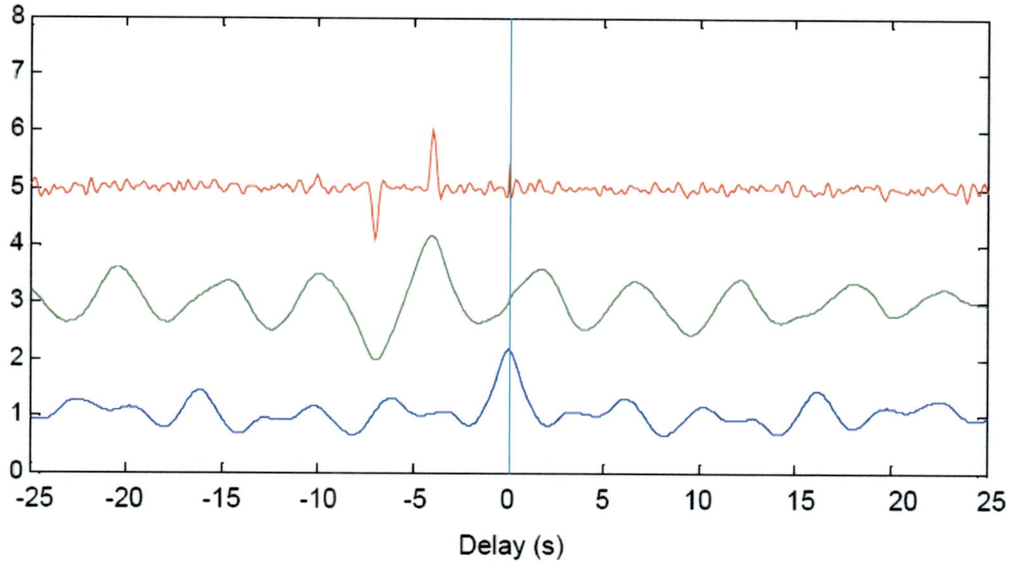

Figure 12. Autonormalized analysis of inhibitory feedback. ACF of input signal (blue), CCF of output with (iterative) inhibitory feedback (green), and autonormalized CCF (red) revealing the excitatory (7 *s*) and inhibitory (4 *s*) delays.

Conclusion

The suite of techniques introduced in this paper can provide a significant enhancement in the ability to resolve the timing and neural signal estimation underlying the BOLD waveforms recorded throughout the cortex. Of course, the precision of the results is inherently limited by the signal/noise ratio of the recordings, but this precision can be enhanced by trade-offs against spatial resolution and by continued technological improvements such as multi-channel coils. The main point of this paper is to show that, given adequate signal/noise ratio, it is possible to develop approaches that overcome the temporal limitations of BOLD signal and are able to reveal the relevant properties of the underlying neural signals. These neural signal estimates may, in turn, be applied to the non-invasive analysis of deficits in the temporal processing of neurological diseases affecting cortical processing in the human brain. The neural delay estimates may, in turn, be applied to revealing the causal relations in understanding the whole-brain functional integration, and in particular to reveal the interactions in cortical networks of activated areas.

Acknowledgements

Supported by RO1 EY 7890 and the Pacific Vision Foundation.

References

Baccala LA, Sameshima K (2001) Partial directed coherence: a new concept in neural structure determination. *Biol. Cybern.* 84: 463-74.

Barlow HB (1958) Temporal and spatial summation in human vision at different background intensities. *J. Physiol.* 141:337-50

Bandettini PA, Ungerleider LG (2001) From neuron to BOLD: new connections. *Nat. Neurosci.* 4:864-6.

Barth M, Norris DG (2007) Very high-resolution three-dimensional functional MRI of the human visual cortex with elimination of large venous vessels. *NMR Biomed.* (in press).

Bellgowan PS, Saad ZS, Bandettini PA (2003) Understanding neural system dynamics through task modulation and measurement of functional MRI amplitude, latency, and width. *Proc. Natl. Acad. Sci. USA.* 10: 1415-9.

Bernasconi C, Konig P (1999) On the directionality of cortical interactions studied by structural analysis of electrophysiological recordings. *Biol. Cybern.* 81: 199-210.

Bernasconi C, von Stein A, Chiang C, Koenig P (2000) Bi-directional interactions between visual areas in the awake behaving cat. *NeuroReport.* 11: 689-92.

Birn RM, Saad ZS, Bandettini PA (2001) Spatial heterogeneity of the nonlinear dynamics in the FMRI BOLD response. *NeuroImage.* 14: 817-26.

Bloch AM (1885) Experiences sur vision. *Comptes Rend. Soc. Biol.* 2, 493-495.

Breiwald WA, Valdes P, Bosch J, Biscay R, Jimenez JC, Rodriguez LM, Rodriguez V, Kreiter AK, Singer W (1999) Testing non-linearity and directedness of interactions between neural groups in the macaque inferotemporal cortex. *J. Neurosci. Methods.* 94: 105-19.

Brovelli A, Ding M, Ledberg A, Chen Y, Nakamura R, Bressler SL (2004) Beta oscillations in a large-scale sensorimotor cortical network: directional influences revealed by Granger causality. *Proc. Natl. Acad. Sci. USA.* 101: 9849-54.

Boynton GM, Engel SA, Glover GH, Heeger DJ (1996) Linear systems analysis of functional magnetic resonance imaging in human V1. *J. Neurosci.* 16: 4207-21.

Buchel C, Friston KJ 1997) Modulation of connectivity in visual pathways by attention: cortical interactions evaluated with structural equation modelling and fMRI. *Cereb. Cortex.* 7: 768-78.

Carandini M, Ferster D (1997) A tonic hyperpolarization underlying contrast adaptation in cat visual cortex. *Science.* 276:949-52.

Carandini M, Ferster D (2000) Membrane potential and firing rate in cat primary visual cortex. *J. Neurosci.* 20:470-84.

Dale AM (1999) Optimal experimental design for event-related fMRI. *Hum. Brain Mapp.* 8:109-14.

Feigl H (1953) Notes on causality. In, Readings in the Philosophy of Science, Eds. H. Feigl and M. Brodbeck, Appleton-Century-Crofts, New York.

Filosa JA, Bonev AD, Nelson MT (2004) Calcium dynamics in cortical astrocytes and arterioles during neurovascular coupling. *Circ. Res.* 95: 73-81.

Friston KJ (2002) Bayesian estimation of dynamical systems: an application to fMRI. *NeuroImage.* 16:513-30.

Friston K (2005) A theory of cortical responses. *Philos. Trans. R. Soc. Lond. B. Biol. Sci.* 360:815-36.

Friston KJ, Buchel C (2000) Attentional modulation of effective connectivity from V2 to

V5/MT in humans. *Proc. Natl. Acad. Sci. USA.* 97: 7591-6.

Friston KJ, Frith CD, Frackowiak RSJ (1993a) Time-dependent changes in effective connectivity measured with PET. *Hum. Brain Mapp.* 1: 69-79.

Friston KJ, Frith CD, Liddle PF, Frackowiak RSJ (1993b) Functional connectivity: the principle component analysis of large (PET) data sets. *J. Cereb. Blood Flow Metab.* 13: 5-14.

Friston KJ, Harrison L, Penny W (2003) Dynamic causal modelling. *NeuroImage.* 19: 1273-302.

Glover G (1999) Deconvolution of impulse response in event-related BOLD fMRI. *Neuroimage.* 9:416-29.

Goebel R, Roebroeck A, Kim DS, Formisano E (2003) Investigating directed cortical interactions in time-resolved fMRI data using vector autoregressive modeling and Granger causality mapping. *Magn. Reson. Imaging.* 21:1251-61.

Goebel R, Roebroeck A, Kim DS, Formisano E (2004) Directed cortical interactions during dynamic sensory-motor mapping. In: Duncan J (ed.), Attention and Performance XX. Oxford University Press, New York, pp. 439-62.

Gorea A, Tyler CW (1986) New look at Bloch's law for contrast. *J. Opt. Soc. Am.* A3, 52-61.

Granger CWJ (1969) Investigating causal relations by econometric models and cross-spectral methods, *Econometrica.* 37:424-438.

Handwerker DA, Ollinger JM, D'Esposito M (2004) Variation of BOLD hemodynamic responses across subjects and brain regions and their effects on statistical analyses. *Neuroimage.* 21:1639-51.

Hansen KA, David SV, Gallant JL (2004) Parametric reverse correlation reveals spatial linearity of retinotopic human V1 BOLD response. *NeuroImage.* 23: 233-41

Harel N, Lin J, Moeller S, Ugurbil K, Yacoub E (2006) Combined imaging-histological study of cortical laminar specificity of fMRI signals. *Neuroimage.* 29:879-87.

Henson RN, Price CJ, Rugg MD, Turner R, Friston KJ (2002) Detecting latency differences in event-related BOLD responses: application to words versus nonwords and initial versus repeated face presentations. *NeuroImage.* 15:83-97.

Hesse W, Moller E, Arnold M, Schack B (2003) The use of time variant EEG Granger causality for inspecting directed interdependencies of neural assemblies. *J. Neurosci. Methods.* 124: 27-44.

Horwitz B (1990) Simulating functional interactions in the brain: a model for examining correlations between regional cerebral metabolic rates. *Int. J. Biomed. Comput.* 26: 149-70.

Horwitz B, Grady CL, Haxby JV, Ungerleider LG, Schapiro MB, Mishkin M, Rapoport SI (1992) Functional associations among human posterior extrastriate brain regions during object and spatial vision. *J. Cogn. Neurosci.* 4: 311-22.

Kelly JP, Van Essen DC (1974) Cell structure and function in the visual cortex of the cat. *J. Physiol.* 238:515-47.

Kraft TW, Schneeweis DM, Schnapf JL (1993) Visual transduction in human rod photoreceptors. *J. Physiol.* 464:747-65.

Levin N, Orlov T, Dotan S, Zohary E (2006) Normal and abnormal fMRI activation patterns

in the visual cortex after recovery from optic neuritis. *Neuroimage.* 33:1161-8.
Likova LT, Tyler CW (2007) Instantaneous stimulus paradigm: Cortical network and dynamics of figure-ground organization. Human Vision and Electronic Imaging XII 6492: 248-255.
Logothetis NK (2002) The neural basis of the BOLD fMRI signal. *Phil. Trans. R. Soc. Lond.* 357:1003-1037.
Logothetis NK (2003) The underpinnings of the BOLD functional magnetic resonance imaging signal. *J. Neurosci.* 23:3963-3971
Logothetis, NK, Wandell BA (2004) Interpreting the BOLD signal. *Annual Review Physiology.* 66:735-769
McIntosh AR, Gonzalez-Lima F (1994) Structural equation modeling and its application to network analysis in functional brain imaging. *Hum. Brain Mapp.* 2:2-22.
McIntosh AR, Grady CL, Ungerleider LG, Haxby JV, Rapoport SI, Horwitz B (1993) Network analysis of cortical visual pathways mapped with PET. *J. Neurosci.* 14: 655-66.
Menon RS, Luknowsky DC, Gati JS (1998) Mental chronometry using latency-resolved functional MRI. *Proc. Natl. Acad. Sci. U S A.* 95:10902-7.
Metea MR, Newman EA (2006) Glial cells dilate and constrict blood vessels: a mechanism of neurovascular coupling. *J. Neurosci.* 26:2862-70.
Miller RG (1964) A trustworthy jackknife. *Ann. Math. Stat.* 35:1594-1605.
Neima D, Regan D (1984) Pattern visual evoked potentials and spatial vision in retrobulbar neuritis and multiple sclerosis. *Arch. Neurol.* 41:198-201.
Pitman, EJG (1937) Significance tests which may be applied to samples from any population, Royal Statistical Society Supplement. 4: 119-130 and 225-32
Regan D, Tyler CW (1971) Temporal summation and its limit for wavelength changes: an analog of Bloch's law for color vision. *J. Opt. Soc. Am.* 61:1414-21.
Regan D, Milner BA, Heron JR (1976) Delayed visual perception and delayed visual evoked potentials in the spinal form of multiple sclerosis and in retrobulbar neuritis. *Brain.* 99:43-66.
Roebroeck A, Formisano E, Goebel R (2005) Mapping directed influence over the brain using Granger causality and fMRI. *NeuroImage.* 25: 230-42.
Russ MO, Cleff U, Lanfermann H, Schalnus R, Enzensberger W, Kleinschmidt A (2002) Functional magnetic resonance imaging in acute unilateral optic neuritis. *J. Neuroimaging.* 12:339-50.
Sato JR, Junior EA, Takahashi DY, Felix MM, Brammer MJ, Morettin PA (2006) A method to produce evolving functional connectivity maps during the course of an fMRI experiment using wavelet-based time-varying Granger causality. *NeuroImage.* 31:187-96.
Schneeweis DM, Schnapf JL (1995) Photovoltage of rods and cones in the macaque retina. *Science.* 268:1053-6.
Schneeweis DM, Schnapf JL (1999) The photovoltage of macaque cone photoreceptors: adaptation, noise, and kinetics. *J. Neurosci.* 19:1203-16.
d'Avossa G, Shulman GL, Corbetta M (2003) Identification of cerebral networks by classification of the shape of BOLD responses. *J. Neurophysiol.* 90:360-71.
Sekiguchi N, Williams DR, Brainard DH (1993) Efficiency in detection of isoluminant and

isochromatic interference fringes. *J. Opt. Soc. Am.* A 10:2118-33.

Shank R, Aprison M (1979) Biochemical aspects of the neurotransmitter function of glutamate. In: Glutamic Acid: Advances in Biochemistry and Physiology. New York: Raven, p. 139–150.

Shmuel A, AugathM, Oeltermann A, Logothetis NK (2006) Negative functional MRI response correlates with decreases in neuronal activity in monkey visual area V1. *Nature Neurosci.* 9, 569-577.

Sims CA (1980) Macroeconomics and reality, *Econometrica.* 48, 1-48

Stefano E, Cupini LM, Rizzo P, Pierelli F, Rizzo PA (1991) Simultaneous recording of pattern electroretinogram (PERG) and visual evoked potential (VEP) in multiple sclerosis. *Acta Neurol. Belg.* 91:20-8.

Tolhurst DJ, Movshon JA, Dean AF (1983) The statistical reliability of signals in single neurons in cat and monkey visual cortex. *Vision Res.* 23:775-85.

Tolhurst DJ, Movshon JA, Thompson ID (1981) The dependence of response amplitude and variance of cat visual cortical neurones on stimulus contrast. *Exp. Brain Res.* 41:414-9.

Uludag K, Yesilyurt B, Ugurbil K (2006) Hemodynamics and nonlinearities of BOLD response to ultrashort visual stimulation (5ms - 1s) Proc ISMRM, 5772.

Vogels R, Spileers W, Orban GA (1989) The response variability of striate cortical neurons in the behaving monkey. *Exp. Brain Res.* 77:432-436

Wang Y, Floor E (1994) Dynamic storage of glutamate in rat brain synaptic vesicles. *Neurosci Lett.* 180:175–178.

Werring DJ, Bullmore ET, Toosy AT, Miller DH, Barker GJ, MacManus DG, Brammer MJ, Giampietro VP, Brusa A, Brex PA, Moseley IF, Plant GT, McDonald WI, Thompson AJ (2000) Recovery from optic neuritis is associated with a change in the distribution of cerebral response to visual stimulation: a functional magnetic resonance imaging study. *J. Neurol. Neurosurg. Psychiatr.* 68:441-9.

In: Brain Mapping Research Progress
Editors: Ines C. Girard and Jade S. Andre

ISBN: 978-1-60456-784-7

Chapter II

DNA Damage Response and Apoptosis of Postmitotic Neurons

Inna I. Kruman[1,*] ***and Elena I. Schwartz***[2]
[1]Sun Health Research Institute, 1015 West Santa Fe Drive, Sun City, AZ 85351;
[2]Department of Pathology and Oncology, Georgetown University Medical Center, 3900 Reservoir RD NW, Washington, DC 20057.

Abstract

Programmed cell death or apoptosis is a relevant process in the physiology and pathology of the nervous system. Apoptosis is an organized form of cell death which is triggered by different factors including DNA damage. A growing body of evidence suggests that DNA damage and genomic instability are involved in neuronal abnormalities and may play a central role in neurodegeneration. DNA strand breaks and DNA lesions have been reported in Parkinson's and Alzheimer's diseases and as an early event after reperfusion of ischemic brain. DNA damage has been found to activate a cell death program in terminally differentiated postmitotic neurons. Since the genome is continuously damaged by a variety of endogenous and exogenous agents and the majority of DNA damage is produced by oxyradicals, generated by normal aerobic metabolism, neurons are particularly susceptible to DNA damage due to the high rate of oxidative metabolism. To maintain genomic integrity, cells are equipped with special defense mechanism, DNA damage response, to remove DNA damage by DNA repair pathways or eliminate damaged cells via apoptosis. Generally, differentiated cells, like neurons, are deficient in DNA repair and more vulnerable to DNA damage-initiated apoptosis. For example, neurons are more vulnerable than astrocytes to DNA-damaging conditions such as ionizing radiation. Breast cancer patients receiving hemotherapy commonly experience long-lasting cognitive impairment. It is known that radiotherapy may cause CNS toxicity. DNA damaging agents including γ-irradiation induce neuronal apoptosis *in vitro*, suggesting the direct adverse effect of these DNA damaging agents on

* Correspondence concerning this article should be addressed to Correspondence to: Inna Kruman, Ph.D.; Sun Health Research Institute, 1015 West Santa Fe Drive, Sun City, AZ 85351; Tel.: 623-876-5607; FAX 623-876-5695; Email: inna.kruman@sunhealth.org.

neurons. The importance of DNA repair for neuronal survival is illustrated by disorders observed in patients with hereditary DNA repair abnormalities. These disorders combine the predisposition to cancer with progressive neurodegeneration. Although indirect evidence suggests that DNA damage and repair mechanisms play critical roles in neuronal survival, the pathways involved are poorly understood. Recently, we have found that cell cycle activation is essential for DNA damage-induced neuronal apoptosis which suggests that the cell cycle machinery is a critical element of the DNA damage response not only in cycling but also in quiescent cells. Here, we discuss the DNA damage response in postmitotic neurons and possible mechanisms by which neurons are forced to apoptosis versus DNA repair thereby controlling cell fate. Elucidation of these mechanisms promises to provide multiple points of therapeutic intervention in neurodegenerative diseases.

Introduction

Neuronal cell death is both a normal developmental process and the result of trauma or degenerative disorders. During development, a significant portion of neurons dies (Oppenheim, 1991), and this death is a part of normal process leading to appropriate matching of pre- and postsynaptic elements Greene et al., 2004). On the other hand, loss of neurons may be a part of the pathological process. Understanding the mechanisms of neuronal death, thus provides insights about nervous system development and anunderstanding of the pathogenesis of neurodegeneration.

Apoptosis is a regulated form of cell death that is often likened to cellular suicide. Unlike necrosis, apoptosis is an active ATP-dependent biochemical process which is regulated through transcriptional, as well as post-translational mechanisms and is not accompanied by inflammation. Apoptotic cells undergo shrinkage, membrane blebbing, chromatin condensation, DNA fragmentation, and cellular disintegration followed by phagocytosis (Wyllie et al., 1980). Many neurons die by apoptosis during early CNS development (Burek and Oppenheim, 1996). In addition, apoptosis contributes to neuronal loss in a number of acute and chronic neurological diseases including stroke, Alzheimer's disease (AD), and amyotrophic lateral sclerosis (ALS) (Friedlander, 2003; Honig and Rosenberg, 2000; Przedborski and Vila, 2003 and Yuan and Yankner, 2000). In general, neuronal apoptosis in these disorders is thought to be caused by toxic insults such as free-radical generation (Klein and Ackerman, 2003). The intracellular end point of many neurotoxic stimuli including excitotoxicity and exposure to amyloid β peptide (Aβ, an essential feature of Alzheimer's disease) is oxidative stress (Butterfield, 2002 and Lewen et al., 2000). Oxidative stress in the form of increased reactive oxygen species (ROS) appears to be a common apoptotic trigger leading to neurodegeneration (Carri et al., 2003; Klein and Ackerman, 2003). ROS include the superoxide anion, hydrogen peroxide, hydroxyl radical, peroxynitrite and lipid peroxides. ROS are constantly produced within the cell, in particular via mitochondrial oxidative metabolism and pathological processes such as inflammation. ROS are also secondary messengers in specific signaling pathways, generated by plasma membrane oxidases in response to growth factors and cytokines (Mahmoudi et al., 2006); they are and therefore, involved in normal cell signaling. The cell has a number of mechanisms of protection against oxidative damage (Offord et al., 2000), including direct interaction with antioxidants such as α-tocopherol, ascorbic acid and glutathione. In general, the balance between ROS levels and the activity of these defense mechanisms determines the degree of oxidative stress encountered by the cell. Neurons are highly susceptible to oxidative stress due to their high rate of oxidative metabolism and low level of antioxidant enzymes (Brook, 2000). ROS are thought to lead to apoptosis by the destruction of lipids, proteins, and nucleic acids (Kannan and Jain, 2000). DNA is perhaps the major target of ROS. In many neurodegenerative disorders, DNA damage is thought to contribute to neuronal loss. DNA damage has been found in chronic neurodegenerative conditions such as Parkinson's (Alam et al., 1997; Jenner and Olanow, 1998) and Alzheimer's diseases (Mecocci et al., 1998; Lovell and Markesbery, 2001), as well as amyotrophic lateral sclerosis (Bogdanov et al., 2000).

The DNA Damage Response

Living cells are continuously exposed to endogenous and environmental DNA-damaging agents. More than 10^4 DNA-damaging events occur in each mammalian cell every day from spontaneous decay, replication errors and cellular metabolism alone (Foray et al., 2003). A major portion of DNA damage occurs via ROS (Williams and Jeffrey, 2000). Exogenous damage may be caused by ultraviolet (UV) radiation from the sun, x- and gamma rays, hydrolysis or thermal disruption, certain plant toxins, such as botulin, or human-made mutagenic chemicals acting as DNA intercalating agents (Jeggo and Lobrich, 2006). If not repaired, some of these lesions are cytotoxic or mutagenic. A cell that has accumulated a large amount of DNA damage, or one that no longer effectively repairs damage, can enter one of three possible states:an irreversible state of dormancy, known as senescence, apoptosis, or mutagenesis and carcinogenesis (Figure1). The protection of genomic integrity, therefore, is a major challenge for living cells. To cope with the deadly consequences of DNA lesions, that interfere with essential DNA-dependent processes such as transcription and replication, cells are equipped with an efficient defense mechanism termed the DNA damage response. The function of the DNA damage response is to eliminate DNA damage through DNA repair or to remove cells with incurred DNA damage by means of apoptosis. DNA damage response mechanisms encompass pathways of DNA repair, cell cycle checkpoint arrest and apoptosis. Thus, two systems are essential for genome integrity, DNA repair and apoptosis (Shiloh, 2006). Cells defective in DNA repair tend to accumulate excess DNA damage, while cells defective in apoptotic process, tend to survive with excess DNA damage. In this regard, the cellular response to DNA damage is crucial for maintaining homeostasis, preventing the development of cancer and neurodegeneration. Defects in this response lead to severe "genomic instability syndromes" (Brooks, 2002). The many types of DNA lesions are rapidly detected, with subsequent activation of a web of signaling pathways which together compose the DNA damage response, culminating in the activation of cell-cycle checkpoints and appropriate DNA repair pathways, or the initiation of apoptotic programs.

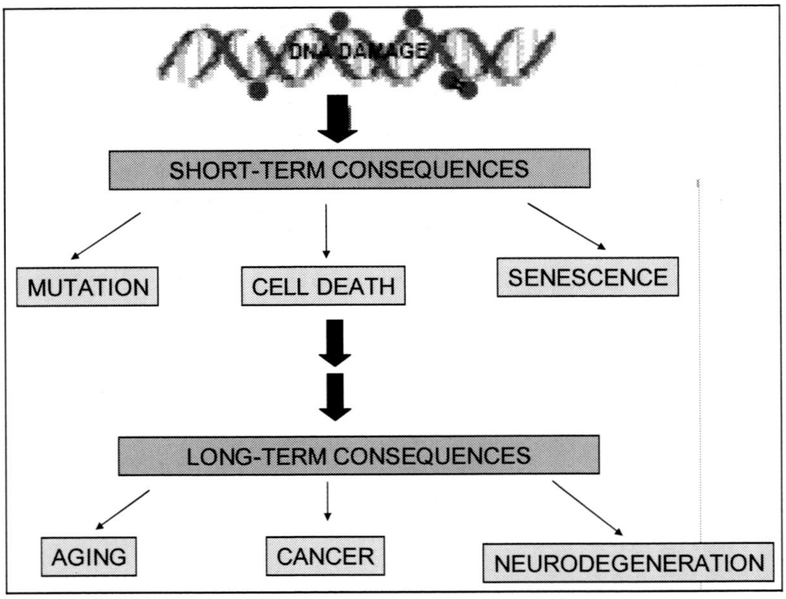

Figure 1. The consequences of non-repaired DNA damage.

DNA Damage Check Points

Checkpoints tightly control progress throughout the cell cycle. Cells may be arrested at any of the checkpoints, and the DNA will be repaired, or alternately cells may die by apoptosis (Sancar et al., 2004). The latter is a mechanism to ensure that non-repairable DNA modifications are not passed on to the progeny of a damaged cell. The same proteins involved in regulating the orderly progression through the cell cycle are also involved in the checkpoint responses (Sancar et al., 2004). The process of DNA replication itself in addition to the usual DNA damaging insults, adds intrinsic risks, such as base misincorporation errors and stalled replication forks, which demand an immediate response from the checkpoint machinery to preserve genomic integrity. If left uncorrected, the errors may lead to the nucleotide sequence alterations and chromosomal rearrangements usually associated with cellular transformation (Kunkel and Bebenek, 2000). The integrity of the S-phase is monitored mainly via two phosphoinositide 3-kinase (PI3)-related kinases ATM (ataxia telangiectasia mutated) and ATR (ATM and Rad 3-related), which play critical roles in early signal transmission (Tibbetts et al, 2000; Abraham, 2003). These two serine/threonine kinases play a central role in signaling DNA damage (Abraham, 2003). G_1- to S-phase transition requires the coordinated action of many proteins including members of the E2F family of transcription factors (Harbour and Dean 2000). E2F activity is required for the transcriptional induction of many genes required for cell cycle progression including cyclins, cyclin dependent kinases (CDKs) and enzymes involved in DNA replication. In addition, E2F functions in apoptosis following DNA damage and regulates expression of pro-apoptotic genes including *apaf-1* and several caspases (DeGregori, 2002). ATM and ATR are thought to be involved in the transmission of signals from stalled replication forks through a multitude of signaling cascades. It has been found that E2F-1 protein levels, DNA binding activity and transcriptional activity are increased following exposure to UV light (O'Connor and Lu, 2000; Blattner et al et al., 1999) or other DNA-damaging agents (Meng et al., 1999). Thus, DNA-damage may induce apoptosis through E2F-1. In turn, the association of this apoptosis with S-phase may result from the fact that E2F-1 is in its free form (i.e. not complexed with retinoblastoma protein Rb (pRb) and thus most active during this phase of the cell-cycle (Harbour and Dean, 2000). The pRb and its related proteins (p107, p130) are thought to act as a checkpoint for G1/S transition in proliferating cells (Niida and Nakanishi, 2006). In its inactive state, pRb is non-phosphorylated and is believed to inhibit cell cycle progression by repressing E2F transcription factors. Upon mitogenic stimulation, pRb is phosphorylated by active cyclin D/CDK4/6 complexes and released from E2F, which results in the derepression and transactivation of E2F-target genes required for S phase entry (Harbour and Dean, 2000; Liu and Greene, 2001). However, there is evidence of the involvement of pRb, possibly activated and recruited to E2F-binding sites, in response to DNA damage (Knudsen et al., 2000). In addition, several genes involved in DNA repair were shown to be regulated by E2F. Deregulation of E2F upregulates the expression of genes involved in the DNA-damage response, e.g. ATM, BRCA1 and RAD51 (Polager et al., 2002; Ren et al., 2002; Berkovich and Ginsberg, 2003). The E2F1 protein has been shown to be stabilized and its levels to rise in response to DNA damage (Blattner et al., 1999; Lin et al., 2001). These findings support a role for E2F transcription factors in the DNA damage response. E2F regulation of DNA repair-associated genes at G1/S transition is consistent with the view that DNA replication is an error-prone process and that DNA repair is tightly linked to DNA synthesis (Boudsocq et al., 2002; Ren et al., 2002). Thus, the DNA damage response, apoptosis and the cell cycle share some common participants such as pRb, E2F, and ATM/ATR (King and Cidlowski, 1995; Stevaux and Dyson, 2002).

The activation of cell cycle checkpoints arrests the cell cycle, while the damage is assessed and repaired. DNA damage response involves alterations in numerous physiological processes such as gene expression and protein synthesis, degradation and trafficking (Shiloh, 2006). The DNA damage response is executed through a series of steps (Figure2). First, the DNA lesions are detected by sensor proteins. Damage to DNA modifies the spatial configuration of the helix and these modifications can be detected by the cell. Transducers initiate a signal transduction cascade that amplifies the signal and conveys the damage signal to downstream effectors. When damage is localized, specific DNA repair molecules, which are part of the whole DNA repair machinery, are recruited and bind at the site of damage, inducing other molecules to bind and form a complex that facilitates the actual DNA repair mechanism. The transducers might also be involved in the assembly of DNA-repair complexes at the sites of DNA damage (Iliakis et al., 2003; Shiloh, 2003; Niida and Nakanishi, 2006). The vast majority of DNA damage affects the primary structure of the double helix. The bases, which are the main component of the double helix, are chemically modified by themselves. These modifications can disrupt the regular helical structure of DNA by introducing non-native chemical bonds or bulky adducts that are not consistent with the standard double helix (Veglia et al., 2003).

There are four main types of chemical DNA damage that arise mainly from endogenous processes that generate ROS, especially superoxide and peroxides: oxidation of bases [e.g. 8-oxo-7,8-dihydroguanine (8-oxoG)] and generation of DNA strand interruptions from reactive oxygen species: alkylation of bases (usually methylation); hydrolysis of bases, such as depurination and depyrimidination;. mismatch of bases, due to DNA replication, in which the wrong DNA base is stitched into place in a newly forming DNA strand (Hoeijmakers, 2001).

Mitochondrial DNA is also vulnerable to damage. In this regard, the attack by oxyradicals especially affects mtDNA due to a highly oxidative environment inside mitochondria (Larsen et al., 2005).

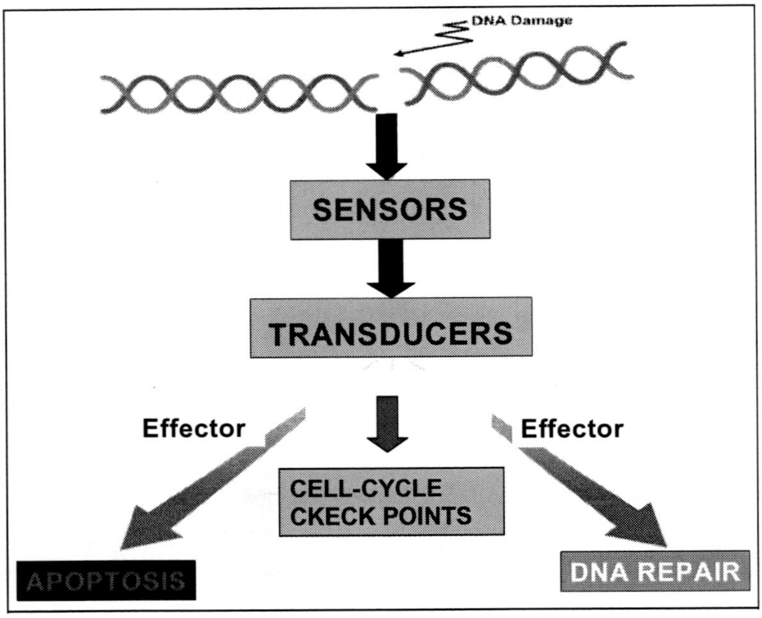

Figure 2. Outline of the DNA damage response pathway in mammalian cells.

DNA Repair

DNA damage initiates various repair mechanisms that recognize and repair specific DNA lesions. The mechanism of DNA repair and the types of molecules involved depend on the type of DNA damage, as well as other factors including the response of signal transduction pathways and the efficiency of DNA repair machinery. Based on all these factors, the consequences for the cell after DNA damage may be variable (Figure3). Various repair mechanisms recognize and repair specific DNA lesions. DNA can be damaged by the introduction of single-strand breaks (SSBs), double-strand breaks (DSBs) and DNA adducts (that is, covalent modifications and crosslinking of individual pyrimidine or purine bases). The efficiency of DNA repair machinery depends on the type of information which is missing or damaged. If damage affects non-essential genes, cells stay superficially functional in contrast to cells with a loss of essential information in the genome. If possible, cells use the unmodified complementary strand of the DNA or the sister chromatid as a template to loosely recover the original information. Without access to a template, cells use an error-prone recovery mechanism known as translesion synthesis as a last resort (Friedberg et al., 2004). A typical DNA-repair pathway might involve DNA lesion detection, signaling to recruit DNA repair factors, the activation of DNA-repair enzymes, and disassembly or degradation of DNA-repair factors after the initial damage is fixed. The main DNA-repair pathways are: nucleotide-excision repair (NER) (which involves global genome repair (GGR) and transcription-coupled repair (TCR), base-excision repair (BER), mismatch repair (MMR), single-strand break (SSB) repair and double-strand break (DSB) repair which includes homologous recombination (HR) and non-homologous end joining (NHEJ) repair. There are two main mechanisms of DNA repair for damaged or inappropriate bases. One of them is direct chemical reversal of the damage. This mechanism is specific to the type of damage incurred. Another well-known mechanism is excision repair. In general, these mechanisms require removal of a damaged region by specialized nuclease systems and then DNA synthesis to fill the gap. NER, BER and MMR lead to the excision of the damaged or mispaired bases, whereas SSBR and DSBR (HR and NHEJ) allow the repair of SSBs and DSBs (Figure3). Although some DNA-repair processes are generally constitutively active, certain ones are activated in response to specific types of DNA lesions (Hoeijmakers, 2001).

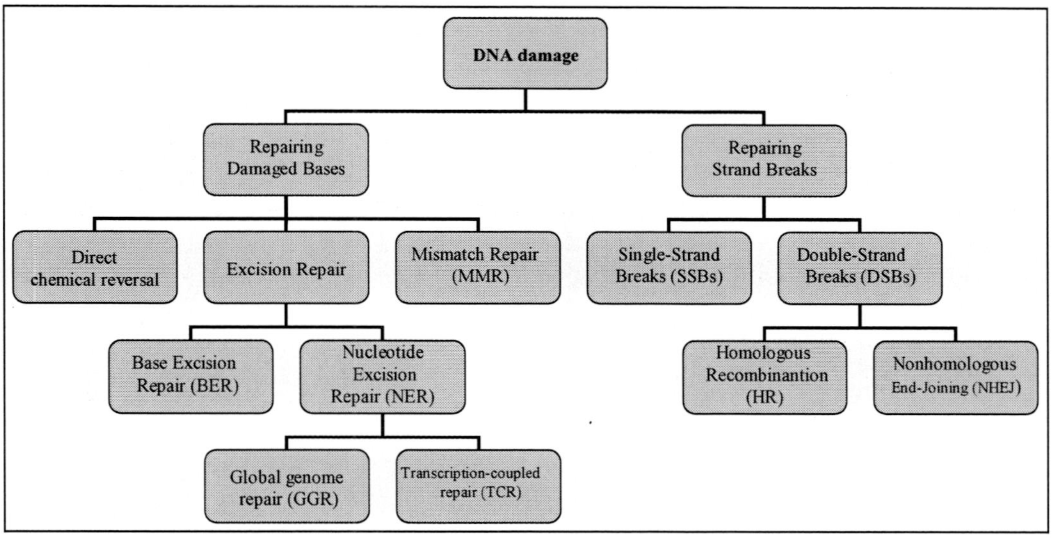

Figure 3. The classification of DNA repair mechanisms.

Base Excision Repair

The most common types of DNA damage are associated with the modificantions of DNA bases, such as uracil, which can arise in genomic DNA by misincorporation of dUMP or by the spontaneous deamination of cytosine to form a premutagenic lesion (Longerich and Storb, 2005). ROS the products of normal cellular respiration, also generate a variety of oxidized DNA base damage, including 8-oxoguanine, that is frequently used as a biomarker for oxidative DNA damage (ESCODD, 2002, 2003). The mutagenic and cytotoxic potential of such DNA base modifications suggests that they may be considered as factors in the induction of cancer and other diseases. These types of DNA damage are so common that they have their own cellular subsystem committed to repairing them. The most important and well-known mechanism is base excision repair (BER). In general, this mechanism requires removal of a damaged region by specialized nuclease systems and then DNA synthesis to fill the gap. BER involves five primary steps: (1) base excision, (2) AP site incision, (3) terminus "cleanup," (4) gap filling, and (5) nick ligation (Parikh et al., 1997). In the process of repair, corresponding DNA glycosylase removes a modified base from the DNA backbone, creating a transient abasic (AP) site (Nilsen et al., 1997; Slupphaug et al., 1991). AP endonuclease 1 (Ape1) cleaves the DNA backbone, which permits incorporation of a correct nucleotide by DNA polymerase β (β-pol) (Srivastava et al., 1998). Completion of BER is accomplished upon ligation (Dimitriadis et al., 1998).

Single-Strand Break Repair

SSBs arise primarily from attack by ROS, whereas indirect SSBs are mainly normal intermediates of DNA BER, as a result of AP endonuclease activity and before they are "handed" to the next enzyme in the BER process, in a molecular relay. In addition to being the most common 'endogenous' lesion (thousands per cell per day) SSBs are also the most common lesions induced by exogenous genotoxins such as ionizing radiation, and alkylating agents (Caldecott, 2004). SSB repair contains four basic steps, beginning with DNA damage binding. SSB detection is largely achieved by the poly (ADP-ribose) polymerases, PARP-1 or PARP-2. A subset of SSBs arising during BER may also require detection or binding by PARPs. These proteins rapidly bind to and are activated by DNA strand breaks, and then covalently modify both themselves and other target proteins with poly (ADP-ribose).

Double-Strand Break Repair

A type of DNA damage particularly hazardous to cells is a break to both strands in the double helix, double strand breaks (DSBs). DSBs are more common than was once expected and are estimated to occur at levels of 10 per cell per day in mammals. This is because they are caused not only by environmental sources, such as ionizing radiation and exposure to genotoxic compounds, but also, and more importantly, from endogenous sources, such as free radicals generated by oxidative respiration (Pfeiffer et al., 2000; Karanjawala et al., 2002). The stability of the mammalian genome therefore relies on efficient repair of DNA DSBs. Two mechanisms exist to repair this damage - non-homologous end-joining (NHEJ) and homologous recombination (HR) (Watson et al., 2004). The NHEJ pathway operates when the cell has not yet replicated the region of DNA on which the lesion has occurred. The process directly joins the two ends of the broken DNA strands without a template, losing sequence information in the process. Thus, this repair mechanism is necessarily mutagenic. However, if the cell is not dividing and has not replicated its DNA, the NHEJ pathway is the cell's only option (Wang et al., 2003). NHEJ involves DNA dependent protein kinase (DNA-PK), a holoenzyme consisting of a catalytic subunit (DNA-PKcs) and a DNA binding and regulatory subunit, Ku heterodimers (Ku 70 and Ku 80), DNA ligase-IV (LIG4), XRCC4 and Artemis (Lieber, 1999; Ma et al., 2002). Mice deficient in LIG4 (or XRCC4) exhibit a pleiotropic phenotype, including late embryonic lethality, cellular growth defects, ionizing-radiation sensitivity, and massive apoptosis of newly generated neurons (Gao et al., 1998; Barnes et al., 1998). Ku70- (Gu et al., 1997) and Ku80- (Nussenzweig et al., 1996) null mice exhibit a similar phenotype. The severe combined immune deficiency (SCID) mice which are deficient in DNA-PK-deficient exhibit severe immunodeficiency, and neurons are hypersensitive to DSB-induced apoptosis (Culmsee et al., 2001; Vemuri et al., 2001), suggesting the importance of NHEJ pathway. One of the very early events following DSBs is the phosphorylation of histone H2AX on serine 139 and simultaneously the autophosphorylation of Ser1981 of the nuclear protein kinase ataxia telangiectasia mutated (ATM) which is the primary DSB transducer (Sedelnikova et al., 2003; Bakkenist and Kastan, 2003). H2AX phosphorylation at serine 139 occurs at sites surrounding DSBs. Recent reports indicate that the dephosphorylation of γH2AX and dispersal of γH2AX foci in γ-irradiated cells correlate with DNA DSB repair (Rothkamm et al., 2003; MacPhail et al., 2003; Nazarov et al., 2003) and numerically correspond to DNA DSBs (Sedelnikova et al.,2002). The ATM function is critical for many aspects of the DSB response (Shiloh, 2003). After DSB induction, ATM is rapidly activated by autophosphorylation (Bakkenist and Kastan, 2003). Active ATM then phosphorylates different substrates, involved in the DNA damage response. An important mediator of cell-cycle checkpoints and damage-induced apoptosis is the tumor suppressor protein p53, which is activated by ATM via various posttranslational modifications (Meek, 2004) or by phosphorylating Mdm2, a ubiquitin ligase of p53, thereby targeting p53 for degradation (Stommel and Wahl, 204). In addition to its role in DNA NHEJ repair, DNA-PK plays important roles in the DNA damage response signaling (Jackson, 2002; Yang et al., 2003). The accumulating data point to an important role of p53 in the DNA-PK-mediated DNA damage signaling pathway (Achanta et al., 2001). Recent observations suggest that in contrast to ATM, DNA-PK is not involved in cell cycle checkpoint regulation through p53, but serves as an upstream regulator of the p53-mediated apoptosis pathway (Burma and Chen, 2004). On the other hand, DSB-induced apoptosis has been reported in p53-deficient cells (Lips and Kaina, 2001). Thus, the mechanisms by which DNA-PK and ATM work in DSB-induced signaling remain unclear. Another transcription factor that has been recently found to be a direct target of ATM is the Ca^{2+}/cAMP response element binding protein (CREB), which is involved in various cellular growth pathways (Shi et al., 2004*)*. The loss of ATM activity is associated with the autosomal recessive disorder ataxia-telangiectasia (A-T), which is characterized by neuronal degeneration, severe neuromotor dysfunction, immunodeficiency, chromosomal fragility, a marked predisposition to cancer, and sensitivity to ionizing radiation (Shiloh, 2003).

DNA Damage in the Nervous System

DNA damage is an important initiator of neuronal cell death and has also been implicated in neurodegenerative conditions. Given that the DNA of postmitotic neurons is particularly susceptible to oxidative stress because of the high rate of oxidative metabolism in the brain, and also due to the fact that postmitotic neurons may live for many decades, DNA damage could be a critical factor in ageing and the progression of some pathologies. DNA strand breaks have been reported in neurons after reperfusion of ischemic tissue, well in advance of DNA fragmentation caused by the apoptotic process (Tobita et al., 1995; Chen et al., 1997; Cui et al., 2000). DNA damage has also been found in various chronic neurodegenerative conditions (Alam et al., 1997; Jenner and Olanow, 1998; Mecocci et al., 1998; Bogdanov et al., 2000; Lovell and Markesbery, 2001). A two-fold higher incidence of single-strand breaks and other alkali-labile DNA lesions are detected in the cerebral cortex of AD versus control brains (Mullaart et al., 1990). In this regard, factors known to be relevant to DNA damage, such as poly (ADP-ribose) polymerase (PARP) and p53, have been implicated in a variety of neurodegenerative diseases (Cosi et al., 1997). Thus, neuronal DNA damage often occurs as a result of oxidative stress (Ratan et al. 1994; Park et al. 1998; Martin et al. 2003). According to our data, elevated levels of oxo8dG in brains of APP mutant transgenic mice, a mouse model of Alzheimer's disease, are correlated with increased levels of soluble Aβ1-42/Aβ1-40 (Kruman et al., 2004a). The amount of oxo8dG was found to be elevated in nuclear and mitochondrial DNA in neurons of diseased brain regions in patients with neurodegenerative disorders (Iida et al., 2002). The importance of DNA damage is illustrated further by the observation that neurological abnormalities are known to accompany defective DNA repair in various human syndromes such as ataxia telangiectasia and Cockayne syndrome (Rolig and McKinnon, 2000). Since neurons have a high metabolic rate and extensive exposure to oxidative stress, it is not surprising that defects in various branches of the DNA damage response lead to severe neurological demise (Brooks, 2002).

In further support, mice deficient in a variety of DNA damage repair pathways display aberrant neuronal loss and impaired neural development (Gao et al., 1998; Sugo et al., 2000), demonstrating connections between DNA damage and neurodegeneration. The importance of DNA repair for the nervous system is illustrated by the fact that many neurological abnormalities and progressive neurodegeneration in patients with hereditary diseases are associated with defects in DNA repair (Rolig and McKinnon, 2000). The nervous system most likely has a DNA repair system largely similar to that found in other tissues (Brooks, 2002; Biton et al., 2006). Terminally differentiated neurons are able to repair DNA damage, although the process is slower than in proliferating cells, and neurons are more prone to DNA damage-initiated apoptosis (Gobbel et al., 1998; Morris and Geller, 1996). A close link between DSB DNA damage and neurodegeneration, essential during nervous system development, appears evident from many pathological data and observations with mouse knockouts. Thus, DNA damage is an important initiator of neuronal cell death implicated in neurodegenerative conditions.

DNA Damage Response in Neurons

Since neurons have an elevated rate of metabolism, particularly oxidative metabolism, which may result in accumulation of numerous lesions in the genome and may compromise transcription (Brooks, 2002), it would be logical to suggest that a mechanism exists to maintain the integrity of those genes needed for viable cell function. Neurons can repair DNA damage, but the process is slower than in proliferating cells, and neurons are known to be more prone to apoptosis (Gobbel et al., 1998). Upon terminal differentiation of neurons, there is a sharp decrease in global genomic repair (GGR). However, repair of active genes has been found to be maintained or even enhanced by differentiation (Ho and Hanawalt, 1991). Differentiated cells have been shown to repair transcribed genes using the specialized repair pathway termed transcription-coupled repair (TCR), which targets repair systems to transcribed genes (Nouspikel and Hanawalt, 2002). The mechanisms of this type of DNA repair are not yet fully understood. Several DNA repair systems, including base excision repair (BER) may be involved in TCR (Larsen et al., 2000).

Role of Cell Cycle Reentry in the DNA Damage Response

The DNA damage response has been investigated mainly in proliferating cells, which integrate cell cycle machinery with DNA damage signaling; the response is involved both in DNA repair and apoptosis (Shiloh, 2003; Lukas et al., 2004). Traditionally, neurons have been considered to be "locked" into the G0 phase of the cell cycle. Normally, the release of a cell from the resting G0 phase results in its entry into the first gap phase (G1), during which the cell prepares for DNA replication in the S phase. This is followed by the second gap phase (G2) and mitosis (M phase). While a number of studies have investigated the responses of proliferating cells to genotoxic agents, little is known about the DNA damage response in neurons and other terminally differentiated cells. Differentiated neurons are characterized by the reduction in the cellular levels of several DNA damage response proteins (Lukas et al., 2004; Nouspikel and Hanawalt, 2002; McMurray, 2005; Biton et al., 2006). While this observation is in keeping with the notion that resting cells must reenter the cell cycle in order to carry out DNA repair, a role for cell cycle activation in terminally differentiated cells remains unclear. This activation may be involved in the DNA damage response, DNA repair and apoptosis (Kruman, 2004; Kruman et al., 2004a). Evidence is emerging that in neurodegenerative diseases, neurons attempt to re-enter the cell cycle and this attempt is followed by programmed cell death (Kruman, 2004; Herrup et al., 2004). However, while terminally differentiated neurons retain the ability to reactivate the cell cycle, it rarely leads to neuronal proliferation but typically induces apoptosis (Wartiovaara et al., 2002; Husseman et al., 2000 and Liu and Greene, 2001). Consistent with this idea are the rare incidence of brain tumors of neuronal origin and the resistance of neurons to oncogenic transformation (Heintz, 1993). On the other hand, aneuploidy was demonstrated to be quite common in the brain of adult animals (Rehen et al., 2001), meaning that DNA replication in terminally differentiated cells may lead to aneuploidy. Nevertheless, re-expression and activation of cell cycle proteins have been observed in dying neurons of brains of patients with neurodegenerative disorders (Nagy et al., 1997; Husseman et al., 2000; Yang et al., 2001). Recently, a direct interaction between cell cycle machinery and the cell-intrinsic apoptotic program was demonstrated in postmitotic neurons with the observation that cdc2, a cell cycle regulator, directly initiates apoptosis via direct activation of Bad, a trigger of apoptosis (Konishi et al., 2002). The suppression of cell cycle-dependent kinase (CDK) activity has been shown to produce a neuroprotective effect both *in vivo* and *in vitro* (Park et al., 1997; O'Hare et al., 2002; Katchanov et al., 2001; Rideout et al., 2003), supporting the idea that cell cycle reentry underlies neuronal apoptosis. The suppression of ATM, a key player in the

DNA damage response, was found to attenuate the damage-induced attempts to reenter cell cycle and consequently apoptosis following DNA damage in neurons (Kruman et al., 2004a). This can be linked to findings that neurons from ATM-deficient mice have demonstrated a striking resistance to DNA damage-induced apoptosis (Herzog et al., 1998; Chong et al., 2000; Macleod et al., 2003; Kruman et al., 2004a). Importantly, ATM deficiency rescued the apoptosis of neurons observed in *Lig4*, *Ku70* or *Ku80*- knockout mice (Nussenzweig et al., 1996; Gu et al., 1997; Lee et al., 1997; Sekiguchi et al., 2001). This suggests that the disturbance of DSB repair resulting from the lack of NHEJ components (Lig4, Ku70 or Ku80) in neurons can be recognized by ATM in a pathway leading to apoptosis. In the developing nervous system, this process may serve to remove cells that suffer irreparable damage from the system (McKinnon, 2001), indicating that ATM may function to eliminate neural cells that have incurred DNA damage. On the other hand, the amount of unrepaired DNA after γ-irradiation was greater in cells from ataxia-telangiectasia patients than in cells from normal individuals (Cornforth and Bedford, 1985), underscoring the importance of ATM for DNA repair. Recently, we and others have shown that the DNA damage response in postmitotic neurons committed to apoptosis involves cell cycle- associated events (Klein et al., 2002; Kruman et al, 2004a). Previously, we found that suppression of the ATM function attenuates apoptosis and abrogates cell cycle reentry in postmitotic cortical neurons exposed to DNA-damaging agents (Kruman et al., 2004a). We have now extended this work by showing that ATM deficiency also affects cell cycle activation associated with DNA repair in neurons (Figure 4), in keeping with the documented reduction in DNA repair efficiency in cells from ataxia-telangiectasia patients (Cornforth and Bedford, 1985). This reflects the intimate relationship between ATM, cell cycle activation, and DNA repair in postmitotic neurons, and further suggests that cell cycle reentry is a requisite component of the response to DNA damage essential for the execution of both apoptosis and DNA repair in neurons. Although it is widely accepted that postmitotic cells and tissues have decreased DNA repair capacity, several findings indicate that postmitotic cells such as muscle cells and neurons may up-regulate the expression of DNA glycosylases in certain conditions (Karahalil et al., 2002). Thus, oxoguanine-DNA glycosylase (OGG1; which recognizes and removes 8-oxoguanine) activity in rat heart increases significantly with age (Souza-Pinto et al., 1999). Up-regulation of mRNA levels of APE/Ref1, a multifunctional enzyme that has both an AP endonuclease activity and is essential for glycosylase initiated BER (Flaherty et al., 2001) in neurons, were shown to be high in certain hypothalamic nuclei, as well as in the hippocampus and cerebellum (Wilson et al., 1996). In brain, up-regulation of BER activity was detected after ischemia-reperfusion injury (Lin et al., 2000). Oxidative stress and oxidative DNA damage induce up-regulation of OGG1 activity associated with this type of DNA damage. In support of these observations, we found up-regulated levels of UNG mRNA in brains of cystathionine-β-synthase-knockout (CBS) mice compared to wild-type mice. CBS mice are characterized by hyperhomocysteinemia (Watanabe et al., 1995), which is associated with one-carbon metabolism impairment (itself associated with uracil misincorporation) (Duthie, 1999). Like the up-regulation of OGG1 in response to oxidative DNA damage, uracil misincorporation mediated by hyperhomocysteinemia induces up-regulation of UNG mRNA. The UNG activity is in general significantly higher in proliferating as compared with nonproliferating tissues (Aprelikova and Tomilin, 1982), and the expression of UNG has been demonstrated to be under cell cycle regulation (Nahelhus et al., 1997; Walsh et al., 1995). The inducibility of the BER enzymes, OGG1, UNG and APE/Ref1 may indicate that BER in general is essential for maintaining genomic integrity in the brain and that up-regulation of expression and/or activity of BER enzymes in brain tissue may be induced by DNA damage during certain challenges (e.g. hyperhomocysteinemia in CBS knockout mice or oxidative stress) and mediated by cell cycle activation in neurons.

In cycling cells, the DNA damage response is comprised of cell cycle arrest at specific checkpoints, presumably to allow time for the damage to be repaired, or to activate the apoptotic program if the damage is too extensive to be repaired (Rhind and Russell, 2000). Cell cycle regulation is integrated with DNA repair mechanisms and even utilizes some common proteins (Slupphaug et al., 2003). ATM activated by DSBs phosphorylates key proteins that lead to cell cycle checkpoint arrest and/or apoptosis (Shiloh, 2003). In postmitotic, terminally differentiated neurons, signaling through cell cycle components is also essential for the response to DNA damage, but in contrast to cycling cells, which undergo growth arrest at specific checkpoints, the signaling in neurons is associated with activation of the cell cycle.

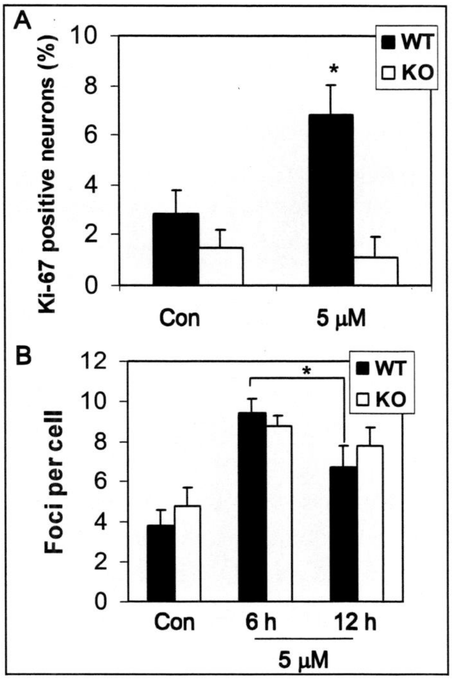

Figure 4. Suppression of ATM function prevents the cell cycle activation in cultured cortical neurons induced by subtoxic (5 μM) concentration of H_2O_2, and inhibits DNA repair. (A) Ki-67-positive neurons are reduced in cultures of cortical neurons derived from ATM knockout (ATM-/-) mice compared with those derived from wild-type (WT) following treatment for 12 h with 5 μM H_2O_2. (B) Cultures were exposed to either saline or subtoxic (5 μM) concentration of H_2O_2, during the indicated periods of time. Immunoreactivity for γ-H2AX was visualized with FITC (488, green). Cells were co-stained with PI. γ-H2AX foci were determined in at least 50 cells. Note significant reduction of γ-H2AX foci in cultures derived from wild-type (WT) mice after 12-h exposure to 5 μM compared to 6-h exposure in contrast to those derived from ATM knockout (ATM-/-) mice. Control (Con) represents the untreated culture. The values are the mean and SD (n=6); *p<0.01.

Cell Cycle Reentry and Neuronal Apoptosis

Traditionally, neurons have been considered to rest in the G0 phase of the cell cycle. However, accumulating evidence suggests that postmitotic neurons re-express cell cycle markers with the occurrence of neuronal apoptosis (Liu and Greene, 2001; Herrup et al., 2004). These markers include cyclin D, which is involved in the G0-G1 transition, phosphorylated at Ser 795 retinoblastoma tumor suppressor protein (Rb) which is critical for activation of the cell cycle, the DNA helicase subunit minichromosome maintenance (Mcm) proteins 2-7 which assemble in the pre-replication complex, a nuclear antigen Ki-67, which is absent from resting (G0) cells, and cyclin E, a marker of G1-S transition (Becker and Bonni, 2004). Moreover, neurons are able to undergo full or partial DNA replication, showing that they have completed the S phase (Yang et al., 2001; Kruman et al., 2004a). DNA replication has been suggested to be lethal for neurons (Herrup et al., 2004). DNA damage-initiated apoptosis was shown to increase the expression of error-prone DNA polymerase β (Copani et al., 2002), whose physiological role appears restricted to DNA repair (Sobol et al., 1996). In neurons entering the S phase, polymerase β-directed DNA replication might produce additional DNA damage, thus contributing to the execution of apoptosis (Klein et al., 2002).

Little is known about the mechanisms of the DNA damage response in terminally differentiated neurons, especially concerning its integration with cell cycle machinery. However, there is both *in vitro* and *in vivo* evidence of a link between DNA damage and cell cycle reentry in dying postmitotic neurons. Analysis of the X-harlequin (Hq) mutation in the gene encoding apoptosis-inducing factor (AIF) which is accompanied by oxidative stress, has demonstrated that in Hq mice, many cerebellar granule cells had newly synthesized nuclear DNA and were positive for oxo8dG, a marker of oxidative DNA damage (Klein et al., 2002). Using flow cytometry and BrdU incorporation analyses, we have demonstrated that cell cycle activation followed by apoptosis is induced by DNA damage and can be blocked along with the DNA damage response (Kruman et al., 2004a). Although these observations imply that induction of unscheduled cell cycle reentry is highly correlated with, and is likely induced by DNA damage, the mechanisms of the DNA damage response, its link to cell cycle machinery and roles of this machinery in DNA repair of postmitotic neurons are poorly defined. Both the cell cycle and apoptosis are controlled by a highly conserved machinery and exhibit morphological similarities of cell rounding and chromatin condensation. They also share some common participants such as ATM, E2F and p53 (King and Cidlowski, 1995; Matsumura et al., 2003). The *in vivo* evidence that cell cycle re-entry in postmitotic terminally differentiated neurons is associated with DNA damage came from the analysis of the X-linked *harlequin* (*Hq*) mutation in the gene encoding apoptosis-inducing factor (AIF) that causes progressive ataxia (Klein et al., 2002). In *Hq* mice, many but not all cerebellar granule cells had newly synthesized nuclear DNA, as demonstrated by BrdU incorporation, and were positive for caspase-3, indicating the association with apoptosis. In cycling cells, whether DNA damaging conditions cause growth arrest or apoptosis may depend in part on where the cell resides in the cell cycle when the insult is delivered. The fact that not all oxo8dG-positive neurons in brains of *Hq* mice were in the S-phase indicates that these neurons may enter the S-phase later and then die by apoptosis; aqlternately, these oxo8dG-positive neurons may repair the DNA and not enter the S-phase, with subsequent apoptosis, but instead continue normal functioning. Using flow cytometry and BrdU incorporation analyses, we have demonstrated that cell cycle activation followed by apoptosis is induced by DNA damage and can be blocked together with the DNA damage response (Kruman et al., 2004a). These observations and the detection of markers for oxidative DNA damage (long before neurodegeneration) demonstrate that induction of unscheduled cell cycle reentry is highly correlated with, and is likely induced by DNA damage. Furthermore, the amount of oxo8dG, a major oxidative DNA lesion that has been found to be elevated in neuronal DNA in brains of patients with neurodegenerative disorders (Migliore and Coppede, 2002). Increases in oxo8dG are also correlated with increased incidence of cancer (Helbock et al., 1998), endorsing the importance of the same factors in the pathogenesis of both types of disorders.

Conclusion

In summary, DNA damage may activate cell cycle machinery in postmitotic neurons as an essential part of the DNA damage response. Like in cycling cells, DNA damage may result in DNA repair or apoptosis if DNA damage is unrepaired, and the consequent loss of neurons by apoptosis could result in neurodegeneration. In addition, neurodegeneration is a hallmark of various diseases observed in patients with hereditary DNA repair disorders. The mechanisms by which a cell is forced into apoptosis versus DNA repair, or instead dies by a nonapoptotic mechanism from unrepaired DNA, are not clear. It is likely that both outcomes are managed by the DNA damage response. Suppression of ATM which is a proximal component of DNA damage response, attenuates both apoptosis and cell cycle reentry, suggesting that both cell cycle activation and apoptosis constitute the DNA damage response. ATM deficiency in humans is characterized by predisposition to cancer and progressive neurodegeneration suggesting the impairment of DNA repair when the main player in the DNA damage response does not act. Cortical neurons from ATM-deficient mice are more resistant to apoptosis initiated by DNA damage, suggesting that ATM may function to eliminate neural cells when they have incurred sufficient DNA damage. ATM suppression in neurons prevent cell cycle reentry, while cycling cells deficient in ATM exhibited defective cell cycle checkpoints, implying that neurons may be influenced by the same cell cycle checkpoints that govern apoptosis in cycling cells.

References

Abraham, RT. (2003). Checkpoint signaling: epigenetic events sound the DNA strand-breaks alarm to the ATM protein kinase. *Bioessays. 25*,627-630.

Achanta, G; Pelicano, H; Feng, L; Plunkett, W; Huang, P. (2001). Interaction of p53 and DNA-PK in response to nucleoside analogues: potential role as a sensor complex for DNA damage. *Cancer Res 61*,8723-8729.

Alam, ZI; Jenner, A; Daniel, SE; Lees, AJ; Cairns, N;Marsden, CD; Jenner, P; Halliwell, B. (1997). Oxidative DNA damage in the parkinsonian brain: an apparent selective increase in 8-hydroxyguanine levels in substantia nigra. *J Neurochem. 69*,1196-1203.

Aprelikova, O N & Tomilin N V. (1982) Activity of uracil-DNA glycosylase in different rat tissues and in regenerating rat liver. *FEBS Lett. 137*,193-195

Bakkenist, CJ & Kastan, MB. (2003). DNA damage activates ATM through intermolecular autophosphorylation and dimer dissociation. *Nature. 421*,499-506.

Barnes, DE; Stamp, G; Rosewell, I; Denzel, A; Lindahl, T. (1998). Targeted disruption of the gene encoding DNA ligase IV leads to lethality in embryonic mice. *Curr Biol. 8*,1395-1398.

Becker, EB & Bonni, A.(2004). Cell cycle regulation of neuronal apoptosis in development and disease. *Prog Neurobiol. 72*,1-25.

Berkovich, E & Ginsberg, D. (2003). ATM is a target for positive regulation by E2F-1. *Oncogene.22*,161-167.

Bernstein, C; Bernstein, H; Payne CM; Garewal H. (2002). DNA repair/pro-apoptotic dual-role proteins in five major DNA repair pathways: fail-safe protection against carcinogenesis. *Mutat Res 511*,145-178.

Biton, S; Dar, I, Mittelman, L; Pereg, Y; Barzilai, A; Shiloh Y. (2006). Nuclear ataxia-telangiectasia mutated (ATM) mediates the cellular response to DNA double strand breaks in human neuron-like cells. *J Biol Chem. 281*,17482-17491.

Blattner, C; Tobiasch, E; Litfen, M; Rahmsdorf, HJ; Herrlich, P. (1999). DNA damage induced p53 stabilization: no indication for an involvement of p53 phosphorylation. *Oncogene. 18*,1723-1732.

Bogdanov, M; Brown, RH; Matson, W; Smart, R; Hayden, D; O'Donnell; H, Flint Beal; M, Cudkowicz, M. (2000). Increased oxidative damage to DNA in ALS patients. *Free Radic Biol Med. 29*,652-658.

Brooks, PJ. DNA repair in neural cells: basic science and clinical implications (2002). *Mut Res. 509*,93.-108

Boudsocq, F; Ling, H; Yang, W; Woodgate, R. (2002). Structure-based interpretation of missense mutations in Y-family DNA polymerases and their implications for polymerase function and lesion bypass. *DNA Repair (Amst). 1*,343-358.

Burek, MJ & Oppenheim, RW (1996). Programmed cell death in the developing nervous system. *Brain Pathol. 6*,427-446.

Burma, S & Chen, DJ. (2004). Role of DNA-PK in the cellular response to DNA double-strand breaks. *DNA Repair (Amst). 3*,909-918.

Butterfield, DA. (2002). Amyloid beta-peptide (1-42)-induced oxidative stress and neurotoxicity: implications for neurodegeneration in Alzheimer's disease brain. *Free Radic Res. 36*,1307-1313.

Caldecott, KW. (2004). DNA single-strand breaks and neurodegeneration. *DNA Repair (Amst). 3*,875-882.

Carri, NG.(2003). Multiple neurotrophic signalling: certain TGF molecules are involved in retinal development and maturation, but do they complement one another's actions? *Cell Biol Int. 27*,1033-1036.

Chen, J; Jin, K; Chen, M; Pei, W; Kawaguchi, K; Greenberg, DA; Simon, RP. (1997). Early detection of DNA strand breaks in the brain after transient focal ischemia: implications for the role of DNA damage in apoptosis and neuronal cell death. *J Neurochem. 69*,232-245.

Chong, MJ; Murray, MR; Gosink, EC; Russell, HR; Srinivasan, A; Kapsetaki, M; Korsmeyer, SJ; McKinnon, P J. (2000). Atm and Bax cooperate in ionizing radiation-induced apoptosis in the central nervous system. *Proc Natl Acad Sci U S A. 97*.889-894.

Copani, A; Sortino, MA; Caricasole A; Chiechio, S; Chisari, M; Battaglia, G; Giuffrida,-Stella, AM; Vancheri, C; Nicoletti F. (2002). Erratic expression of DNA polymerases by beta-amyloid causes neuronal death. *FASEB J. 16*,2006-2008.

Cornforth; M N & Bedford, JS. (1985). On the nature of a defect in cells from individuals with ataxia-telangiectasia. *Science. 227*,1589-1591.

Cosi, C; Suzuki, H; Skaper, SD; Milani, D; Facci, L; Menegazzi, M; Vantini, G; Kanai, Y; Degryse, A; Colpaert, F; Koek, W; Marien MR. (1997). Poly(ADP-ribose) polymerase (PARP) revisited. A new role for an old enzyme: PARP involvement in neurodegeneration and PARP inhibitors as possible neuroprotective agents. *Ann N Y Acad Sci. 825*,366-379.

Cui, J; Holmes, EH; Greene, TG; Liu, PK. (2000). Oxidative DNA damage precedes DNA fragmentation after experimental stroke in rat brain. *FASEB J. 14*,955-967.

Culmsee, C; Bondada, S; Mattson, MP. (2001). Hippocampal neurons of mice deficient in DNA-dependent protein kinase exhibit increased vulnerability to DNA damage, oxidative stress and excitotoxicity. *Brain Res Mol Brain Res. 87*,257-262.

DeGregori J. (2002). The genetics of the E2F family of transcription factors: shared functions and unique roles. *Biochim Biophys Acta. 1602*,131-150.

Foray, N; Marot, D; Gabriel, A; Randrianarison, V; Carr, AM; Perricaudet, M; Ashworth, A; Jeggo, P. (2003). A subset of ATM- and ATR-dependent phosphorylation events requires the BRCA1 protein. *EMBO J. 22*,2860-28671.

Dimitriadis, EK; Prasad, R; Vaske, MK; Chen, L; Tomkinson, AE; Lewis, MS; Wilson, SH. (1998). Thermodynamics of human DNA ligase I trimerization and association with DNA polymerase beta. *J Biol Chem. 273*,20540-20550.

Duthie, G G. (1999) Determination of activity of antioxidants in human subjects.*Proc. Nutr. Soc. 58*,1015-1024

European Standards Committee on Oxidative DNA Damage (ESCODD). (2002). Comparative analysis of baseline 8-oxo-7,8-dihydroguanine in mammalian cell DNA, by different methods in different laboratories: an approach to consensus. *Carcinogenesis. 23*,2129-2133.

European Standards Committee on Oxidative DNA Damage (ESCODD). (2003). Measurement of DNA oxidation in human cells by chromatographic and enzymic methods. *Free Radic Biol Med. 34*,1089-1099.

Flaherty, DM; Monick, MM; Hunninghake, GW. (2001). AP endonucleases and the many functions of Ref-1. *Am J Respir Cell Mol Biol. 25*,664-667.

Friedberg, EC; McDaniel, LD; Schultz, RA. (2004). The role of endogenous and exogenous DNA damage and mutagenesis. *Curr Opin Genet Dev. 14*,5-10.

Friedlander, RM. (2003). Apoptosis and caspases in neurodegenerative diseases. *N Engl J Med. 348*,1365-1375.

Gao, Y; Sun, Y; Frank, KM; Dikkes, P; Fujiwara, Y; Seidl, KJ; Sekiguchi JM; Rathbun, GA; Swat, W; Wang, J; Bronson, RT; Malynn BA; Bryans, M; Zhu, C; Chaudhuri J; Davidson, L; Ferrini, R J. (1998). *Cell Biol. 119*,493-501.

Gobbel, GT; Bellinzona, M; Vogt, AR; Gupta, N; Fike, JR; Chan, PH. (1998). Response of postmitotic neurons to X-irradiation: implications for the role of DNA damage in neuronal apoptosis. *J Neurosci. 18*,147-55.

Greene, LA; Biswas, SC; Liu, DX. (2004). Cell cycle molecules and vertebrate neuron death: E2F at the hub. *Cell Death Diffe*r. *11*,49-60.

Gu, Y; Seidl, K J ; Rathbun, G A; Zhu, C; Manis, J P; van der Stoep, N; Davidson, L; Cheng, H L; Sekiguchi, J M; Frank, K; Stanhope-Baker, P; Schlissel, MS; Roth, DB; Alt, FW. (1997) Growth retardation and leaky SCID phenotype of Ku70-deficient mice. *Immunity 7*,653-665.

Harbour, JW & Dean, DC. (2000). The Rb/E2F pathway: expanding roles and emerging paradigms. *Genes Dev.14*,2393-2409.

Heintz, N. (1993). Cell death and the cell cycle: a relationship between transformation and neurodegeneration? *Trends Biochem Sci. 18*,157-159.

Helbock, HJ; Beckman, KB; Shigenaga, MK; Walter, PB; Woodall, AA; Yeo, HC; Ames, BN.(1998). DNA oxidation matters: the HPLC-electrochemical detection assay of 8-oxo-deoxyguanosine and 8-oxo-guanine. *Proc Natl Acad Sci U S A. 95*,288-293.

Herrup, K; Neve, R; Ackerman, SL; Copani, A. (2004). Divide and die: cell cycle events as triggers of nerve cell death. *J Neurosci. 24*,9232-9239.

Herzog, KH; Kapsetaki, M; Morgan, JI; McKinnon, P.J., (1998). Requirement for ATM in ionizing radiation-induced cell death in the developing central nervous system. *Science 280*,1089-1091.

Herzog, KH; Chong, MJ; Kapsetaki, M; Morgan, JI; McKinnon PJ. (1998). Requirement for Atm in ionizing radiation-induced cell death in the developing central nervous system. *Science. 280*,1089-1091.

Ho, L & Hanawalt, PC. (1991).Gene-specific DNA repair in terminally differentiating rat myoblasts. *Mutat Res. 255*,123-141.

Hoeijmakers, JH. (2001). Genome maintenance mechanisms for preventing cancer. *Nature. 411*,366-374.

Honig, LS & Rosenberg, RN.(2000). Apoptosis and neurologic disease. *Am J Med.108*,317-330.

Husseman, JW; Nochlin, D; Vincent, I. (2000). Mitotic activation: A convergent mechanism for a cohort of neurodegenerative disease. *Neurobiol. Aging. 21*,815-828.

Iida, T; Furuta, A; Nishioka, K; Nakabeppu, Y; Iwaki, T. (2002). Expression of 8-oxoguanine DNA glycosylase is reduced and associated with neurofibrillary tangles in Alzheimer's disease brain. *Acta Neuropathol (Berl). 103*,20-25.

Iliakis, G; Wang, Y; Guan, J; Wang, H. (2003). DNA damage checkpoint control in cells exposed to ionizing radiation. *Oncogene. 22*,5834-5847.

Jackson, S. (2002). Sensing and repairing DNA double strand breaks. *Carcinogenesis. 23*, 687-696.

Jeggo, PA & Lobrich M. (2006). Contribution of DNA repair and cell cycle checkpoint arrest to the maintenance of genomic stability. *DNA Repair (Amst).* [Epub ahead of print]

Jenner, P & Olanow, CW. (1998). Understanding cell death in Parkinson's disease. *Ann Neurol. 44* (Suppl 1),S72-84

Johnson, RT; Gotoh, E; Mullinger, AM; Ryan, AJ; Shiloh, Y; Ziv, Y; Squires, S. (1999). Targeting in double-strand breaks to replicating DNA identifies a subpathway of DSB repair that is defective ataxia-telangiectasia cells. *Biochem Biophys Res Commun. 261*,317-325.

Kannan, K & Jain, SK. (2000). Oxidative stress and apoptosis. *Pathophysiology. 7*,153-163.

Karahalil, B; Hogue, BA; de Souza-Pinto; NC; Bohr, VA. (2002). Base excision repair capacity in mitochondria and nuclei: tissue-specific variations. *FASEB J. 16*,1895-1902.

Karanjawala, ZE; Adachi, N; Irvine, RA; Oh, EK; Shibata, D; Schwarz, K; Hsieh, CL; Lieber, MR. (2002). The embryonic lethality in DNA ligase IV-deficient mice is rescued by deletion of Ku: implications for unifying the heterogeneous phenotypes of NHEJ mutants. *DNA Repair (Amst). 1*, 1017-1026.

Katchanov; J; Harms; C; Gertz; K; Hauck; L; Waeber; C; Hirt; L; Priller; J; von Harsdorf; R; Bruck, W; Hortnagl, H; Dirnagl, U; Bhide, PG; Endres, M. (2001). Mild cerebral ischemia induces loss of cyclin-dependent kinase inhibitors and activation of cell cycle machinery before delayed neuronal cell death. *J Neurosci. 21*,5045-5053.

King, KL & Cidlovski, JA (1995). Cell cycle and apoptosis: common pathways to life and death. *J Cell Biochem. 58*,175-180.

Klein, JA & Ackerman, SL. (2003). Oxidative stress, cell cycle, and neurodegeneration. *J Clin Invest. 111*,785-793.

Klein, JA; Longo-Guess, CM; Rossmann, MP; Seburn, KL; Hurd, RE; Frankel, WN; Bronson, RT; Ackerman, SL. (2002). The harlequin mouse mutation downregulates apoptosis-inducing factor. *Nature. 419*,367-374.

Knudsen, KE; Booth, D; Naderi, S; Sever-Chroneos, Z; Fribourg, AF; Hunton, IC; Feramisco, JR; Wang, JY; Knudsen; ES. (2000). RB-dependent S-phase response to DNA damage. *Mol Cell Biol. 20*,7751-63.

Konishi, Y; Lehtinen, M; Donovan, N; Bonni, A. (2002). Cdc2 phosphorylation of BAD links the cell cycle to the cell death machinery. *Mol Cell. 9*,1005-1016.

Kruman, II (2004). Why do neurons enter the cell cycle? *Cell Cycle. 3*,769-773.

Kruman, II; Wersto, RP; Cardozo-Pelaez, F; Smilenov, L; Chan, SL; Chrest, FJ; Emokpae, R Jr; Gorospe, M; Mattson, MP. 2004a. Cell cycle activation linked to neuronal cell death initiated by DNA damage. *Neuron. 41*,549-561.

Kruman, I; Schwartz, E; Kruman, Y; Cutler, RG; Zhu, X; Greig, NH; Mattson, MP.(2004). Suppression of uracil-DNA glycosylase induces neuronal apoptosis. *J Biol Chem. 279*,43952-60.

Kunkel, TA & Bebenek, K. (2000). DNA replication fidelity. *Annu Rev Biochem. 69*,497-529.

Larsen, NB; Rasmussen, M; Rasmussen, LJ. (2005). Nuclear and mitochondrial DNA repair: similar pathways? *Mitochondrion. 5*,89-108.

Larsen, E; Kwon, K; Coin, F; Egly, JM; Klungland, A. (2004). Transcription activities at 8-oxoG lesions in DNA. *DNA Repair (Amst). 3*,1457-1468.

Lee, SE; Mitchell, RA; Cheng, A; Hendrickson, EA. (1997). Evidence for DNA-PK-dependent and -independent DNA double-strand break repair pathways in mammalian cells as a function of the cell cycle. *Mol Cell Biol. 17*,1425-1433.

Lewen, A; Matz, P; Chan, PH.(2000). Free radical pathways in CNS injury. *J Neurotrauma. 17*,871-890.

Lieber, MR. (1999). The biochemistry and biological significance of nonhomologous DNA end joining: an essential repair process in multicellular eukaryotes. *Genes Cells. 4*, 77-85.

Lin, LH; Cao, S; Yu, L; Cui, J; Hamilton, WJ; Liu, PK.(2000). Up-regulation of base excision repair activity for 8-hydroxy-2'-deoxyguanosine in the mouse brain after forebrain ischemia-reperfusion. *J Neurochem. 74*,1098-10105.

Lin, SC; Skapek, SX; Papermaster, DS; Hankin, M; Lee, EY. (2001). The proliferative and apoptotic activities of E2F1 in the mouse retina. *Oncogene. 20*,7073-7084.

Lips, J & Kaina, B. (2001). DNA double-strand breaks trigger apoptosis in p53-deficient fibroblasts. *Carcinogenesis. 22*,579-585.

Liu, DX & Greene, LA.(2001). Regulation of neuronal survival and death by E2F-dependent gene repression and derepression. *Neuron. 32*,425-438.

Longerich, S & Storb, U. (2005). The contested role of uracil DNA glycosylase in immunoglobulin gene diversification. *Trends Genet. 21*,253-256.

Lovell, MA & Markesbery, WR. (2001). Ratio of 8-hydroxyguanine in intact DNA to free 8-hydroxyguanine is increased in Alzheimer disease ventricular cerebrospinal fluid. *Arch Neurol. 58*,392-396.

Lukas, J; Lukas, C; Bartek, J. (2004). Mammalian cell cycle checkpoints: signalling pathways and their organization in space and time. *DNA Repair (Amst). 3*,997-1007.

Ma, Y; Pannicke, U; Schwarz, K; Lieber, MR. (2002). Hairpin opening and overhang processing by an Artemis/DNA-dependent protein kinase complex in nonhomologous end joining and V(D)J recombination. *Cell. 108*,781-794.

Macleod, MR; Ramage, L; McGregor, A; Seck, JR. (2003). Reduced NMDA-induced apoptosis in neurons lacking ataxia telangiectasia mutated protein. *NeuroReport. 14*,215-217.

MacPhail, S; Banath, J; Yu, T; Chu, E; Lambur, H; Olive, P. (2003). Expression of phosphorylated histone H2AX in cultured cell lines following exposure to X-rays. *Int J Radiat Biol, 79*,351–358.

Mahmoudi, M; Mercer, J; Bennett, M. (2006). DNA damage and repair in atherosclerosis. *Cardiovasc Res. 71*,259-268.

Martin, FL; Williamson, SJ; Paleologou, KE; Hewitt, R; El-Agnaf, OM; Allsop, D. (2003). Fe(II)-induced DNA damage in alpha-synuclein-transfected human dopaminergic BE(2)-M17 neuroblastoma cells: detection by the Comet assay. *J Neurochem. 87*,620-630.

Matsumura, S; Matsumura, T; Ozeki, S,; Fukushima, S; Yamazaki, H; Inoue, T; Inoue, T; Furusawa, Y; Eguchi-Kasai, K.(2003). Comparative analysis of G2 arrest after irradiation with 75 keV carbon-ion beams and 137Cs gamma-rays in a human lymphoblastoid cell line. *Cancer Detect Prev. 27*,222-228.

McKinnon, PJ.(2001). Ataxia telangiectasia: new neurons and ATM. T*rends Mol Med. 7*,233-4.

McMurray, CT.(2005). To die or not to die: DNA repair in neurons. *Mutat Res. 577*,260-274

Mecocci, P; Polidori, MC; Ingegni, T; Cherubini, A; Chionne, F; Cecchetti, R; Senin, U. (1998). Oxidative damage to DNA in lymphocytes from AD patients. *Neurology. 51*,1014-1017.

Meek, DW. (2004). The p53 response to DNA damage. *DNA Repair (Amst). 3*,1049-1056.

Meng, RD; Phillips, P; El-Deiry, WS (1999). p53-independent increase in E2F-1 expression enhances the cytotoxic effects of etoposide and of adriamycin. *Int J Oncol. 14*,5-14.

Migliore, L & Coppede, F. (2002). Genetic and environmental factors in cancer and neurodegenerative diseases. *Mutat Res. 512*,135-153.

Morris, EJ & Geller, HM. (1996). Induction of neuronal apoptosis by camptothecin, an inhibitor of DNA topoisomerase-I: evidence for cell cycle-independent toxicity. *J Cell Bio*l. *134*, 757-770.

Mullaart, E; Boerrigter, ME; Ravid, R; Swaab, DF; Vijg, J. (1990). Increased levels of DNA breaks in cerebral cortex of Alzheimer's disease patients. *Neurobiol Aging. 11*,169-173.

Nahelhus, TA; Haug, T; Singh, KK; Keshav, KF; Skorpen, F; Otterlei, M; Bharati, S; Lindmo, T; Benichou, S; Benarous, R; Krokan, HE. (1997). A sequence in the N-terminal region of human uracil- DNA glycosylase with homology to XPA interacts with the C-terminal part of the 34-kDa subunit of replication protein A. *J Biol Chem. 272*,6561-6566.

Nagy, Z; Esiri, MM; Cato, AM; Smith, AD.(1997). Cell cycle markers in the hippocampus in Alzheimer's disease. *Acta Neuropathol (Berl). 94*,6-15.

Nazarov, I; Smirnova, A; Krutilina, R; Svetlova, MP; Solovjeva, LV; Nikiforov, AA; Oei, SL; Zalenskaya, IA; Yau, PM.; Bradbury, EM; Tomilin, NV. (2003). Dephosphorylation of histone g-H2AX during repair of DNA double-strand breaks in mammalian cells and its inhibition by calyculin A. *Radiat Res. 160*,309–317.

Niida, H & Nakanishi, M. (2006). DNA damage checkpoints in mammals. *Mutagenesis. 21*,3-9.

Nilsen, H; Otterlei, M; Haug, T; Solum, K; Nagelhus, TA; Skorpen, F; Krokan, HE (1997). Nuclear and mitochondrial uracil-DNA glycosylases are generated by alternative splicing and transcription from different positions in the UNG gene. *Nucleic Acids Res. 25*,750-755.

Nouspikel, T & Hanawalt, PC. (2002). DNA repair in terminally differentiated cells. *DNA Repair (Amst). 1*,59-75.

Nussenzweig, A; Chen, C; da Costa Soares, V; Sanchez, M; Sokol, K; Nussenzweig, MC; Li, GC.(1996) Requirement for Ku80 in growth and immunoglobulin V(D)J recombination. *Nature. 382*,551-555.

O'Connor, DJ & Lu, X. (2000). Stress signals induce transcriptionally inactive E2F-1 independently of p53 and Rb. *Oncogene. 19*,2369-2376.

Offord, E; van Poppel, G; Tyrrell, R. (2000). Markers of oxidative damage and antioxidant protection: current status and relevance to disease. *Free Radic Res. 33* Suppl, S5-19.

O'Hare, M; Wang, F; Park, DS. (2002). Cyclin-dependent kinases as potential targets to improve stroke outcome. *Pharmacol Ther. 93*,135-143.

Oppenheim, RW. (1991). Cell death during development of the nervous system. *Annu Rev Neurosci. 14*,453-501.

Parikh, SS; Mol, CD; Tainer, JA, (1997). Base excision repair enzyme family portrait: integrating the structure and chemistry of an entire DNA repair pathways. *Structure 5*,1543-1550.

Park, DS; Levine, B; Ferrari, G; Greene, L (1997). Cyclin dependent kinase inhibitors and dominant negative cyclin dependent kinase 4 and 6 promote survival of NGF-deprived sympathetic neurons. *J. Neurosci. 17*,8975-8983.

Park, DS; Morris, EJ; Padmanabhan, J; Shelanski, MI; Geller, HM; Greene LA. (1998). Cyclin-dependent kinases participate in death of neurons evoked by DNA-damaging agents. *J.Cell. Biol. 143*,457-467.

Pfeiffer, P; Goedecke, W; Obe, G. (2000). Mechanisms of DNA double-strand break repair and their potential to induce chromosomal aberrations. *Mutagenesis. 15*,289-302.

Polager, S; Kalma, Y; Berkovich, E; Ginsberg, D. (2002). E2Fs up-regulate expression of genes involved in DNA replication, DNA repair and mitosis. *Oncogene. 21*,437-446.

Przedborski, S & Vila, M. (2003). The 1-methyl-4-phenyl-1,2,3,6-tetrahydropyridine mouse model: a tool to explore the pathogenesis of Parkinson's disease. *Ann N Y Acad Sci. 991*,189-198.

Ratan, RR; Murphy; TH; Baraban, JM. (1994). Oxidative stress induces apoptosis in embryonic cortical neurons. *J Neurochem. 62*,376-379.

Rehen, SK; McConnell, MJ; Kaushal, D; Kingsbury, MA; Yang, AH;Chun, J.(2001). Chromosomal variation in neurons of the developing and adult mammalian nervous system. *Proc Natl Acad Sci U S A. 98*,13361-13366.

Ren, J; Datta, R; Shioya, H; Li, Y; Oki, E; Biedermann, V; Bharti, A; Kufe, D. (2002). p73beta is regulated by protein kinase Cdelta catalytic fragment generated in the apoptotic response to DNA damage. *J Biol Chem. 277*,33758-33765.

Rhind, N & Russell, P. (2000). Checkpoints: it takes more than time to heal some wounds. *Curr Biol. 10*,R908-R911.

Rideout, HJ; Wang, Q; Park, DS; Stefanis, L. (2003). Cyclin-dependent kinase activity is required for apoptotic death but not inclusion formation in cortical neurons after proteasomal inhibition. *J Neurosci 23*,1237-1245.

Rolig, RL & McKinnon, PJ.(2000). Linking DNA damage and neurodegeneration. *Trends Neuroscie. 23*,417- 424.

Rothkamm, K & Lobrich, M. (2003). Evidence for a lack of DNA double-strand break repair in human cells exposed to very low x-ray doses. *Proc Natl Acad Sci USA. 100*:5057–5062.

Sancar A, Lindsey-Boltz LA, Unsal-Kacmaz K, Linn S. (2004). Molecular mechanisms of mammalian DNA repair and the DNA damage checkpoints. Annu Rev Biochem. *73*,39-85.

Sedelnikova, OA; Rogakou, EP; Panyutin, IG; Bonner, WM. (2002). Quantitative detection of (125)IdU-induced DNA double-strand breaks with gamma-H2AX antibody. *Radiat Res. 158*,486-492.

Sedelnikova, OA; Pilch, DR; Redon, C; Bonner, WM. (2003). Histone H2AX in DNA damage and repair. *Cancer Biol Ther. 2*,233-235.

Sekiguchi, J; Ferguson, DO; Chen, HT; Yang, EM; Earle, J; Frank, K; Whitlow, S; Gu, Y; Xu, Y; Nussenzweig, A; Alt, FW. (2001). Genetic interactions between ATM and the nonhomologous end-joining factors in genomic stability and development. *Proc Natl Acad Sci U S A. 98*,3243-3248.

Shi, Y; Venkataraman, SL; Dodson, GE; Mabb, AM; LeBlanc, S; Tibbetts, RS. (2004). Direct regulation of CREB transcriptional activity by ATM in response to genotoxic stress. *Proc Natl Acad Sci U S A. 101*,5898-903.

Shiloh, Y. (2006). The ATM-mediated DNA-damage response: taking shape. *Trends Biochem Sci. 31*,402-410.

Shiloh, Y. (2003). ATM and related protein kinases: safeguarding genome integrity. *Nat Rev Cancer. 3*,155-168.

Slupphaug, G; Kavli, B; Krokan, HE (2003). The interacting pathways for prevention and repair of oxidative DNA damage. *Mutat Res. 531*,231-251.

Sobol, RW; Horton, JK; Kuhn, R; Gu, H; Singhal, RK; Prasad, R; Rajewsky, K, Wilson, SH. (1996). Requirement of mammalian DNA polymerase-beta in base-excision repair. *Nature. 379*, 183-186.

Sonoda, E; Hochegger, H; Saberi, A; Taniguchi, Y; Takeda, S. (2006). Differential usage of non-homologous end-joining and homologous recombination in double strand break repair. *DNA Repair (Amst).* Jun 23; [Epub ahead of print]

Souza-Pinto, NC; Croteau, DL; Hudson, EK; Hansford, RG; Bohr VA.(1999). Age-associated increase in 8-oxo-deoxyguanosine glycosylase/AP lyase activity in rat mitochondria. *Nucleic Acids Res. 27*,1935-1942.

Stevaux, O & Dyson, NJ.(2002). A revised picture of the E2F transcriptional network and RB function. *Curr Opin Cell Biol. 14*,6846-6891.

Stommel, JMn & Wahl, GM. (2004). Accelerated MDM2 auto-degradation induced by DNA-damage kinases is required for p53 activation. *EMBO J. 23*,1547-1556.

Tibbetts, RS; Cortez, D; Brumbaugh, KM; Scully, R; Livingston, D; Elledge, SJ; Abraham, RT. (2000). Functional interactions between BRCA1 and the checkpoint kinase ATR during genotoxic stress. *Genes Dev. 14*,2989-3002.

Tobita, M; Nagano, I; Nakamura, S; Itoyama, Y; Kogure, K. (1995). DNA single-strand breaks in postischemic gerbil brain detected by in situ nick translation procedure. *Neurosci Lett. 200*,129-132.

Veglia, F; Matullo, G; Vineis, P. (2003). Bulky DNA adducts and risk of cancer: a meta-analysis. *Cancer Epidemiol Biomarkers Prev. 12*,157-160.

Vemuri, MC; Schiller, E; Naegele, R. (2001). Elevated DNA double strand breaks and apoptosis in the CNS of scid mutant mice. *Cell Death Differ. 8*,245-255.

Verdaguer, E; Jorda, EG; Stranges, A; Canudas, AM; Jimenez, A; Sureda, FX;, Pallas, M; Camins, A. Inhibition of CDKs: a strategy for preventing kainic acid-induced apoptosis in neurons. *Ann N Y Acad Sci 1010*,671-674.

Walsh, MJ; Shue, G; Spidoni, K; Kapoor, A. (1995). E2F-1 and a cyclin-like DNA repair enzyme, uracil-DNA glycosylase, provide evidence for an autoregulatory mechanism for transcription. *J. Biol. Chem. 270*,5289-5298.

Wang, H; Perrault, AR; Takeda, Y; Qin, W; Wang, H; Iliakis, G. (2003). Biochemical evidence for Ku-independent backup pathways of NHEJ. *Nucleic Acids Res. 3*,5377-5388.

Wartiovaara, K; Barnabe,-Heider, F; Miller, FD; Kaplan, DR. (2002). N-myc promotes survival and induces S-phase entry of postmitotic sympathetic neurons. *J Neurosci. 22*,815-824.

Watanabe, M; Osada, J; Aratani, Y; Kluckman, K; Reddick, R; Malinow, MR; Maeda, N.(1995). Mice deficient in cystathionine beta-synthase: animal models for mild and severe homocyst(e)inemia. *Proc Natl Acad Sci U S A. 92*,1585-1589.

Williams, GM & Jeffrey, AM. (2000). Oxidative DNA damage: endogenous and chemically induced. *Regul Toxicol Pharmacol. 32*,283-292.

Wilson, TM; Rivkees, SA; Deutsch, WA; Kelley, MR.(1996). Differential expression of the apurinic / apyrimidinic endonuclease (APE/ref-1) multifunctional DNA base excision repair gene during fetal development and in adult rat brain and testis. *Mutat Res. 362*,237-248.

Wyllie, AH; Kerr, JF; Currie, AR. (1980). Cell death: the significance of apoptosis. *Int Rev Cytol. 68*,251-306.

Yang, Y; Geldmacher, DS; Herrup, K. (2001). DNA replication precedes neuronal cell death in Alzheimer's disease. *J Neurosci 21*,2661-2668.

Yang, J; Yu, Y; Hamrick, HE; Duerksen-Hughes, PJ. (2003). ATM, ATR and DNA-PK: initiators of the cellular genotoxic stress responses. *Carcinogenesis. 24*,1571-1580.

Yuan, J & Yankner, BA. (2000). Apoptosis in the nervous system. *Nature. 407*,802-809.

In: Brain Mapping Research Progress
Editors: Ines C. Girard and Jade S. Andre

ISBN: 978-1-60456-784-7

Chapter III

Hallmarks of Apoptotic-Like Cell Death in Response to Hypoxic Injury in Various Developmental Models Are Closely Related to Brain Immaturity

***Jean-Luc Daval*[1,*] *and Christiane Charriaut-Marlangue*[2]**

[1]INSERM U.724, Université Henri Poincaré, Faculté de Médecine, 9 avenue de la Forêt de Haye, F-54500 Vandoeuvre-lès-Nancy, France;

[2]Groupe Hypoxie et Ischémie du Cerveau en Développement, Université Pierre et Marie Curie-Paris6, UMR-CNRS 7102, 9 quai St-Bernard, Paris, F-75005 France.

Abstract

With regard to the specificity of the developing brain, a better understanding of cellular mechanisms involved in perinatal hypoxic-ischemic injury would help to prevent neurological impairments. We therefore examined temporal features of brain injury in three different developmental models of oxygen deprivation capable of inducing apoptotic cell death. Nuclear staining by DAPI (4,6-diamidino-2-phenylindole) was used to identify healthy, apoptotic and necrotic nuclei as well as for cell counting in cultures and brain sections. DNA fragmentation was monitored by in situ terminal dUTP nick end labeling (TUNEL) and electrophoresis on agarose gels. Also, the expression profile of apoptosis-related proteins Bax and Bcl-2 was studied by immunohistochemistry. In all cases, oxygen deprivation induced significant delayed cell death with morphological features of apoptosis and a progressive increase in the Bax/Bcl-2 protein ratio, except in the penumbra of the ischemic infarct where Bcl-2 remained predominant. As in the control newborn brain that still exhibited physiological death, hypoxia-associated DNA breakdown led to small fragments of ~200 bp in the cortex of hypoxic rat pups. Ladder pattern and TUNEL-positive cells exhibiting apoptotic bodies were only present in the

* Correspondence concerning this article should be addressed to Dr. Jean-Luc Daval, INSERM U.724, Université Henri Poincaré, Faculté de Médecine, 9 avenue de la Forêt de Haye, F-54500 Vandoeuvre-lès-Nancy, France. E-mail: Jean-Luc.Daval@nancy.inserm.fr.

penumbra of 7 day-old ischemic rats. These data indicate that hallmarks of hypoxia-induced apoptosis may vary according to brain maturity, possibly through specific nuclease activities. While retaining a part of the developmental death program, the newborn brain seems to be prone to an apoptotic-like response that resembles physiological programmed death.

Introduction

Apoptosis is considered as the ubiquitous form of naturally occurring cell death that plays a fundamental role in brain development, as about half of the cells in the immature brain are eliminated by apoptosis (Oppenheim, 1991). This physiological process needs the activation of an intrinsic 'death program' requiring time and energy (Richter et al., 1996) as well as gene transcription and translation (Pittman et al., 1993). Indeed, the apoptotic cascade involves the participation of 'killer' proteins (e.g., Bax) generally present constitutively in the cell but normally repressed by their survival counterparts (e.g., Bcl-2). Morphologically, apoptosis is typified by cell shrinkage, chromatin condensation and subsequent nucleus fragmentation, with a specific pattern of DNA breakdown leading usually to multiple segments of approximately 200 bp in length. By contrast, the second form of cell death, namely necrosis, which has been implicated in cell destruction consecutive to severe trauma, induces cellular swelling, membrane disruption with leakage of cell contents to the extracellular space, and leads to random DNA degradation (Wyllie, 1981). In response to a variety of insults, all cells seem to be able to undergo apoptosis but there is compelling evidence to suggest that developing brain cells are more prone to programmed death by retaining a part of the developmental cell death program (Blaschke et al., 1996; Sidhu et al., 1997).

Perinatal hypoxic-ischemic injury remains a major cause of mortality and cerebral morbidity, susceptible to generate permanent neurological sequelae (Volpe, 1987; Berger and Garnier, 1999). Whereas necrotic cell damage was first considered prevalent in response to hypoxia-ischemia, the participation of apoptosis has been largely documented, including in the developing brain (Beilharz et al., 1995; Charriaut-Marlangue et al., 1996; Bossenmeyer et al., 1998, Bossenmeyer-Pourié et al., 2002; Daval et al., 2004). In addition, some studies suggest an apoptotic-necrotic continuum in the consequences of acute cerebral ischemia (Nakajima et al., 2000; Benchoua et al., 2001).

Since the developing brain displays specific properties and sensitivity to oxygen supply (Grafe, 1994), hallmarks of cell injury may thus vary according to brain maturity, and the present study was designed to gain a better understanding of the cellular mechanisms triggered by a severe hypoxic insult at various ages of the perinatal period. For this purpose, we compared hypoxia-associated features of cell death in three different developmental models of oxygen deprivation capable of inducing brain apoptosis, i.e. in cultured neurons from the embryonic rat forebrain exposed to 95% $N2$/5% $CO2$ (Bossenmeyer et al., 1998), in the rat neonate exposed to 100% N2, a model corresponding to birth asphyxia (Grojean et al., 2003), and in the 7-day-old rat pup subjected to transient unilateral focal ischemia followed by reperfusion (Renolleau et al., 1998). In contrast, exposure to 100% N2 in 7 day-old rat induced mainly necrosis and did not enter this study (JLD, unpublished results).

Experimental Procedures

Animals

Experiments were conducted in respect to the French (Statement N° 04223) and European Community guidelines for the care and use of experimental animals. Sprague-Dawley female rats (R. Janvier, Le Genest-St-Isle, France) in the proestrus period, as shown by daily vaginal smears, were housed together with males for 24 h, and then maintained during gestation in separate cages under standard laboratory conditions on a 12:12 h light/dark cycle (lights on at 6:00 a.m.) with food and water available ad libitum.

Hypoxia in Neuronal Cell Cultures

Primary cultured neurons were obtained from the embryonic rat brain as previously described (Bossenmeyer et al., 1998; Chihab et al., 1998; Bossenmeyer-Pourié et al., 1999a; Grojean et al., 2000). Forebrains of 14-day-old embryos were carefully collected, dissected free of meninges and dispersed in culture medium consisting of a mixture of Dulbecco's modified Eagle's medium (DMEM) and Ham's F12 medium (50:50, ICN Pharmaceuticals, Costa Mesa, CA) supplemented with 5% inactivated fetal calf serum (Valbiotech, Paris, France). After centrifugation at 700 g for 10 min, the pellet was dispersed in the same medium and passed through a 46 µm-pore size nylon mesh. Aliquots of the cell suspension were transferred into 35 mm Petri dishes (Falcon, Becton Dickinson, Le Pont-de-Claix, France) precoated with poly-L-lysine in order to obtain a final density of 10^6 cells/dish. Cultures were then placed at 37°C in a humidified atmosphere of 95% air/5% CO2. The following day, the culture medium was replaced with a fresh hormonally defined serum-free medium corresponding to the DMEM/Ham's F12 mixture enriched with human transferrin (1 mM), bovine insulin (1 mM), putrescine (0.1 mM), progesterone (10 nM), estradiol (1 pM), Na selenite (30 nM), and also containing fibroblast growth factor (2 ng/ml) and epidermal growth factor (10 ng/ml) (Sigma Chemicals, St Louis, MO). Two days later, the culture medium was renewed with serum-free medium in the absence of growth factors.

After 6 days in vitro, neuronal cells were exposed to hypoxia for 6 h by transferring culture dishes to a humidified incubation chamber thermoregulated at 37°C and filled with 95% N2/5% CO2. Cultures were then returned to normoxic atmosphere, at 37°C, whereas control cells were constantly maintained under standard conditions. When used, 1 µM cycloheximide (CHX, Sigma Chemicals) was added to the culture medium prior to hypoxia and removed by changing the medium as soon as reoxygenation began. Cells were studied as a function of time until 96 h post-reoxygenation to assess the effects of hypoxia.

In Vivo Birth Hypoxia

Between 8 to 24 h after delivery, the litter size was reduced to 10 pups for homogeneity, and 5 neonates were placed for 20 min in a thermostated plexiglas chamber flushed with

100% N2, whereas the remaining 5 pups were taken as matched controls and exposed to 21% O2/79% N2 for the same time. The rate of gas delivery inside the box was calculated to prevent any overpressure, and was fixed to 3 liters/min. Gas in excess was evacuated through a central lengthwise split on the top of the box. The temperature inside the chamber was adjusted to 36°C to maintain body temperature in the physiological range. Following exposure to gas, all rats were allowed to recover for 20 min in normoxic conditions, and they were then returned to their dams. In these conditions, the final rate of mortality in the hypoxia group was 4%, and surviving animals did not display significant suckling problems. Hypoxic and control rats were finally sacrificed by decapitation at various time intervals between 1 day and 13 days post-exposure. Their brains were rapidly collected and immediately frozen in methylbutane previously chilled to -30°C, and stored at -80°C in plastic bags until used. Thereafter, the brains were coated with embedding medium (4% carboxymethylcellulose in water), and cut at -20°C in a cryostat (Reichert Jung, Frigocut 2800, Les Ulis, France) to generate 5-μm coronal sections at the level of the rostral hippocampus, according to the developing rat brain atlas of Sherwood and Timiras (1970), and tissue sections were mounted onto glass slides for subsequent analyses.

In Vivo 7-Day Ischemia

Ischemia was performed in 7 day-old rats (17-21 g) of both sexes, as previously described (Renolleau et al., 1998). Rat pups were anaesthetized with intraperitoneal injection of chloral hydrate (300 mg/kg). After 15 min, rats were positioned on their back and a median incision was made in the neck to expose left common carotid artery. Rats were then placed on the right side and an oblique skin incision was made between the ear and the eye. After excision of the temporal muscle, the cranial bone was removed from the frontal suture to a level below the zygomatic arch. Then, the left middle cerebral artery, exposed just after its apparition over the rhinal fissure, was coagulated at the inferior cerebral vein level. After this procedure, a clip was placed to occlude the left common carotid artery and was removed after 1 h. Carotid blood flow restoration was verified with the aid of a binocular loupe. Both neck and cranial skin incisions were then closed. During surgery, body temperature was maintained at 37-38°C. After awake, rat pups were transferred to their mother for time survival at 6, 24 and 48 h and 3 to 5 days after reperfusion.

Evaluation of Cell Damage

Cell viability was measured in cultured neurons by the spectrophotometric method using 3-[4,5-dimethylthiazol-2-yl]-2,5-diphenyltetrazolium bromide (MTT), according to Hansen et al. (1989). Neurons were incubated for 3 h at 37°C with MTT (500 μg/mL, Sigma Chemicals), washed twice with ice-cold phosphate-buffered saline (PBS), and lysed in dimethyl sulfoxide (DMSO) which solubilizes the residual formazan salt for subsequent quantification. Optical density was measured at 519 nm and data were compared to those obtained from sister control cells to which 100% viability was assigned.

In vivo cell counts were performed to determine the percentage of damaged neurons in cerebral cortex. For this purpose, brain sections were fixed for 10 min in a mixture of ethanol:acetic acid (3:1), washed for 30 seconds in distilled water, air-dried, and then stained for 10 min with the fluorescent dye 4,6-diamidino-2-phenylindole (DAPI, Sigma Chemicals) in phosphate-buffered saline (0.5 μg/ml) (Wolvetang et al., 1994). Sections were washed twice with distilled water, air-dried, and treated with anti-fading medium (10 mg/ml p-phenyldiamine in 90% glycerol, pH 9.0). The number of cell nuclei which were labeled by DAPI was scored at an excitation wavelength of 365 nm under fluorescence microscopy (Zeiss Axioscop, Strasbourg, France). Cell density was measured in the infragranular part of the parietal cortex (layers III-V) at a 40 x magnification in at least 3 separate experiments by counting cells in 3 distinct section areas delineated by an ocular grid of 1/400 mm2. For each selected field, only cells with their nuclei present in the focal plane were counted. Numbers of cells were calculated per mm2 and finally reported as percentages of change from matched controls.

Monitoring of Apoptosis and Necrosis

Morphological hallmarks of apoptosis and necrosis were analyzed both in cultured neurons and tissue sections after nuclear labeling by DAPI, as previously documented (Bossenmeyer et al., 1998; Chihab et al., 1998; Bossenmeyer-Pourié et al., 1999b; Grojean et al., 2000; Park et al., 1997). Indeed, it has been demonstrated that healthy cells exhibit intact round-shaped nuclei with diffuse fluorescence, indicative of homogeneous chromatin. Necrotic cells are characterized by highly refringent smaller nuclei with uniformly dispersed chromatin, while condensation and fragmentation of chromatin lead to typically shrunken nuclei in apoptotic cells, along with apoptotic bodies. Characteristic nuclei were scored under fluorescence microscopy (Zeiss Axioscop, Strasbourg, France) at an excitation wavelength of 365 nm in at least 3 separate experiments by counting concerned cells in at least 3 distinct areas of 100 cells.

Electrophoretic Detection of DNA Fragmentation

At 48 h and 96 h post-reoxygenation, hypoxic and control cultured neurons were washed twice with PBS, scraped off in 2 ml PBS, and the contents of 5 dishes were pooled to be centrifuged for 5 min at 700 g. Following in vivo birth hypoxia or ischemia, rat pups were sacrificed at various time intervals and the brains were rapidly removed, dissected on a cold plate and stored at -80° C. Cell pellets or tissue samples from separate brains were processed for DNA isolation according to Laird et al. (1991).They were gently homogenized and lysed in 0.5 ml of lysis buffer (100 mM tris-HCl at pH 8.5, 5 mM EDTA, 0.2% sodium dodecyl sulfate (SDS), and 200 mM NaCl) containing 100 μg/ml proteinase K. After 16 h incubation at 55°C, DNA was precipitated by adding one volume isopropanol with continuous agitation for 15 min at room temperature. Following centrifugation at 13000 g for 5 min the pellet was air dried and dissolved in TE buffer (several hours), treated with RNAse A (20 μg/ml) for 2 h at 37°C and DNA content determined spectrophotometrically. DNA (10 μg/lane) was electrophoresed on a 1% agarose gel in 100 mM tris borate (60 V for 4 h) in the presence of 0.3 mg/ml ethidium bromide and visualized with UV illumination.

Detection of DNA Breaks by Nick End-Labeling

Sections were processed for DNA strand breaks (TUNEL assay) using the in situ Cell Death Detection Kit, Fluorescein (Roche, Meylan, France) according to the manufacturer's instructions. TUNEL assay reveals apoptosis and necrosis as previously reported (Charriaut-Marlangue and Ben-Ari, 1995).

Bax and Bcl-2 Immunohistochemistry

The expression of the two prototypic apoptosis-related proteins Bax and Bcl-2 was analyzed in cultured neurons and rat brain coronal sections. In vitro neuronal cells were rinsed twice with PBS, then fixed for 10 min in methanol at -10°C, and rinsed again with PBS. Non-specific binding sites for IgG were blocked by incubating the cells for 20 min with 10% horse serum (Gibco-BRL, Inchinnan, U.K.) in PBS. Thereafter, cultures were incubated for 60 min at room temperature in buffer containing the primary antibody., i.e. a rabbit polyclonal antibody against Bax (N-20, Santa Cruz, Tebu, France) diluted at 1/20 or a goat polyclonal antibody against Bcl-2 (N-19, Santa Cruz) diluted at 1/40. Following two washing steps to remove unfixed antibody, the cells were incubated for 120 min in the presence of a second-step antibody corresponding to either an anti-rabbit IgG conjugated to indocarbocyanine (Cy3, dilution 1/80) or an anti-goat IgG conjugated to rhodamine (TRITC, dilution1/100), both from Jackson ImmunoResearch Laboratories (West Grove, PA). Cultured cells were finally washed 3 times with PBS, coverslipped using mounting medium (Aquapolymount), and kept in the dark until fluorescence analysis by means of a Zeiss Axioscop microscope.

For quantitative analysis, cell fluorescence activity was computerized from microphotographs, and mean intensity was calculated by using Adobe Photoshop® software and expressed as arbitrary units of mean emission per 1 000 pixels (Bossenmeyer-Pourié et al., 2002; Bossenmeyer-Pourié and Daval, 1998). The results were finally reported as Bax/Bcl-2 protein ratios as a function of time after reoxygenation as well as in normoxic control cultures processed in parallel.

Both proteins were also analyzed in rat brain coronal sections of 7 μm-thickness previously fixed by incubating the slides for 10 min at 4°C in acetic acid:ethanol (1:3) in the presence of 30% hydrogen peroxide. In these conditions, brain sections were incubated at 4°C for 48 h with the primary antibody against Bax (dilution 1/20) or Bcl-2 (dilution 1/30), and secondary antibodies were used at 1/50 and 1/100, respectively, for subsequent measurements as described above. In the case of coronal sections from 7 day-old ischemic pups, Bax and Bcl-2 immunoreactivity was visualized by the avidin-biotin peroxidase (Elite ABC kit, Vecstastain, Vector, AbCys, France). The peroxidase activity was evidenced with the use of 3,3'-diaminobenzidin (DAB) and 0.02 % hydrogen peroxide. The counting of Bax- and Bcl-2 positive cells within the core and penumbra was performed in 3-5 sections (at the level of the anterior commissure) using a x40 objective, and results were reported as indicated above.

Results

Hypoxia in Neuronal Cell Cultures

As illustrated in Table 1, a hypoxic episode in cultured neurons from the embryonic rat brain induced delayed cell death inasmuch as cell viability was not yet different from controls at 48 h post-reoxygenation. Thereafter, the number of living cells gradually decreased to reach 64% from controls at 96 h. At this experimental time point, a significant number of cell nuclei stained by the fluorescent dye DAPI exhibited characteristic apoptosis-related morphological features, such as condensed chromatin, whereas the presence of apoptotic bodies could be seen. Necrotic cells were also depicted, but the percentage of apoptotic nuclei increased more markedly, as revealed by cell counts. Moreover, a concomitant treatment with cycloheximide, a potent inhibitor of protein synthesis, had beneficial effects. In the presence of CHX, cell viability was not significantly affected and the number of apoptotic nuclei remained within control values (Table 1), suggesting that hypoxia triggers a programmed death process in cultured neurons. When DNA fragmentation was monitored on agarose gel, no significant degradation was observed at 48 h, in good agreement with viability and morphology data, whereas DNA fragmentation was shown at 96 h after the hypoxic insult (Figure 1). However, DNA alteration was only reflected by a smear, without visualization of a ‘ladder pattern’. Finally, immunohistochemical studies revealed detectable baseline values of the prototypic apoptosis-related proteins Bcl-2 and Bax. Following exposure to hypoxia, expression of the survival Bcl-2 protein transiently increased above control values at 48 h post-insult without apparent change in Bax expression, leading to a significantly reduced Bax/Bcl-2 ratio (Figure 2). At 96 h, Bcl-2 levels abruptly declined, while the expression of Bax was markedly stimulated, resulting in a robust increase of the final Bax/Bcl-2 ratio (Figure 2).

Table 1. Effects of a 6-h exposure to hypoxia of cultured rat forebrain neurons on cell viability and nuclear hallmarks of necrosis and apoptosis at 48 h and 96 h post-reoxygenation. Influence of cycloheximide.

	Cell viability *(% from controls)*	Necrosis *(% of total neurons)*	Apoptosis *(% of total neurons)*
Controls 48 h	100.0 ± 4.6	4.9 ± 1.2	1.6 ± 0.6
+ 1 μM CHX	90.6 ± 5.3	9.1 ± 2.3*	1.2 ± 0.9
Hypoxia 48 h	96.6 ± 4.3	5.2 ± 1.1	1.9 ± 0.9
+ 1 μM CHX	92.0 ± 6.1	11.0 ± 2.6*°°	1.3 ± 0.8
Controls 96 h	100.0 ± 5.8	5.6 ± 1.5	2.7 ± 0.8
+ 1 μM CHX	86.4 ± 6.0*	13.4 ± 2.6**	2.8 ± 1.0

Table 1. (Continued).

	Cell viability *(% from controls)*	Necrosis *(% of total neurons)*	Apoptosis *(% of total neurons)*
Hypoxia 96 h	63.6 ± 6.2**	10.8 ± 2.8**	21.2 ± 5.7**
+ 1 μM CHX	88.5 ± 5.1*°°	16.1 ± 3.0**°	3.0 ± 1.2°°

Cell viability as well as rates of necrosis and apoptosis were analyzed as described in the method section. Data are reported as means ± S.D. obtained from 3 separate experiments. Statistically significant differences from controls: *$p<0.05$ and **$p<0.01$; Statistically significant differences from hypoxia alone: °$p<0.05$ and °°$p<0.01$ (Dunnett's test for multiple comparisons).

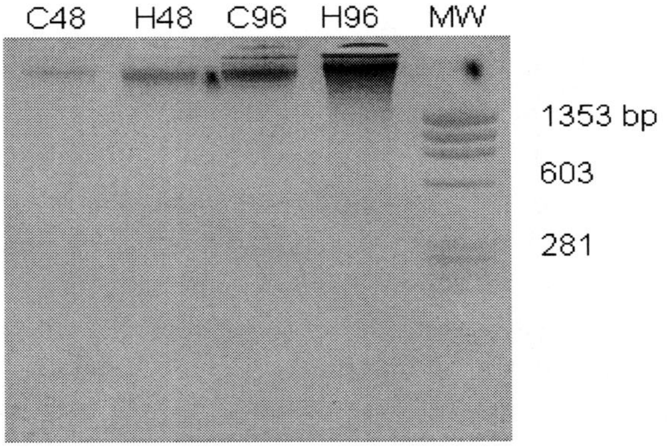

Figure 1. Temporal analysis on agarose gel of DNA isolated from control and hypoxic cultured neurons from the embryonic rat forebrain. DNA was isolated from cultured cells at 48 h (H48) and 96 h post-reoxygenation (H96) and from matched controls (C48 and C96). One representative example is presented for illustration, and similar profiles were obtained from 5 separate experiments. (Size marker: Superladder mid 1-500 bp, Eurogentec, Paris, France).

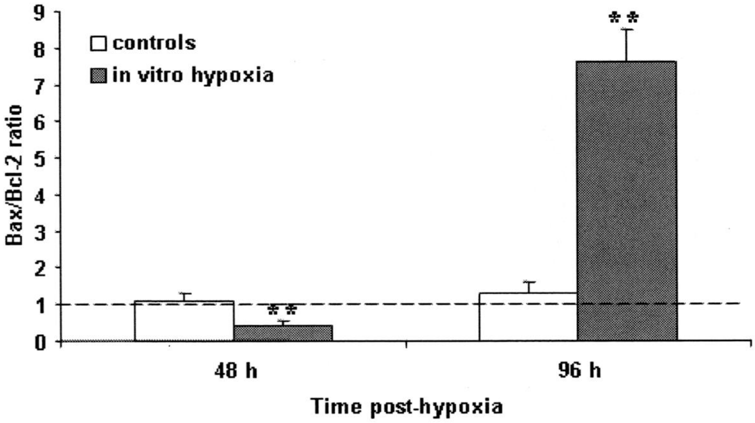

Figure 2. Evolution of the Bax/Bcl-2 protein ratio in cultured neurons exposed to hypoxia for 6 hours and their normoxic controls. Immunohistochemical studies were performed at 48 h and 96 h post-hypoxia and in matched controls. Fluorescence activity was computerized by means of Adobe Photoshop software, and the protein ratio was calculated at each time point. The data represent mean values (± S.D.) obtained from 3 separate experiments. Statistically significant difference from controls: ** $p<0.01$ (Dunnett's test for multiple comparisons).

In Vivo Birth Hypoxia

When rat pups were subjected to hypoxia within 24 h after birth, no histopathological alteration of the cerebral cortex could be noticed by the four ensuing days. Then, a progressive decline of the total number of cells labeled by DAPI was observed in this brain structure, and maximal cell loss was seen around 6 days post-reoxygenation (Table 2). Whereas examination of nuclear morphology depicted a significant number of cells exhibiting the characteristic hallmarks of both necrosis and apoptosis during early postnatal life in control animals, birth hypoxia was associated with a gradual elevation of the percentage of affected cells, with a peak observed at 6 days post-reoxygenation. The number of altered nuclei was then shown to decrease during the second week after hypoxia, and only the proportion of necrotic cells remained significantly augmented by comparison with controls at 13 days after the insult (Table 2). Surprisingly, no TUNEL-positive nuclei were detected on coronal sections tested at various time intervals after hypoxia (not shown). As illustrated in Figure 3, where only representative time-points are presented, analysis of DNA on agarose gel revealed similar fragmentation in control and hypoxic rat cortex during the first 3 days following exposure to gas. In these conditions, only one spot could be repeatedly visualized, and the size marker indicated that such fragments corresponded to ~200 bp. Between 5 and 7 days post-exposure, DNA fragmentation was exclusively seen in the cortex of hypoxic rats, with the absence of alteration in controls. Again, hypoxia led to DNA fragments of ~200 bp. At 13 days post-insult, no DNA fragmentation could be observed.

Table 2. Temporal evolution of the number of cells and their nuclear morphological features of necrosis and apoptosis in the cerebral cortex of rats exposed to birth hypoxia for 20 min.

Time post-reoxygenation	Number of total cells *(% from controls)*	Necrosis (%)		Apoptosis (%)	
		Controls	Hypoxia	Controls	Hypoxia
1 day	98.3 ± 5.7	5.3 ± 0.5	4.8 ± 1.7	6.7 ± 1.3	4.8 ± 1.7
2 days	98.3 ± 1.5	3.2 ± 1.0	2.9 ± 1.0	4.3 ± 0.9	4.7 ± 0.8
3 days	95.6 ± 1.7	1.4 ± 1.2	1.8 ± 1.2	2.2 ± 0.8	2.2 ± 0.6
4 days	86.5 ± 3.6**	1.2 ± 0.1	3.6 ± 0.8**	2.4 ± 0.7	6.0 ± 0.5**
5 days	80.6 ± 6.2**	0.8 ± 1.1	4.7 ± 0.6**	2.0 ± 0.3	6.0 ± 0.5**
6 days	77.1 ± 9.2**	2.7 ± 0.8	8.7 ± 0.7**	3.1 ± 0.1	9.0 ± 0.6**
7 days	78.7 ± 7.1**	1.3 ±1.1	4.3 ± 0.1**	2.2 ± 0.2	6.9 ± 0.6**
13 days	78.5 ± 7.3**	3.7 ±0.6	5.6 ± 0.3*	2.9 ± 0.6	3.1 ± 0.5

Total number of cells was measured in the cerebral cortex as a function of time after hypoxia by cell counting following nuclear staining by DAPI and is expressed as a percentage from matched controls. Proportions of necrotic and apoptotic nuclei were calculated after DAPI labeling according to morphological hallmarks and are expressed as a percentage of total cells in both control and hypoxic rats. Data were obtained from 3 to 5 separate experiments using animals from different litters, and are given as means ± S.D. Statistically significant differences from controls: *$p<0.05$ and **$p<0.01$; Statistically significant differences from hypoxia alone: °$p<0.05$ and °°$p<0.01$ (Dunnett's test for multiple comparisons).

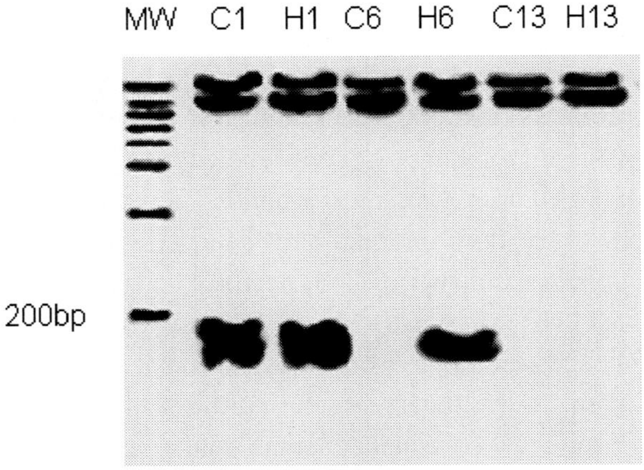

Figure 3. Temporal analysis on agarose gel of DNA isolated from the cerebral cortex of control and hypoxic rats. Cortical DNA was isolated at 1 day (H1), 6 days (H6) and 13 days (H13) after birth hypoxia and from matched controls (C1, C6 and C13). One representative example is presented for illustration, and similar profiles were obtained from 5 separate experiments.

Regarding Bax and Bcl-2, a significant basal expression of both proteins was detected in the cortex of control animals of 1-4 days of age, and their levels tended to decrease thereafter. The resulting Bax/Bcl-2 ratio was globally maintained around 1 during the period examined (Figure 4). Following birth hypoxia, Bcl-2 was transiently overexpressed at 3 days post-insult, and its expression gradually declined as a function of time, to be reduced by 38% by comparison to matched controls at 13 days. Bax expression was similar to controls at 3 days, and then markedly increased in response to birth hypoxia, depicting a significant elevation of the Bax/Bcl-2 protein ratio at the final stage (Figure 4).

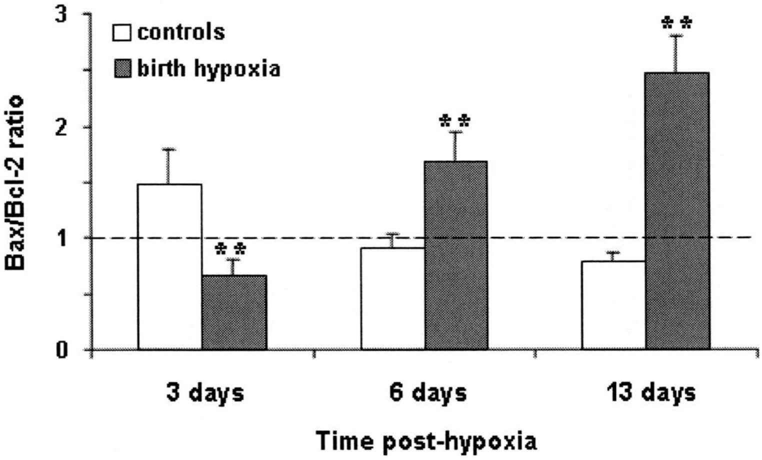

Figure 4. Evolution of the Bax/Bcl-2 protein ratio in the cerebral cortex of rats exposed to birth hypoxia and their matched controls. Immunohistochemical studies were performed at 3 days, 6 days and 13 days post-hypoxia and in control rat pups. Fluorescence activity was analysed as described in the legend of Figure 2. The data represent mean values (± S.D.) obtained from 3 separate experiments. Statistically significant difference from controls: ** $p<0.01$ (Dunnett's test for multiple comparisons).

In Vivo 7-Day Ischemia

When 7-day old rat pups were subjected to ischemia, a cortical infarct was clearly delineated at 48 h of reperfusion, as previously documented (Renolleau et al., 1998). At this time point of recovery, a decline in the number of cells was recorded. Three zones were depicted, the core of the infarct, penumbra close to the core and distant penumbra in which 13, 34 and 52 % of surviving cells were respectively counted, as compared to the contralateral cortex (Table 3). With DAPI staining and examination of the nuclear morphology, cells exhibiting the characteristic hallmarks of apoptosis were significantly detected in the 2 penumbral zones, whereas nuclei with a necrotic profile were mainly observed in the core of the infarct (Table 3). Similar findings were obtained by the TUNEL assay. Whereas the presence of necrotic nuclei with flocculent chromatin was shown in the core (Figure 5 A, B), all of the TUNEL-positive nuclei in the penumbra demonstrated chromatin condensation and apoptotic body formation (Figure 5 C). Analysis of DNA fragmentation on agarose gel demonstrated DNA laddering in the ipsilateral cortex, which mainly corresponded to penumbral tissue, 5 days after the onset of ischemia, which was not present in the contralateral cortex (Figure 5D).

Table 3. Temporal evolution of the number of cells and their nuclear morphological features of necrosis and apoptosis in the cerebral cortex of 7 day-old rats exposed to ischemia and killed at 48 h of reperfusion.

	Number of total cells *(per 0.01 mm^2)*	**Necrosis** *(% of total cells)*	**Apoptosis** *(% of total cells)*
Contralateral cortex	72.0 ± 1.4	2.1 ± 0.5	0.7 ± 0.1
	Table 3 (continued)		
	Number of total cells *(per 0.01 mm^2)*	**Necrosis** *(% of total cells)*	**Apoptosis** *(% of total cells)*
Ischemic Core	12.3 ± 1.1**	82.3 ± 1.9**	13.3 ± 0.5**
Ischemic Penumbra (a)	31.5 ± 0.7**	6.3 ± 0.3**	58.1 ± 0.2**
Ischemic Penumbra (b)	48.5 ± 0.7**	4.2 ± 0.1	30.6 ± 0.5**

Cell density as well as rates of necrosis and apoptosis were analyzed as described in the method section. Data are reported as means ± S.D. obtained from 3 separate experiments. Statistically significant differences from contralateral cortex (control): **$p<0.01$ (Dunnett's test for multiple comparisons). Penumbra (a) = close to the core; Penumbra (b) = distant from the core.

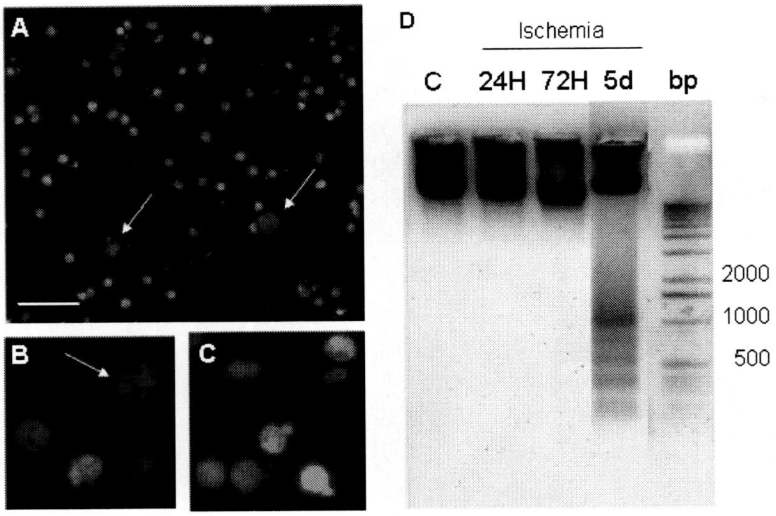

Figure 5. Typical illustration of DNA fragmentation by the TUNEL assay and agarose gel of genomic DNA from ischemic rat pups. A-C: Nuclei exhibited flocculent chromatin in the core (white arrows in A and B) and chromatin condensation and apoptotic bodies in both core (A, B) and penumbra (C). D: Temporal analysis on agarose gel of DNA isolated from ipsilateral (i) and contralateral (c) cortex. Cortical DNA was isolated at 48 h (H48), 4 days (D4) and 5 days (D5) post-ischemia and compared to control (C). Note DNA fragmentation with formation of a ladder at 5 days post-injury. One representative example is presented for illustration, and similar profiles were obtained from 4 separate experiments. Bar represents 100 (A) and 20 μm (B, C).

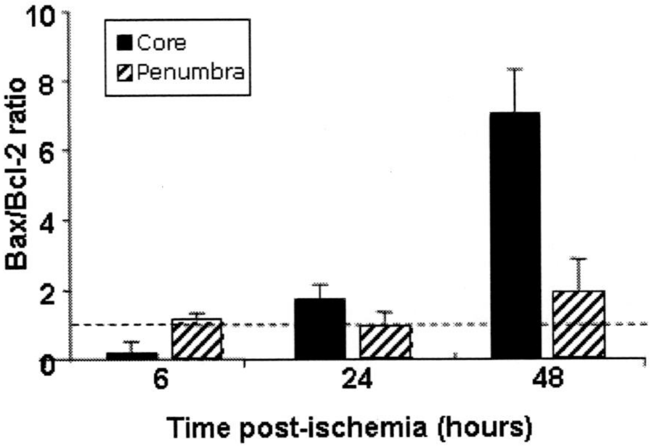

Figure 6. Evolution of the Bax/Bcl-2 positive cell ratio in the cerebral cortex of 7-day-old rats exposed to ischemia. Immunohistochemical studies were performed at 6, 24 and 48 h post-ischemia. No Bcl-2 positive cells and a few (2 to 4) Bax positive cells have been detected in controls. The data represent mean values ± S.D. obtained from 3 separate experiments.

A basal Bax immunoreactivity was observed in a few cells scattered in the control cortex and in the contralateral side of ischemic brains whereas no Bcl-2-positive cells was detected. Quantification of the number of Bax-positive cells indicated a gradual elevation of their number after reperfusion in the core of the infarct in which a slight number of Bcl-2-positive cells were present. The resulting Bax/Bcl-2 ratio progressively increased between 6 and 24 h and was conspicuous at 48 h of reperfusion (Figure 6) in the core of the infarct. In contrast, Bcl-2-positive cells were still detected in the penumbra (close and distant from the core), leading to a similar Bax/Bcl-2 ratio at 24 h. Cell death in the penumbra began to be effective, as the Bax/Bcl-2 ration increased, at 48 h of recovery (Figure 6).

Conclusion

During development, apoptosis is a crucial event for maintaining the brain homeostasis and setting up appropriate neuron-target cell connections (Oppenheim, 1991). In the rat brain, the physiological death program does not take place exclusively during embryogenesis but is also present during early postnatal development. Consistently, characteristic features of programmed cell death were observed during the life span of cultured neurons isolated from the forebrain of 14-day-old embryos as well as in the brains of rat pups by the first days of postnatal life. For example, baseline levels of Bax and Bcl-2 proteins were routinely detected in control samples, and higher Bax levels depicted by the first days of postnatal age are indicative of active apoptosis in the rat brain, although other members of the Bcl-2 family may play a critical role (Isenmann et al., 1998; Otter et al., 1998). In good agreement, the numbers of DAPI-labeled nuclei exhibiting morphological features of condensed chromatin were more elevated in the cortex of rats at 1 and 2 days of age. By contrast to the newborn brain, Bcl-2 was not detectable at baseline in the cerebral cortex of 7-day-old rats. Indeed, it is known that the expression of Bcl-2 in rodents is developmentally regulated, with highest levels present in the antenatal brain (Abe-Dohmae et al., 1993) where it would participate to the selection of surviving neurons during the period of physiological death. Finally, when DNA fragmentation was monitored by electrophoresis, significant amounts of small fragments corresponding to ~200 bp were repeatedly observed, in the absence of typical ladder pattern, in the cortex of control rats until 3 days of age, before to disappear in older animals. According to our criteria, necrotic cells were also detected in cultured neurons and even in the cortex of rat pups in the early postnatal period. It is known, however, that necrosis may appear as an ultimate feature of apoptosis (Nakajima et al., 2000; Benchoua et al., 2001), especially in culture condition where dying cells are not submitted to active phagocytosis (Bonfoco et al., 1995). All the above observations confirm the high propensity of developing brain cells to undergo apoptosis.

The participation of apoptotic-like cell death has been widely described in various pathological states, including in post-mitotic neurons (see Sastry and Rao, 2000 for review). Exposure to hypoxia elicited delayed cell death in the three models examined. Programmed death was confirmed by the beneficial effects of cycloheximide in cultured neurons, as previously documented (Bossenmeyer et al., 1998; Papas et al., 1992), and was shown to require activation of caspases, especially caspase-3 in the various models (Bossenmeyer-Pourié et al., 1999; 2000; Grojean et al., 2003; Benjelloun et al., 2003). Also, apoptotic death is known to be associated with an elevated Bax/Bcl-2 ratio within the cells (Otter et al., 1998). In this respect, Bcl-2 was transiently predominant at 48 h post-insult in cultured neurons. Then, Bcl-2 level decreased, in parallel with a substantial stimulation of Bax expression. By the same time, the presence of typically shrunken nuclei and a reduced number of viable cells were recorded. Such a temporal profile of protein expression was also depicted in the cortex of the asphyxiated newborn rat as well as in the core of the infarct following ischemia in the 7-day-old rat, and these findings are consistent with the view of an apoptotic-necrotic continuum in response to severe neuronal injury (Martin, 2001). In the penumbral area, a long-lasting stimulation of Bcl-2 was recorded, probably due to more effective homeostatic mechanisms and higher availability of energy compared to the core of the infarct where necrosis developed more rapidly.

In the present study, DAPI staining, TUNEL assay and gel electrophoresis of extracted DNA were used to investigate alterations of nuclear DNA in response to hypoxia. Although chromatin condensation and formation of apoptotic bodies were visualized by DAPI in all cases, DNA fragmentation was demonstrated by the TUNEL assay following ischemia in 7 day-old rat pups but not after birth hypoxia. Similarly, DNA laddering was found in the former model but not in the latter, except fragments of ~200 bp. These results suggest that DNA fragmentation occurred in a different manner, probably dependent on the age of injured animals. DNA digestion at internucleosomal linker regions was recognized in 1980 as a characteristic feature of apoptosis, resulting in small double-stranded fragments of DNA that migrate in a ladder pattern (Wyllie, 1980). The fragmentation of ladder type has been attributed to the activities of Ca^{2+}/Mg^{2+}-activated endonucleases (Kyprianou et al., 1988), DNAse I (Arends et al., 1990) or DNAse II (Barry ane Eastmann, 1993). However, less extensive digestion of DNA to sizes of 50 and 300 kbp, corresponding to the loop and rosette structures of higher-order chromatin, occurs in several examples of apoptosis without or prior to processing to oligonucleosome-sized fragments and can be recognized by fractionation of genomic DNA on pulse field gel electrophoresis (Walker et al., 1991; Brown et al., 1993; Oberhammer at al., 1993). Such high molecular weight fragments have been shown following ischemia in the P7 rat pup as early as 4 h of recovery (Charriaut-Marlangue et al., 1999). They appeared prior to the detection of TUNEL-positive nuclei and DNA laddering, and have been previously reported in the brain of P7 rat subjected to the Rice model of hypoxia-ischemia (Hou et al., 1997). Taken together, our results suggest that birth hypoxia may induce high molecular weight DNA fragments which cannot be detected on agarose gels, and 200 bp fragments were probably the result of an endogenous exonuclease activity. When neuronal cultures were submitted to hypoxia, a DNA smear was observed on agarose gels. Consistently, serum deprivation of PC12 cells was reported to induce apoptosis along with a DNA degradation as a smear which was prevented by aurintricarboxylic acid, an endonuclease inhibitor (Dessi et al., 1993). Furthermore, there is at least one in vitro example of apoptotic death in which DNA digestion is not detectable by sensitive methods, consistent with experimental evidence that nuclear events may not be required for apoptosis (Ucker et al., 1992). Finally, it is noteworthy that no DNA degradation could be seen at 13 days after birth asphyxia, along with the lack of apoptotic nuclei as depicted by DAPI staining. Such observations suggest the possibility of repair processes, in line with the remarkable plasticity of the juvenile brain.

In conclusion, oxygen deprivation triggered delayed cell death that mainly corresponds to apoptosis, according to morphological and biochemical criteria, in the three experimental models investigated in the present study. The consequences of hypoxia in cultured neurons, which were shown to be dependent upon protein neosynthesis, are comparable to those observed in the newborn rat brain, these two models being theorically matched with regard to their developmental stages (Dichter, 1978). Furthermore, we have shown that when it was monitored by 4-6 days post-reoxygenation, DNA fragmentation elicited by birth asphyxia exhibited the same characteristics as DNA fragmentation consecutive to naturally occurring cell death in the newborn brain (i.e., TUNEL-negative in situ and leading solely to small fragments of approximately 200 bp on agarose gels). Conversely, hypoxia-ischemia in the 7-day-old rat induced apotic cell death in the penumbra with characteristics closer to those reported in the adult brain, but with reduced level of necrosis compared to the adult (Li et al., 1998). Therefore, our results suggest that a shift may occur in the rat brain by the end of the first week of postnatal age with respect to the hallmarks of apoptotic-like cell injury in response to hypoxia, with brain manifestations in the neonate mainly corresponding to the developmental death pattern. These findings might account, at least partly, for the relative resistance of the immature brain to hypoxic insults.

References

Abe-Dohmae, S., Harada, N., Yamada, K., Tanaka, R. Bcl-2 gene is highly expressed during neurogenesis in the central nervous system. *Biochem Biophys Res Commun*, 1993, 191, 915-921.

Arends, M.J., Morris, R.G., Wyllie, A.H. Apoptosis. The role of the endonuclease. *Am J Pathol*, 1990, 136, 593-608.

Barry, M.A. and Eastmann, A. Identification of deoxyribonuclease II as an endonuclease involved in apoptosis. *Arch Biochem Biophys*, 1993, 300, 440-450.

Beilharz, E.J., Williams, C.E., Dragunow, M., Sirimanne, E.S., Gluckman, P.D. Mechanisms of delayed cell death following hypoxic-ischemic injury in the immature rat: evidence for apoptosis during selective neuronal loss. *Mol Brain Res*, 1995, 29, 1-14.

Berger, R., and Garnier, Y. Pathophysiology of perinatal brain damage. *Brain Res Rev*, 1999, 30, 107-134.

Benchoua, A., Guégan, C., Couriaud, C., Hosseini, H., Sampaïo, N., Morin, D., Onténiente, B. Specific caspase pathways are activated in the two stages of cerebral infarction. *J Neurosci*, 2001, 21, 7127-7134.

Benjelloun, N., Joly, L.M., Palmier, B., Plotkine, M., Charriaut-Marlangue, C. Apoptotic mitochondrial pathway in neuron and astrocyte after neonatal hypoxia-ischemia in the rat brain. *Neuropathol & Applied Neurobiol,* 2003, 29, 350-360.

Blaschke, A.J., Staley, K., Chun, J. Widespread programmed cell death in proliferative and postmitotic regions of the fetal cerebral cortex. *Development*, 1996, 122, 1165-1174.

Bonfoco, E., Kraine, D., Ankarcrona, M., Nicotera, P., Lipton, S.A. Apoptosis and necrosis: two distinct events induced, respectively, by mild and intense insults with N-methyl-D-aspartate or nitric oxide/superoxide in cortical cell cultures. *Proc Natl Acad Sci (USA)*, 1995, 92, 7162-7166.

Bossenmeyer, C., Chihab, R., Muller, S., Schroeder, H., Daval, J.L. Hypoxia/reoxygenation induces apoptosis through biphasic induction of protein synthesis in central neurons. *Brain Res*, 1998, 787, 107-116.

Bossenmeyer-Pourié C., Daval, J.L. Prevention from hypoxia-induced apoptosis by preconditioning: a mechanistic approach in cultured neurons from fetal rat forebrain. *Mol Brain Res*, 1998, 58, 237-239.

Bossenmeyer-Pourié, C., Chihab, R., Schroeder, H., Daval, J.L. Transient hypoxia may lead to neuronal proliferation in the developing mammalian brain: from apoptosis to cell cycle completion. *Neuroscience*, 1999a, 91, 221-231.

Bossenmeyer-Pourié, C., Koziel, V., Daval, J.L. CPP32/CASPASE-3-like proteases in hypoxia-induced apoptosis in developing brain neurons, *Mol. Brain Res*, 1999b 71, 225-237.

Bossenmeyer-Pourié, C., Koziel, V., Daval, J.L. Involvement of caspase-1 proteases in hypoxic brain injury. Effects of their inhibitors in developing neurons, *Neuroscience*, 2000, 95, 1157-1165.

Bossenmeyer-Pourié, C., Lièvre V, Grojean S, Koziel, V., Pillot T., Daval, J.L. Sequential expression patterns of apoptosis- and cell cycle-related proteins in neuronal response to severe or mild transient hypoxia. *Neuroscience*, 2002, 114, 869-882.

Brown, D., Sun, X., Cohen, G. Dexamethasone-induced apoptosis involves cleavage of DNA to large fragments prior to internucleosomal fragmentation. *J Biol Chem*, 1993, 268, 3037-3039.

Charriaut-Marlangue, C., Ben-Ari, Y. A cautionary note on the use of TUNEL stain to describe apoptosis, *NeuroReport*, 1995, 7, 61-64.

Charriaut-Marlangue, C., Aggoun-Zouaoui, D., Represa, A., Ben-Ari, Y. Apoptotic features in ischemia, epilepsy and gp 120 toxicity. *Trends in Neurosci*, 1996, 19, 109-114.

Charriaut-Marlangue, C., Richard, E., Ben-Ari, Y. DNA damage and DNA damage-inducible protein Gadd45 following ischemia in the P7 neonatal rat. *Dev Brain Res*, 1999, 116, 133-140.

Chihab, R., Ferry, C., Koziel, V., Monin, P., Daval, J.L. Sequential activation of activator protein-1-related transcription factors and JNK protein kinases may contribute to apoptotic death induced by transient hypoxia in developing brain neurons. *Mol Brain Res*, 1998, 63, 105-120.

Daval, J.L., Pourié, G., Grojean, S., Lièvre, V., Strazielle, C., Blaise, S., Vert, P. Neonatal hypoxia triggers transient apoptosis followed by neurogenesis in the rat CA1 hippocampus. *Pediatr Res*, 2004, 55, 561-567.

Dessi, F., Charriaut-Marlangue, C., Khrestchatisky, M., Ben-Ari, Y. Glutamate-induced neuronal death is not a programmed cell death in cerebellar culture. *J Neurochem*, 1993, 60, 1953-1955.

Dichter, M.A. Rat cortical neurons in cell culture: culture methods, cell morphology, electrophysiology and synapse formation. *Brain Res*, 1978, 149, 279-293.

Grojean, S., Koziel, V., Vert, P., Daval, J.L. Bilirubin induces apoptosis via activation of NMDA receptors in developing rat brain neurons. *Exp Neurol*, 2000, 166, 334-341.

Grojean, S., Schroeder, H., Pourié, G., Charriaut-Marlangue, C., Koziel, V., Desor, D., Vert, P., Daval, J.L. Histopathological alterations and functional brain deficits after transient hypoxia in the newborn rat pup: a long term follow-up. *Neurobiol Dis*, 2003, 14, 265-278.

Grafe MR. Developmental changes in the sensitivity of the neonatal rat brain. *Brain Res*, 1994, 653,161-166.

Hansen, M.B., Nielsen, S.E., Berg, K. Re-examination and further development of a precise and rapid dye method for measuring cell growth/cell kill. *J Immunol Meth*, 1989, 119, 203-210.

Hou, S., Tu, Y., Buchan, A., Huang, Z., Preston, E., Rasquinha, I., Robertson, G., MacManus, J. Increase in DNA lesions and the DNA damage indicator Gadd45 following transient ischemia. *Biochem Cell Biol*, 1997, 75,383-392.

Isenmann, S., Stoll, G., Schroeter, M., Krajewski, S., Reed, J.C., Bahr, M. Differential regulation of Bax, Bcl-2, and Bcl-X proteins in focal cortical ischemia in the rat. *Brain Pathol*, 1998, 8, 49-63.

Kyprianou, N., English, H.F., Isaacs, J.T. Activation of a Ca2+-Mg2+-dependent endonuclease as an early event in castration-induced prostatic cell death. *Prostate*, 1988, 13, 103-117.

Laird, P., Zijderveld, A., Linders, K., Rudnicki, M., Jaenisch, R., Berns, A. Simplified mammalian DNA isolation procedure. *Nucleic Acids Res*, 1991, 19, 4293.

Li, Y., Powers, C., Jiang, N., Chopp, M. Intact, injured, necrotic and apoptotic cells after focal cerebral ischemia in the rat. *J Neurol Sci*, 1998, 156, 119-132.

Martin, L.J. Neuronal cell death in nervous system development, disease, and injury. *Int J Mol Med*, 2000, 7, 455-478.

Nakajima, W., Ishida, A., Lange, M.S., Gabrielson, K.L., Wilson, M.A., Martin, L.J., Blue, M.E., Johnston, M.V. Apoptosis has a prolonged role in the degeneration after hypoxic ischemia in the newborn rat. *J Neurosci*, 2000, 20, 7994-8004.

Oberhammer, F., Wilson, J., Dive, C., Morris, I., Hickman, J., Wakeling, A., Walker, P., Sikorska, M. Apoptotic death in epithelial cells: cleavage of DNA to 300 and/or 50 kb fragments prior to or in the absence of internucleosomal fragmentation. *EMBO J*, 1993, 12, 3679-3684

Oppenheim, R.W. Cell death during development of the nervous system. *Ann Rev Neurosci*, 1991, 14, 453-501.

Otter, I., Conus, S., Ravn, U., Rager, M., Olivier, R., Monney, L., Fabbro, D., Borner, C. The binding properties and biological activities of Bcl-2 and Bax in cells exposed to apoptotic stimuli. *J Biol Chem*, 1998, 273, 6110-6120.

Papas, S., Crépel, V., Hasboun, D., Jorquera, I., Chinestra, P., Ben-Ari, Y. Cycloheximide reduces the effects of anoxic insult in vivo and in vitro. *Eur J Neurosci*, 1992, 4, 758-765.

Park, D.S., Morris, E.J., Greene, L.A., Geller, H.M. G1/S cell cycle blockers and inhibitors of cyclin-dependent kinases suppress camptothecin-induced neuronal apoptosis. *J Neurosci*, 1997, 17, 1256-1270.

Pittman, R.N., Wang, S., DiBenedetto, A.J., Mills, J.C. A system for characterizing cellular and molecular events in programmed neuronal cell death. *J Neurosci*, 1993, 13, 3669-3680.

Renolleau, S., Aggoun-Zouaoui, D., Ben-Ari, Y., Charriaut-Marlangue, C. A model of transient unilateral focal ischemia with reperfusion in the P7 neonatal rat: morphological changes indicative of apoptosis. *Stroke*, 1998, 29, 1454-1461.

Richter C, Schweizer M, Cossarizza A, Franceschi C. Control of apoptosis by the cellular ATP level. *FEBS Lett*, 1996, 378:107-110.

Sastry, P.S., Rao, K.S. Apoptosis and the central nervous system. *J Neurochem*, 2000, 74, 1-20.

Sherwood, N.M., Timiras, P.S. A stereotaxic atlas of the developing rat brain. Berkeley: *University of California Press*, 1970

Sidhu RS, Tuor UI, Del Bigio MR. Nuclear condensation and fragmentation following cerebral hypoxia-ischemia occurs more frequently in immature than older rats. *Neurosci Lett*, 1997, 223, 129-132.

Ucker, D., Obermiller, P., Eckhart, W., Apgar, J., Berger, N., Meyers, J. Genome digestion is a dispensable consequence of physiological cell death mediated by cytotoxic T lymphocytes. *Mol Cell Biol*, 1992, 12, 3060-3069.

Volpe, J.J. Neurology of the newborn. In: Volpe J.J. (Ed) *Neurology of the Newborn.* WB Saunders, Philadelphia, 1987, 236-280.

Walker, P., Smith, C., Youdale, T., Leblanc, J., Whitfield, J., Sikorska, M. Topoisomerase II-reactive chemotherapeutic drugs induce apoptosis in thymocytes. *Cancer Res*, 1991, 51, 1078-1085.

Wolvetang, E.J., Johnson, K.L., Krauer, K., Ralph, S.J., Linnane, A.W. Mitochondrial respiratory chain inhibitors induce apoptosis. *FEBS Letters*, 1994, 339, 40-44.

Wyllie, A.H. Glucocorticoid-induced thymocyte apoptosis is associated with endogenous endonuclease activation. *Nature*, 1980, 284, 555-556.

Wyllie, A.H. Cell death: a new classification separating apoptosis from necrosis. In: Bowen ID, Lockshin RA (eds) *Cell Death in Biology and Pathology*. London: Chapman and Hall, 1981, 9-34.

In: Brain Mapping Research Progress
Editors: Ines C. Girard and Jade S. Andre

ISBN: 978-1-60456-784-7

Chapter IV

The Use of Neural Stem Cells in Treating Traumatic Brain Injury in Rats

Shu-Yuan Yang** and Hui Liu
Department of Neurosurgery, Tianjin Medical University,
General Hospital, Tianjin 300052; People's Republic of China

Abstract

Objective

In this study we investigated the neuroprotective effect of transplants of Neural Stem Cells (NSCs) after experimental traumatic brain injury.

Methods

NSCs were derived from human fetal hippocampi. The cells were injected into the cerebral cortex of rats subjected to experimental traumatic brain injury. The effect on the motor function scores of the rats was assessed. The techniques of immunohistochemistry and TUNEL were applied to define the NSCs' differentiation and neuroprotection.

Results

Brain injured animals that received transplants of NSCs had marked and significantly improved motor scores compared with control groups. Animals that received NSCs transplants had significantly more surviving neurons compared with the vehicle treated brain injured rats.

---

* Address for reprints and correspondence: Professor Shu-Yuan Yang, M.D., Department of Neurosurgery, Tianjin Medical University, General Hospital, 154 An-Shan Road, Tianjin 300052, People's Republic of China. Phone: +86-22-6036-2621; Fax: +86-22-6036-2386; Email:dhcan@public.tpt.tj.cn

In situ TUNEL assay demonstrated fewer apoptotic cells in animals that received NSCs transplants than those of the control group.

Conclusions

These results demonstrate the neuroprotective and functional efficacy of NSC transplants after experimental traumatic brain injury.

Key Words: Neural stem cells Traumatic brain injury Neurotransplantation

Introduction

The limited capacity for structural repair in the mammalian brain is in part explained by the inability of the mature CNS to generate new cellular elements in response to damage. Over the last few decades neurotransplantation has been used to explore the processes of development, plasticity and regeneration in the central nervous system. Further, it has been used for the repair and functional restoration of diseased and damaged nervous tissue.

As an example of neurotransplantation a series of patients with Parkinson's disease have been treated with mesencephalic cells from human fetuses, obtained from 6 to 9 weeks old abortuses. These grafts send out processes and make dopamine after implantation. In models of traumatic spinal cord injury, transplanted neural tissue has been shown to survive, bridge gaps in the injured spinal cord, decrease glial scarring, and even make functional connections with the host. Studies involving transplantation of fetal tissue into traumatically damaged adult rodent brain have demonstrated good graft survival, neurite outgrowth across the graft-host interface, attenuation of host neuronal cell death, and improvement in posttraumatic behavioral function. [1-6]

However, inherent limitations of fetal CNS transplants, such as their cellular heterogeneity, limited availability, the limited migratory capacity of differentiated cells, and potential ethical dilemmas, have led investigators to search for an alternative source of transplantable neural cells that can be charactered, expanded and genetically manipulated.

The recent discovery of stem cell population in the central nervous system has generated intense interest, since the brain has long been regarded as incapable of regeneration. Neural stem cells (NSCs) have been propagated in vitro by a variety of equally effective and safe means - both epigenetic and genetic. A population of dividing progenitors is capable of differentiating into both neurons and glia. These plastic cells migrate and differentiate in a temporally and regionally appropriate manner, particularly following implantation into germinal zones (the subventricular zone and the hippocampal dentate gyrus). Intermingling nondisruptively with endogenous progenitors, responding similarly to local cues for their phenotypic determination, and differentiating appropriately into diverse neuronal and glial types, they participate in normal development along the rodent neuraxis. In this way NSCs are raising the possibility of therapeutic potential. [7-16]

Using a model of diffuse brain injury in rats results in well defined outcomes that reproduce many components of human head injury. Novel treatment strategies for traumatic brain injury (TBI) have been directed at reducing secondary or delayed injury by rescuing neural tissue, promoting synaptic reorganization, and ultimately restoring functional recovery.

In the present study we explored the possibility that the transplantation of neural stem cells (NSCs) could be used as a means to reduce the effects of traumatic brain injury (TBI).

Materials and Methods

1. Culture of Human Neural Stem Cells

Embryonic brain tissue was obtained from one 12 weeks and one 16 weeks aborted human embryo. Tissue from the hippocampus was dissected in sterile saline and transferred to N2 medium, a defined DMEM/F12-based medium (Life Technologies) containing 0.6% glucose, 25μg/ml human insulin, 100μg/ml human transferrin, 20nM progesterone, 60μM putrescine, 30nM selenium chloride, 2nM glutamine, 3mM sodium bicarbonate. The tissues were cut up with scissors and dissociated by gentle trituration in DMEM/F12, and filtered through a sterile 200 mesh steel net. The dissociated cells were grown on uncoated plastic T75 flasks in N2 medium containing human EGF (20ng/ml), human basic FGF (20ng/ml), at a density of 10^5 cells / ml. The cells were passaged by mechanical dissociation every week.

2. Brain Injury

35 adult male Wistar rats, each weighting 300-350g, underwent diffuse brain injury as previously described [17,18]. Under general anesthesia a midline scalp incision was made followed by periosteal elevation to expose the central area of the skull vault between the coronal and lambdoid sutures. A stainless steel disc 1cm in diameter was firmly fixed by dental acrylic to the centre of the skull vault. The rat was placed in the prone position on a foam bed with the disc centered immediately under the lower end of the tube of the trauma device. Two belts were fastened around the trunk of the rat to prevent it from falling off the foam bed with the trauma induction. The weight was allowed to drop freely from the selected height through the Plexiglas tube onto the disc. The foam bed together with the rat were removed from underneath the tube immediately after the impact to make sure there was only one hit. The rat was then transferred back to the operating table and was allowed to recover from anesthesia. Rats that died on impact and those with skull fractures were excluded from the morphological study.

3. Cell Transplantation

At 24 hours postinjury, all animals were reanesthetized by intraperitoneal injection of 10% chloralium hydrate and placed in a stereotactic frame (Stoelting, USA). Rats received 5 μl cell suspension in DMEM/F12 according to the following coordinates calculated from the bregma (A and L) and dura(V). Site1, A=-3 mm, L=2mm, V=3mm; site 2, A=-3mm, L=-2mm, V=3mm. The tooth bar was set at –2.3, and all ventral coordinates were taken from dura.

5 μl (1×10^5cells) of the cell suspension were injected over 5 minutes into each of the two sites. The needle was left in place for 5 minutes, and then gradually withdrawn over 5 minutes. The hole then was sealed with bone wax.

Four groups of rats were used. The first group was the control group (sham group). The second was the injured group (TBI group). In the third (TBI+NSCs group) NSCs were injected stereotacticly 24h after the injury. In the last one (TBI+DF group) DF were injected.

4. Assessment of Neurological Motor Deficits [19]

The rats were scored without reference to their group with regard to neurological recovery. Behavioural tests included the ability to maintain position on a inclined plane (vertical, right horizontal, and left horizontal positions), left and right forelimb flexion after suspension by the tail, and degree of resistance to right and left lateral pulsion. The seven individual scores, each graded from 0 (severely impaired) to 5 (normal function), were added to yield a composite neurological score ranging from 0 to 35.

The baseline neurological score was calculated immediately before injury. After injury neurological motor function was assessed in each rat at 48 hours, and one week and two weeks after injury.

5. Histological Evaluation

At either 3 or 7 days after transplantation, rats were terminally anaesthetized with 10% chloral hydrate and transcardially perfused with 0.1 M phosphate buffer saline (PBS) followed by 5 min rapid fixation with ice-cold 4% paraformaldehyde in 0.1 M PBS. Brains were removed and placed in paraformaldehyde overnight, before being transferred to 25% sucrose in PBS.

For light microscopy studies, brains were sectioned in the coronal plane, before being embedded in paraffin. Sections 5μm thick were cut with a rotary microtome and stained with haematoxylin and eosin (HandE).

Sections were first rinsed in 0.1 M PBS three times for 10 minutes each. Blocking of nonspecific binding was achieved with 10% normal horse serum. The blocking solution contained 0.3% Triton X-100. The sections were incubated with primary antibody, diluted 1:100 in PBS, for 16 to 18 hours at 4℃. Subsequently, after three 10 minute rinses with PBS, the sections were reincubated for 60 minutes in biotinylated antimouse immunoglobulin G, diluted 1:100 in PBS. After a brief rinse with PBS, the sections were immersed in avidin-biotin peroxidase complex at room temperature for 60 minutes. Immunolabeled peroxidase was visualized by DAB.

For BrdU labeling, all sections were pretreated with 1M HCL for 30 min at 65℃. For all immunohistochemical procedures, adjacent sections served as negative controls and were processed using identical procedures, except for incubation without the primary antibody in each case.

6. Detection of Apoptosis

Apoptotic cells were visualized using an Insitu Cell Death Detection kit (Roche, Germany). Briefly, after routine dewax, rehydration and washing in PBS, tissue was digested with proteinase K for 15 minutes at room temperature and washed. Endogenous peroxidase activity was blocked by freshly prepared 3% H_2O_2 for 10 minutes at room temperature. After washing with PBS 50μl TUNEL reaction mixture was pipetted onto the sections, which were then incubated in a humidified chamber at 37℃ for one hour. The reaction was stopped by adding wash buffer. The slides were then incubated with 50μl Converter-POD in the humidified chamber for thirty minutes. After washing the slides were then stained with diaminobenzidine substrate and mounted under a glass coverslip. They were examined under a light microscope. As a negative control Label solution was substituted for the TUNEL reaction mixture.

6. Statistical Analysis

Motor scores are ordinal measurements and therefore were evaluated using Kruskal-Wallis analysis of variance(ANOVA) followed by individual Mann-Whitney U-tests. A probability value of less than 0.05 was considered statistical significant.

Results

1. The Proliferation and Ultrastructural Properties of Neural Precursors

At first some cells which were attached to the bottom of wells became larger and began to divide, forming small neurospheres. At seven days larger spheres could be found, some floating freely and others remaining attached to the bottom of the plates. In the medium containing EGF/FGF-2 after every passage the precursor cells proliferated and formed new spheres.

Cultures were examined by TEM. The NSCs were of a relatively small round shape, with large nuclei and little cytoplasm. The nuclei were round, with several indentations and prominent nucleoli. The cytoplasm contained many free ribosomes, but few polysomes, MIT and RER (figure 1).

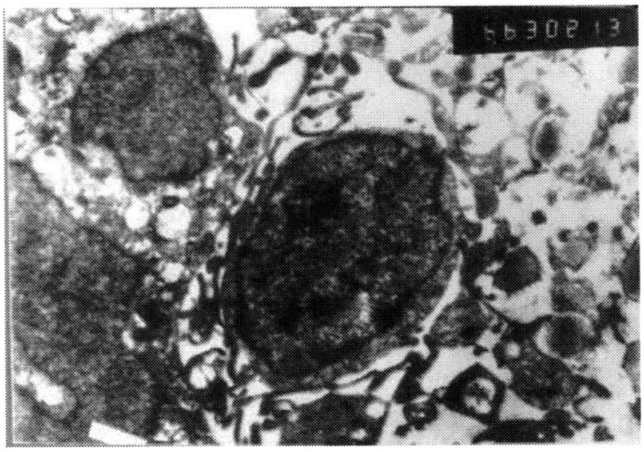

Figure 1. Ultrastructure of precursor cells in vitro. The NSCs exhibited a relatively small round morphology, with large nuclei and little cytoplasma.

2. Antigenic Character and Differentiation of Neural Precursors

Virtually all of the cells within the neurospheres were immmunoreactive for neuroepithelial antigen nestin. The neurospheres were dissociated to a single cell suspension and plated onto poly-l-lysine coated cover slips, where they rapidly attached to the surface of the slips. Two days later, many cells had developed the morphological properties of neurons or astrocytes. At 7 days the cultures were fixed and stained for Tubulin, and also GFAP. Examined by confocal microscopy an even layer of surviving cells was present across the cultural cover slips. Many cells were immunoreactive for Tubulin or GFAP.

3. Neurological Assessment

The motor function scores of rats 48 hours after definitive injury and at one week were significantly lower than those of the sham-injured group. ($P<0.05$). At 48 hours after injury animals that had received NSCs transplants did not show significant improvement compared to the untreated group. However one week after injury, rats of TBI+NSCs group had marked and significant improved scores compared with rats of both TBI group and TBI+DF group.

Table

	2d	1w
Sham-injured	33.13±1.46	35.63±0.52
TBI	15.50±4.04	20.75±1.49
TBI+DF	15.00±3.16	20.63±1.41
TBI+NSCs	17.38±3.85	27.13±3.98

4. Engraftment of Cells

To examine the engraftment of these cells in brain tissue, we repeated the injections using BrdU-labeled NSCs. NSCs were found in and around the grafted site and had the morphological characteristics of round, small-medium sized mononuclear cells, which appeared yellow or brown (figure 2).

Sections from the cortex contained cells that were positive for Tubulin, and other cells that were positive for GFAP (figure 3). Positive staining for neuronal and astrocytic markers was poorly seen when viewing 3-day-old specimens, but was clearly visible in 7-day-old specimen or specimens obtained later.

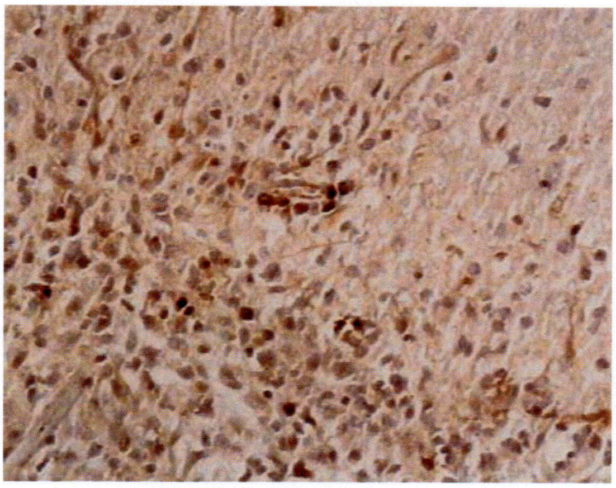

Figure 2. BrdU immunochemical staining of transplanted NSCs(x400). NSCs were found in and around the grafted site and had the morphological characteristics of round, small-medium sized mononuclear cells, which appeared yellow or brown.

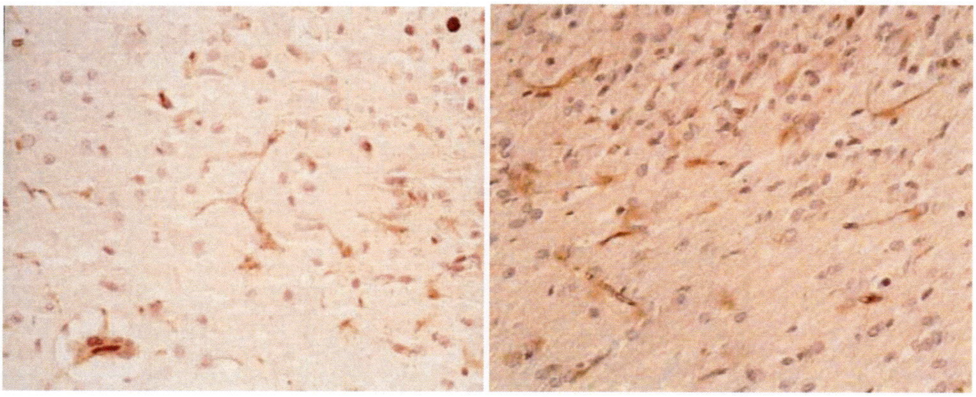

A. **B.**

Figure 3. Immunohistochemical staining of NSCs. (x400); A: Tubulin(+) immunochemical staining; B: GFAP(+) immunochemical staining.

Brain sections were stained with hematoxylin and eosin(HandE). Pink shrunken neurons could be observed in the injured cortex. The brain injured group showed significant neuronal loss compared with uninjured controls. Brain-injured animals that had received NSCs transplants had significantly more surviving pyramidal cells compared with the vehicle-treated brain-injured rats.

An in situ TUNEL assay demonstrated intense nuclear staining of apoptotic cells, which showed less nuclear staining in the treatment group than in the control group (figure 4).

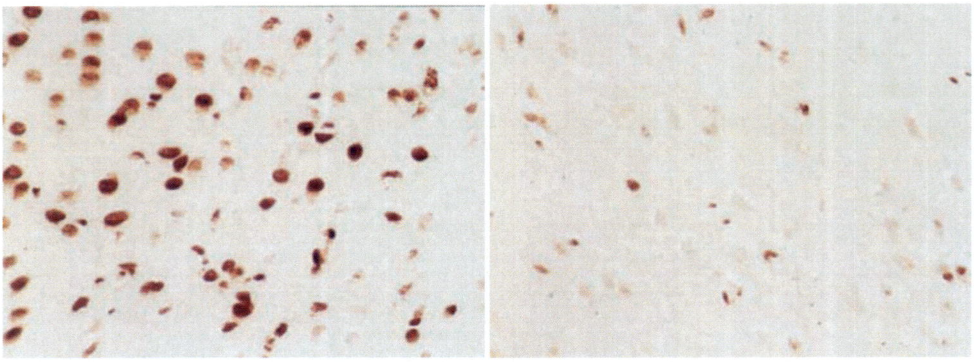

A. B.

Figure 4. TUNEL assay of injured brain. (x400); A: Control group; B: Treatment group; There is less nuclear staining of apoptosis cells in the treatment group.

Discussion

NSCs are defined as undifferentiated cells possessing both the capacity for self-renewal which extends throughout their adult life, and the ability to generate a wide variety of differentiated progeny such as neurons and astrocytes. Their division is asymmetric, one daughter being a stem cell which retains the potential to proliferate, while the other is a progenitor cell which produces terminally differentiated neural cells through a limited proliferation. Reynolds and Gage isolated similar multipotent cells from both striatum and hippocampi. Although the precise location of the CNS stem cells is not known, we do know that they are present in the hippocampi, the striatum and the ventricular zone in both the embryonic and adult brain. Stem cell therapy is the new strategy to treat a variety of diseases. NSCs have many useful properties, such as potential for normal reintegration into host cytoarchitecture and circuitry, the ability to migrate, and the ability to carry multiple transgenes [7,8,15,20,21].

It is difficult to survive in the hostile environment of the acutely injured cortex, where many of the cellular and molecular components responsible for secondary brain injury are most highly expressed. By 24 hours after experimental TBI, a marked increase in extracellular excitatory amino acids, calcium, free radicals, and cytokines, as well as recruited inflammatory cells, renders the transplantation milieu highly cytotoxic. Reactive astrocytes and activated microglia line the injury cavity and can be found throughout the subcortical white matter tracts and ipsilateral hippocampus, and these cells produce cytokine molecules, which further exacerbates blood-brain-barrier disruption and proinflammatory effects. In one study, the dissociation of fetal cells prior to transplantation resulted in uniform failure of all transplants [22-24].

Studies demonstrating survival and appropriate migration of Purkinje cells transplanted into adult animals lacking normal Purkinje cells also suggest that a window may exist during which an organism may permit ingrowth of fibers or cells that are attempting to replace a missing cell type [25]. Some work in TBI demonstrated expression of the embryonic intermediate filament protein nestin, as well as the cellular repair protein cyclin D1 after TBI. Therefore the lesioned CNS may well provide a microenvironment similar to embryonic life [26-28].

The fate of stem cells in vivo is heavily influenced by contextual cues, and stem cells retain the capacity to respond to local epigenetic signals. Our result showed NSCs could differentiate into neurons and astrocytes in cortical tissue. Several factors known to induce neuronal progenitors to differentiate are also expressed in injured brain. For example, levels of FGF-2 expression increase during early stages after injury in rodent brain, and this polypeptide growth factor also has shown to promote self-renewal in vitro of NSCs derived from the neuroepithelium of the developing cortex, and the adult subventricular zone. Other neurotrophic factors for which NSCs express receptors, such as nerve growth factor, may facilitate their differentiation into neural cells lineages.

Our finding showed neurological motor function in brain-injured animals receiving fetal transplants was significantly improved compared with control animals. Functional benefit obtained from CNS transplantation may be due to two different mechanisms, one from functional integration of transplanted tissue into the neural circuitry and secondly from the production of trophic factor, cytokines, and other neuroprotective factors.

Neuronal regeneration may fail to occur in the adult brain because of a tonic inhibition and/or a lack of postmitotic trophic and migratory support rather than because of a lack of precursor cells. Factors that inhibit neuronal regeneration have been identified within the CNS, and it is likely that the balance between neurotropic and inhibitory factors determines the extent of neural regeneration. Thus transplantation of NSCs into brain may alter the balance toward regeneration. During the last two decades, it has been suggested that CNS transplantation also induces a neuroprotective effect by means of specific trophic factors and by other mechanisms such as modification of ionic milieu, remyelination, and the glial transfer of sodium channels to axons [29-31].

NSCs could differentiate into GFAP(+) cells after injection into the cortex. In previous studies it has been demonstrated that grafted cells differentiated in vivo into a predominantly immature glial morphological cell type manifesting staining for GFAP. Previous transplant studies in which isolated astrocyte suspensions were used have demonstrated both neurobehavioral improvements and evidence of CNS regeneration in both acute and chronic neurodegenerative processes. Transplantation of juvenile astrocytes after postcommissural fornix transsection also resulted in significantly increased anterogradely labeled fibers at the lesion site, which is indicative of axonal regeneration. Whereas mature astrocytes appear to inhibit neurite outgrowth and neuronal regeneration, immature astrocytes do not seem to express these inhibitory molecules to the same extent, which may account for their neuroprotective and regeneration-promoting effects. Astrocytes may also serve as a source of trophic factors, and the molecular signals induced in TBI may specifically stimulate host astrocytes to produce trophic factors such as NGF. Other mechanisms underlying the beneficial effect of transplanted HiB5 may be related to the ability of astrocytes to remove extracellular excitotoxic amino acids, free radical, and excess cytopathic ions from the synaptic cleft [32-35].

Our results demonstrate the neuroprotective and behavioral efficacy of NSCs transplants after experimental traumatic brain injury. Being further studied in depth they may be useful vehicles for treating a variety of CNS disorders.

Acknowledgment

We are grateful to Mr. Philip Wrightson FRACS for his advice in preparing this paper for publication.

References

[1] Wictorin K, Brundin P, Sauer H, et al. Long distance directed axonal growth from human dopaminergic mesencephalic neuroblasts implanted along the nigrostriatal pathway in 6-hydroxydopamine lesioned adult rats. *J. Comp. Neural.* 32:475-494,1992

[2] Anderson DK, Reier PJ, Witth ED, et al. Delayed grafting of fatal CNS tissue into chronic compression lesions of the adult cat spinal cord. *Comp. Neural. Neurosci.* 2:309-325,1991

[3] JakemanLB, Reier PJ. Axonal projections between fetal spinal cord transplants and the adult rat spinal cord: a neuroanatomical tracing study of local interactions. *J. Comp. Neural.* 307:311-334,1991

[4] Soares HD, Hicks RR, Smith D, et al. Inflammatory leukocytic recruitment and diffuse neuronal degeneraion are separate pathological processes resulting from traumatic brain injury. *J. Neurosci.* 15:8223-8233,1995

[5] Reier PJ, Stokes BT, Thompson FJ, et al. Fetal cell grafts into resection and contusion /compression injuries of the rat and cats spinal cord. *Exp. Neurol.* 115:177-188,1992

[6] Soares H, McIntosh TK. Fetal cortical transplants in adult rats subjected to experimental brain injury. *J. Neural. Transplant Plast.* 2:207-220,1991

[7] Reynolds BA, Tetzlaff W, Weiss S. A multipotent EGF-responsive striatal embryonic progenitor cell produces neurons and astrocytes. *J. Neurosci.* 12:4565-4574, 1992.

[8] Reynolds BA, Weiss S. Generation of neurons and astrocytes from isolated cells of the adult mammalian central nervous system. *Science.* 255:1707-1710, 1992.

[9] Svendsen CN, Melanic G, Richard JE et al. A new method for the rapid and long term growth of human neural precursor cells. *J. Neurrosci. Methods.* 85:141-152, 1998.

[10] Svendsen CN, Fawcett JW, Bentlage C et al. Increased survival of rat EGF-generated CNS precursor cells using B27 supplemented medium. *Exp. Brain Res.* 102:407-414, 1995.

[11] Gritti A, Parati EA, Cova L et al. Multipotential stem cells from the adult mouse brain proliferate and self-renew in response to a basic fibroblast growth factor. *J. Neurosci.* 16:1091-1100, 1996.

[12] Carpenter MK, Cui X, Hu Z et al. In vitro expansion of a multipotent population of human neural progenitor cells. *Exp. Neurology.* 158:265-278, 1999.
[13] Johansson CB, Svensson M, Wallstedt L et al. Neural stem cells in the adult human brain. *Exp. Cell Res.* 253:733-736, 1999.
[14] Villa A, Snyder EY, Vesccovi A et al. Establishment and properties of a growth factor dependent, perpetual neural stem cell line from the human CNS. *Exp. Neurology.* 161:71-83, 1999.
[15] Gage FH, Coates PW, Palmer TD et al. Survival and differentiation of adult neuronal progenitor cells transplanted to the adult brain. *Proc. Natl. Acad. Sci. USA.* 92: 1179-1183, 1995.
[16] Rubio FJ, Bueno C, Villa A et al. Genetically perpetuated human neural stem cells engraft and differentiate into the adult mammalian brain. *Molecular and Cellular Neurosci.* 16:1-13, 2000.
[17] Marmarou A, Montasser A, Wimer B, et al. A new model of diffuse brain injury in rats. Part I: Pathophysiology and biomechanics. *J. Neurosurg.* 80:291-300,1994
[18] Montasser A, Marmarou A. A new model of diffuse brain injury in rats. Part II: Morphological characterization. *J. Neurosurg.* 80:301-313,1994
[19] Sinson G, Voddi M, McIntosh TK. Combined fetal neural transplantation and nerve growth factor infusion: effects in neurological outcome following fluid-percussion brain injury in the rat. *J. Neurodury.* 84:655-662,1996
[20] Weiss S, Reynolds BA, Vescovi AL et al. Is there a neural stem cell in the mammalian forebrain? *Trends Neurosci.* 19:387-93, 1996.
[21] Ourednik V, Ourednik J, Park KA et al. Neural stem cells - a versatile tool for replacement and gene therapy in the central nervous system. *Clin. Genet.* 56:267-78, 1999.
[22] McIntosh TK, Juhler M, Wieloch T, et al: Novel pharmacologic strategies in the treatment of experimental traumatic brain injuiry. *J. Neurotrauma.* 15: 731-769, 1998
[23] Hill SJ, Barbarese E, McIntosh TK. Regional heterogeneity in the response of astrocytes following traumatic brain injury in the adult rat. *J. Neuropathol. Exp. Neurol.* 55:1221-1229,1996
[24] Rothwell NJ, Strijbos PJ. Cytokines in neurodegeneration and repair. *Int. J. Dev. Neurosci.* 13:179-185,1995
[25] Sotelo C, Alvarado-Mallaart RM, Frain M, et al. Molecular plasticity of adult Bergmannn fibers is associated with radial migration of grafted Purkinje cells. *J. Neurosci.* 14:124-133,1994
[26] Kaya SS, Mahmood A, Li Y, et al. Apoptosis and expression of p53 response proteins and cyclin D1 after cortical impact in rat brain. *Brain Res.* 818:23-33,1999
[27] Kaya SS, Mahmood A, Li Y, et al. Expression of cell cycle proteins (cyclin D1 and cdk4) after controlled cortical impact in rat brain. *J. Neurotrama.* 16:1187-1196,1999
[28] Kaya SS, Mahmood A, Li Y, et al. Expression of nestin after traumatic brain injury in rat brain. *Brain Res.* 840:153-157,1999
[29] Fisher LJ, Gage FH: Grafting in the mammalian central nervous system. *Physiol. Rev.* 73: 583-615, 1993

[30] Reier PJ, Anderson DK, Thompson FJ, et al: Neural tissue transplantation and CNS trauma: anatomical and functional repair of the injurd spinal cord. *J. Neurotrauma.* 9: s223-s248,1992

[31] Stokes BT, Reier PJ. Oxygen transport in intraspinal fetal grafts-graft-host relations. *Exp. Neurro.* 111:312-323,1991

[32] Lundberg C, Martinez-Serrano A, Cattaneo E, et al. Survival, integration, and differentiation of neural stem cell lines after transplantation to the adult rat striatum. *Exp.Neurol.* 145:342-360,1997

[33] Bradbury EJ, Kershaw TR, Marchbanks RM, et al. Astrocyte transplants alleviate lesion induced memory deficits independently of cholinergic recovery. *Neuroscience.* 65:955-972,1995

[34] Kesslak JP, Walencewicz A, Calin L, et al. Hippocampal but not astrocyte transplants enhance recovery on a forced choice alternation task after kainate lesions. *Brain Res.* 454:347-354,1988

[35] Wunderlich G, Stichel CC, Schroeder WO, et al. Transplants of immature astrocytes promote axonal regeneraion in the adult rat brain. *Glia.* 10:49-58,1994

In: Brain Mapping Research Progress
Editors: Ines C. Girard and Jade S. Andre

ISBN: 978-1-60456-784-7

Chapter V

Subdural Interictal EEG Analysis for Extracting Discriminating Features towards Electrode Classification Using Artificial Neural Networks

Mercedes Cabrerizo [*] [1], ***Malek Adjouadi*** [1], ***Melvin Ayala*** [1] ***and Prasanna Jayakar*** [2]

[1] Department of Electrical & Computer Engineering, Florida International University, 10555 West Flagler Street, Miami FL 33174, USA.

[2] Brain Institute, Miami Children's Hospital, 3100 S.W. 62nd Avenue, Miami, Fl 33155

Abstract

This study introduces an algorithm dedicated at discriminating between electrodes that lead to a seizure onset from those electrodes that do not, using interictal subdural EEG data. The significance of this study is in classifying among all of these channels, all containing interictal spikes that are asynchronous and independent of location, which are selected randomly, those channels that lead to seizure from those that do not with the purpose of focusing the attention on those electrodes during epileptogenic focus localization. The main epileptogenic focus is supposed to evolve from the tissue located at the channels that present interictal activity, but sometimes this is no the case. The purpose is to gain a better understanding of the dynamics of subdural EEG, while characterizing the common behaviors of interictal EEG channels prior to an ictal activity. The merits of this algorithm are: (a) its fast computational time and (b) its integrated signal processing design that identifies based on different parameters, electrodes leading or not to seizure. EEG signals were transformed into quantitative measures to account for

[*] Emails: cabreriz@fiu.edu, adjouadi@fiu.edu, ayalam@fiu.edu

those morphological characteristics of interictal signals deemed important in the classification process of channels leading or not to a seizure.

Keywords: Ictal activity, Interictal spike, Signal processing, and Epileptogenic focus

1. Introduction

Epilepsy surgery is now being increasingly performed in children. Seizures are related to a malformed pathologic substrate that is more extensive than the lesion evident on MRI scans. Pre-surgical evaluation is therefore more difficult than in adults and relies heavily on EEG data including interictal spike discharges (Blume et al. 2001; Glover et al. 1989). The EEG interictal data recorded inside the brain can be processed to define similar patterns evident in those electrodes that lead to a given seizure to further facilitate surgical planning (Greenstein et al. 2000).

This study provides a mathematical framework for the study of interictal EEG leading or not to an epileptic seizure. The EEG of epileptic subjects can be divided into two main categories, interictal and ictal. The interictal EEG is the EEG signal recorded when the patient is not having seizures or in between seizures (Gotman 1985; Martini 2001). Interictal activity is characterized by the presence of interictal spikes and it is considered to be abnormal if it can occur in a patient with epilepsy in the absence of an actual seizure. The ictal EEG activity on the other hand is when the actual seizure occurs.

The study of this application elicits how different patients react prior to a seizure in view of the collected EEG data such as to better localize such neurological disorders. The main objectives of this study are as follows: (1) to extract features that best characterize those EEG electrodes that lead to an ictal activity; (2) to establish mathematical derivations that provide not only quantitative measures, but also describes and locates the focus of an ictal activity;(3) to identify and formulate those patterns in EEG recordings that are inherent to those electrodes that lead to a seizure; (4) to correlate the clinical features with the EEG findings in order to determine whether the patient has a consistent source of ictal activity, which is coming from the location concerning the group of channels that present interictal activity; (5) to classify and to group those EEG channels that are known in advance to lead to seizures in order to extract similarities in their behavior, in order to find a common behavioral pattern; (6) to find a suitable classifier that discriminates in the feature space the two regions of electrodes leading and not leading to an ictal state .

The significance of identifying electrodes that lead or don't to seizure relies in allowing the physicians to take a closer look at those electrodes that are identified as leading to seizure in advance so as to better localize the epileptogenic focus.

2. Methods

2.1. Participants

Eight children from 2 to 15 years old with medical refractory partial seizures that underwent pre-surgical evaluation have been analyzed in this study. The epileptic patients recorded were inpatients at the hospital for long-term EEG monitoring. EEG data sets in this study were selected randomly, and contained or may not contain interictal spikes. The EEG data segments varied in their length, with a minimum duration of 20 seconds. Each interictal EEG segment was visually inspected to avoid artifact in the data.

2.2. Recording System

The subdural EEG data was recorded using XLTEK Neuroworks Ver.3.0.5 (equipment manufactured by Excel Tech Ltd. Ontario, Canada). The EEG data was obtained using a sampling rate (sampling frequency) of 500 Hz. A bandpass filter with cut-off frequencies of 0.1 and 70 Hz was used to record the EEG data as well as 12 bits A/D conversion rate.

2.3. Algorithm Development Process

To classify the electrodes, a program was developed in order to quantify the patterns that are inherent to each class of electrode. Input data in this study was subdural EEG segments from 20 to 3600 seconds of duration of epileptic patients. The first step in the procedure involved identifying the pertinent electrodes in the overall interictal EEG recordings in which the seizures occurred. The physicians performed this task initially through visual inspection of the recorded data. A computer program was earlier (Adjouadi et al. 2005; Adjouadi et al. 2004; Adjouadi et al. 2006 and Ayala et al. 2004) developed in order to detect automatically interictal spikes so as to provide more accurate and consistent input data to the proposed classification algorithm. Then, after the input EEG data was selected, the subsequent algorithm to categorize the two classes of electrodes was conducted, as depicted in figure 1.

The classification algorithm consists of the following steps:

Step 1- Filtering the Input EEG Data

The EEG data is first decomposed into signal and noise subspaces using Singular Value Decomposition (SVD). This allows removing the noise in order to extract the dominant EEG patterns.

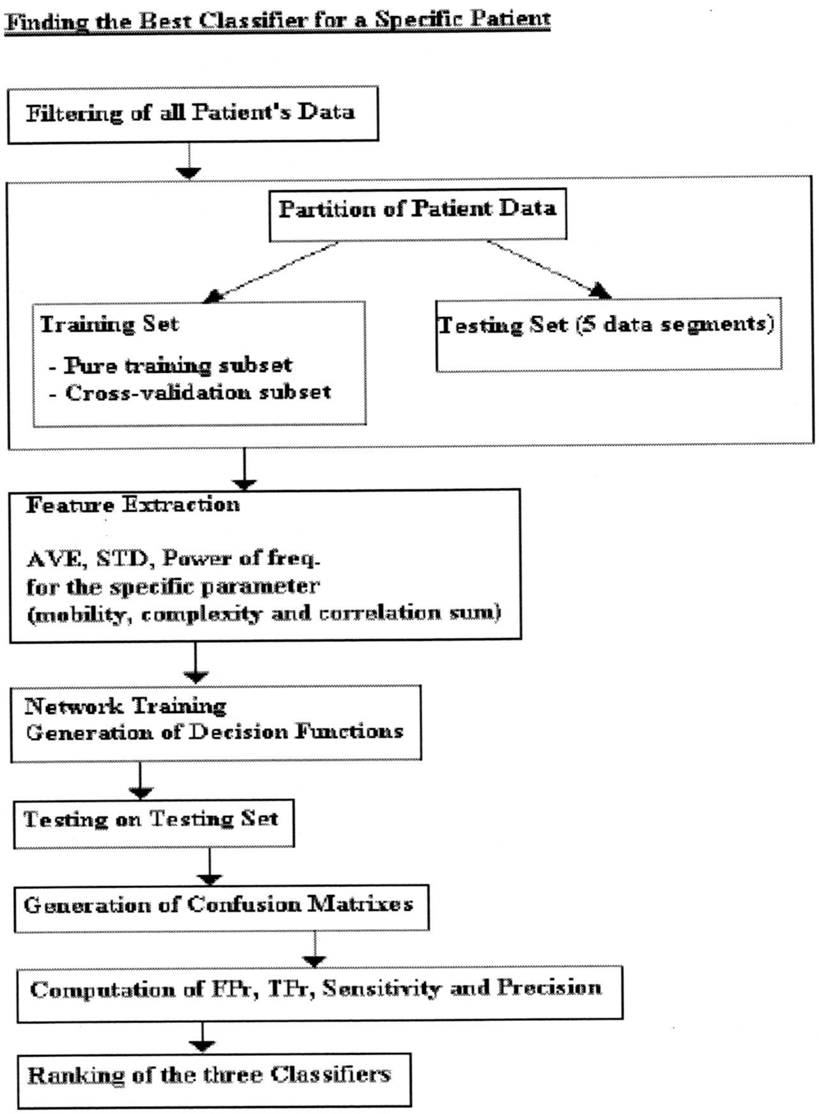

Figure 1. Flow chart describing the basic steps for finding the best classifier for a specific patient.

As illustrated in figure 2, there is a fairly rapid drop over the first few SVD components (the significant ones), and the remaining ones approach zero more slowly (the ones in the noise range).

When EEG is digitally recorded, it is possible to represent it in a matrix form. In this case the input EEG data matrix M, whose columns correspond to the electrodes and whose rows to the time samples, is decomposed into three different matrices as follows:

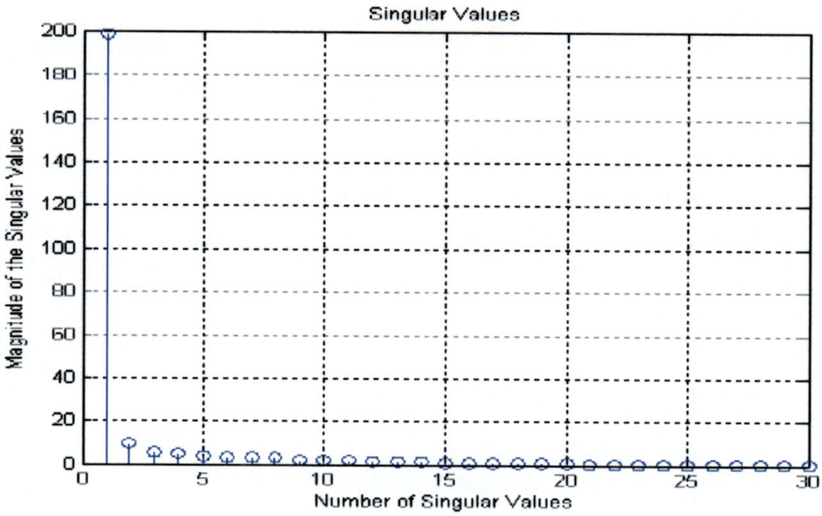

Figure 2. Singular values of an EEG data segment, sorted in decreasing order.

$$M = USV^T \quad (1)$$

with $S = diag(\sigma_i)$. Matrices U and V are orthogonal and S is a diagonal matrix containing singular values in descending order as its elements (Adjouadi et al. 2005; Cabrerizo et al. 2005).

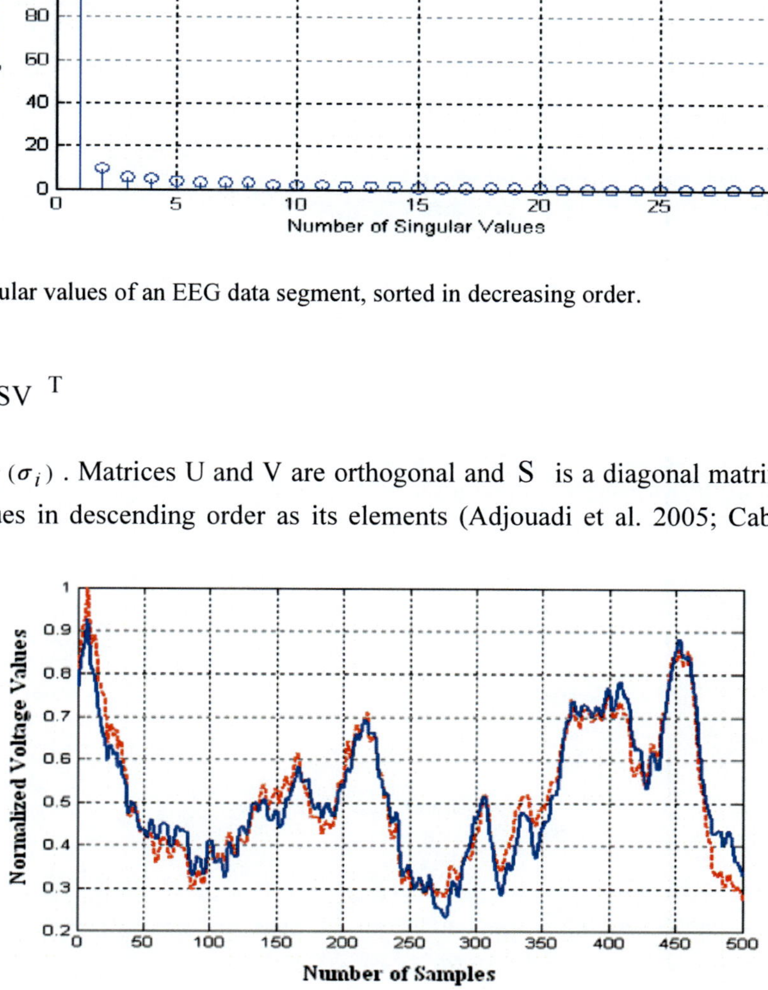

Figure 3. SVD decomposition applied to the EEG signal (original signal is shown in red and the resulting signal after filtering is shown in blue).

From the diagonal matrix S , the larger singular values were retained (in this case the first five were deemed sufficient for the analysis), so a better approximation is obtained, or equivalently, more information is contained in that approximation and the other values are set to zero, thus a new matrix S was created. Instead of using the whole input matrix, only the columns of matrix U , rows of matrix V^T and the new matrix S corresponding to the quality of approximation are used to reconstruct the original input matrix using equation 1. An example is shown in figure 3. The approximated matrix M, containing less noise was used in the subsequent steps. This implementation concluded the filtering preprocessing step.

Step 2- Extraction of Features from the EEG Data

Although there is a variety of parameters that can be used to represent the dynamics of the brain activity, many of them have failed in being suitable for electrode analysis, such as the activity parameter, Lyapunov exponent, coherence, auto correlation, among others (Tito et al. 2007). Therefore the investigation focused on three key measures: correlation sum, EEG mobility and EEG complexity.

The discerning of brain activity, in particular EEG events such as interictal spikes lies on the characterization of the dynamics of the neural activities (Popescu 1998; Gevins et al. 1987 and Birkemeier et al. 1978). The theory of non-linear dynamics provides a frame of digital signal analysis techniques, which may give new information on the behavior of such activities. Since brain dynamics are nonlinear, this study investigated methods such as the calculation of correlation sum, mobility and complexity.

The correlation sum $R(r)$ is given in equation (2) and measures the spatial organization, where the space is occupied by a set of random points. It determines the degree of complexity in the EEG signal.

$$R(r) = \frac{2}{N(N-1)} \sum_{j=1}^{N-1} \sum_{i=j+1}^{N-1} \theta\left(r - \left|X_i - X_j\right|\right) \tag{2}$$

where, r is the threshold value used to evaluate the similarity between two reconstructed vectors X_i and X_j. This threshold could represent 1 or 2 standard deviation of the original EEG signal. N is the total number of points in the time series. The vector X_i is a point in the embedded phase constructed from the input EEG signal $y = (y_1, y_2, \ldots)$ as a single time series according to:

$$X_i = \left(y_i, y_i + \tau, y_i + 2\tau, \ldots. y_i + (m-1)\tau\right),$$

where m is the so called embedding dimension and τ is a time delay. The counting of the distances between the chosen points in the phase space is symbolized by the so called Heaviside unit step function $\theta(x)$, where $\theta(x) = 0$ for $x \leq 0$, and $\theta(x) = 1$ for $x > 0$. The correlation sum averages the probability of measuring a distance smaller than r between two randomly chosen points X_i and X_j.

Additionally, the Hjorth's parameters, mobility and complexity were calculated using equations 3 and 4.

Mobility (equation 3) gives a measure of deviation of the voltage changes with respect to deviation of the EEG voltage amplitude, while complexity (equation 4) provides a measure of excessive details with regard to the slightest possible signal's shape (Proakis et al. 1996 and Gonzalez et al. 1993). The mobility M(y) is computed using the following formula.

$$M(y) = \sqrt{\sigma(y') / \sigma(y)} \tag{3}$$

where σ is the variance and y' is the first derivative of the primary signal y. The complexity $C(y)$ involves the first derivative $M(y')$ of the mobility and the mobility M(y) of the signal itself and is expressed as:

$$C(y) = \sqrt{M(y')/M(y)} \tag{4}$$

All these three parameters were computed for each electrode separately using successive epochs or non-overlapping windows of 1 second for all the recorded subdural EEG data. By doing this, a behavior for each parameter over time was established for each electrode (Le Van Quen et al. 2001 and Yaylali et al. 1996).

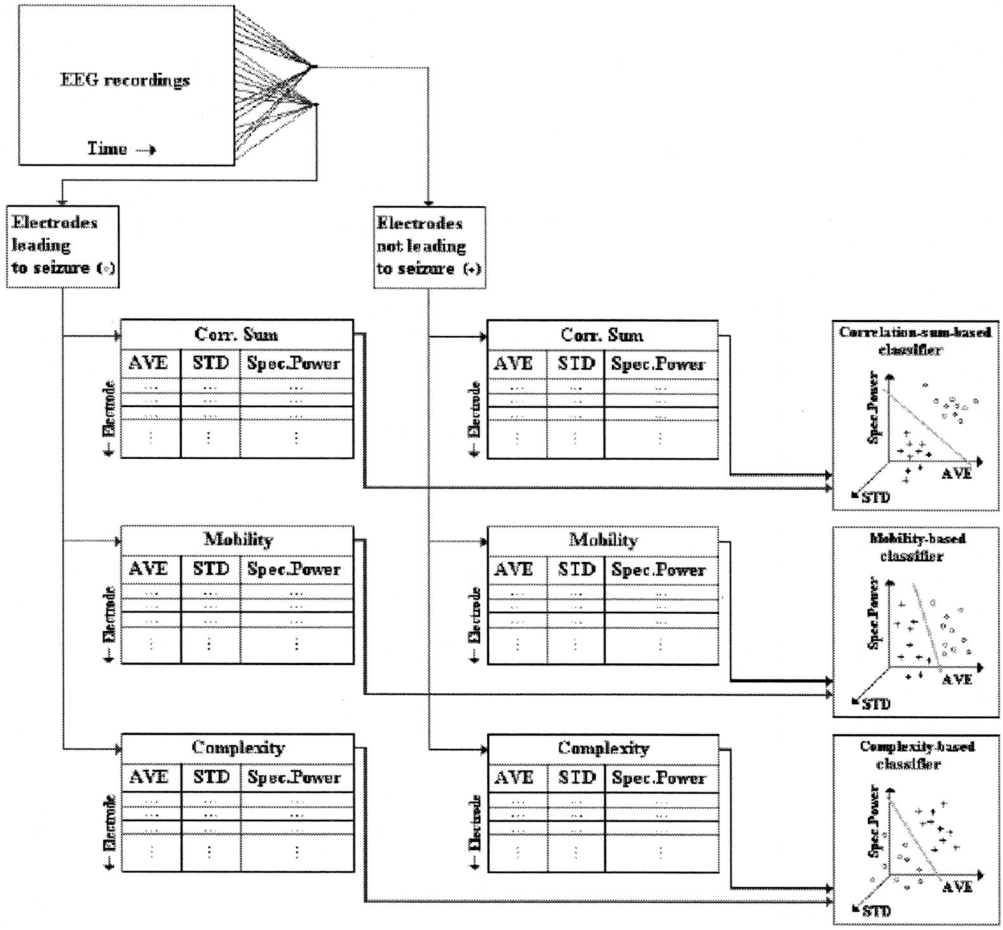

Figure 4. Process of feature extraction in detail. Note how the influence of time has been removed in the dot-plot representation of the parameters.

To make the classifier independent on the number of time windows of the EEG data segments, the parameters (correlation sum, complexity and mobility) of each electrode were aggregated into the following three features:

The electrode average (AVE) along time windows of 1 second each
The electrode standard deviation (STD) along time windows of 1 second each
The electrode spectral power along time windows of 1 second each.

This procedure was performed on the entire recording and done separately on the two groups of electrodes. Thus, for each one of the two groups of electrodes, three 3D data sets were extracted from the recordings, namely a 3D data set for the correlation sum, a 3D data set for the complexity, and another 3D data set for the mobility. The general process is illustrated in figure 4.

Step 3- Implementation of Regression Lines for Each Electrode and Parameter

As all the different parameters were represented in time, regression lines were generated in order to keep a suitable track of the behavior of each electrode with respect to the computed parameter. This also could help in determining a linear classifier that separates in the parameter vs. time space the two different classes of electrodes. One condition to make this study more relevant from a clinical point of view was to require from these two classes of electrodes to be totally independent in terms of source location, and synchronicity of the spike firing. After obtaining regression lines for all electrodes, two groups of regression lines per parameter were created. Regression lines provide for an easier way to track the changes that took place in the signals with respect to the parameters analyzed prior to and after an ictal state. The mathematics for a regression line is based on deriving the equation of line Y'. It is a linear approximation that simply consists of a line such that it approximates the data points with minimum cumulative error. For each point (x_i, y_i), approximation y_i' is given by $y_i' = \alpha + \beta x_i$, where $|y_i - y_i'|$ is the error in estimation, that yields a minimized error E given by $E = \sum_{i=1}^{n} (y_i - y_i')^2$. In these two equations, y_i is the value for the actual data point, and y_i' is its approximation in the y-axis. The values α and β are calculated as follows:

$$\alpha = \bar{y} - \beta \bar{x} \tag{5}$$

with,

$$\beta = \frac{\sum_{i=1}^{n} (x_i - \bar{x})(y_i - \bar{y})}{\sum_{i=1}^{n} (x_i - \bar{x})^2},$$

where $\bar{x} = \frac{1}{n}\sum_{i=1}^{n} x_i$ and $\bar{y} = \frac{1}{n}\sum_{i=1}^{n} y_i$ (6)

These computed linear approximations were used for each electrode to facilitate a 2D visualization of the overall trend of each electrode.

Step 4- Implementation of an Artificial Neural Network for Linear Classification

At this stage, a plot of the three selected features revealed well defined electrodes clusters. No other features produced class clusters so compact and separated from each other. But extrapolation of this mechanism of classification in time did not work as anticipated since the time dynamics of the parameters strongly changed from one recording to the other, despite visible class clustering. In a parameter vs. time plot, the separating points between the two electrode groups changed from one recording to another.

This is best illustrated in figure 5. Note that each plot is represented only for 20 seconds in two different segments of the EEG data.

In order to consider this relative change and yet make real classification possible, time independent analysis was performed by computing for each parameter three statistical features, namely the average (AVE) of the regression line that represents the feature behavior, the standard deviation (STD) of the parameter over time and the spectral power of the feature over time.

These statistical features were computed for each group of electrodes and then inputted to an artificial neural network (ANN) in order to obtain a linear classifier for each parameter. One reason for using ANNs as classifiers (instead of other types of discriminants) was their undisputable simplicity and versatility (Rosenblat 1958; Gurney 1997 and Haykin 1999). Another reason was the availability of a programming tool (Ayala et al., 2004) that was developed at FIU, which provides different settings to enable a cross-validation technique. This technique was setup during training so as to avoid memorization of the network. One linear decision function was created exclusively for each of the three parameters (correlation sum, mobility, and complexity) to classify the electrodes. These specific decision functions would find the optimum separating plane between the two classes of electrodes in a 3D space where the axis are represented by the statistical features used (AVE, STD, and spectral power).

Establishing an artificial neural network (ANN) that is trained to extract seizure-leading features of interictal EEG is a significance outcome, since this ANN

1) can help to overcome the subjective factor associated with human classification;
2) can serve as a second expert for decision process validation; and
3) can be used for fast automated seizure leading channels detection, even for on-line recordings, sparing EEG technicians the tedious task of long-term monitoring.

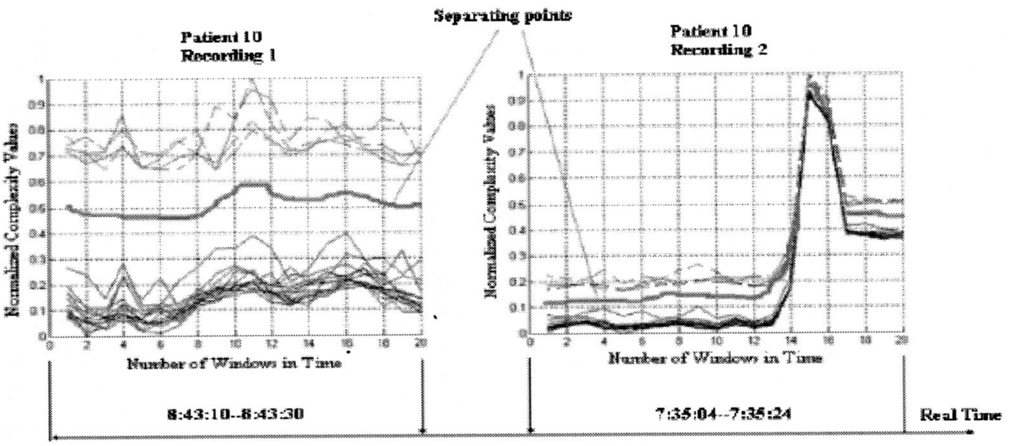

Note: Starting end ending recording times are displayed at the bottom of the two plots.

Figure 5. Electrode clusters changing their relative location in the feature vs. time plot.

The classifiers for each patient are three decision functions of the form:

$$f_{\xi}(\underline{X}) = w_1 \cdot \mu_{\xi}(\underline{X}) + w_2 \cdot \sigma_{\xi}(\underline{X}) + w_3 \cdot \Phi_{\xi}(\underline{X}) + w_4 \qquad (7)$$

The subscript ξ is defined as follows:

$$\xi = \begin{cases} R & for\ Correlation\ Sum \\ M & for\ Mobility \\ C & for\ Complexity \end{cases}$$

In (7), $\underline{X}$ is a vector containing the values of the specific parameter (correlation sum, complexity, or mobility) computed from non overlapping windows of 500 samples; w_1, w_2, w_3, and w_4 are coefficients and $\mu(\underline{X})$, $\sigma(\underline{X})$, and $\phi(\underline{X})$ are the mean, the standard deviation, and the spectral power of vector $\underline{X}$, respectively.. Electrodes are classified as leading to seizure only if $f_{\xi}(\underline{X}) > 0$ for a specific parameter.

Note how the influence of time has been removed from consideration. This allows classifying electrodes regardless of the time the features were extracted and in which sequence they were used.

The decision functions are feed-forward multilayer perceptrons consisting of 3 input neurons and one output neuron (see figure 6) with linear activation functions. The inputs correspond to the mean, standard deviation, and spectral power (μ,σ,Φ) of the parameter analyzed for a given channel. Training targets are 1 and -1, indicating if the channel leads to seizure or not, respectively. The networks were trained via backpropagation. This type of structure produces a linear classifier (Iasemidis et al. 1994).

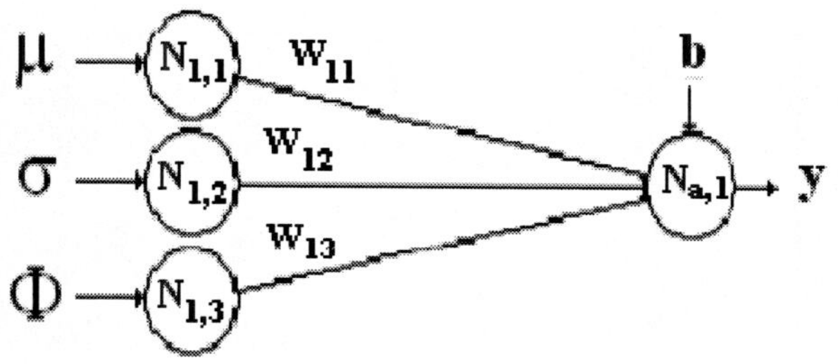

Figure 6. Neural network topology used to create the classifiers.

In order to avoid network memorization, training was performed on a randomly selected recording (data segment #1) of a patient with electrodes properly labeled as leading to seizure or not, while the remaining recordings were kept for testing purposes. The data segment #1 used for training was subsequently partitioned into pure training (66%) and testing (34%) patterns so as to perform cross-validation during network training.

The backpropagation algorithm is an optimization technique based on the gradient descent method in which the aim is to minimize the square error between outputs and targets. The algorithm is called backpropagation because the errors are backpropagated from the last layer back to the first one in order to compute a new (better) set of weights. This operation is done several times on the data base containing the training patterns until a stop condition is found. The influence a neuron output has to the total net error is obtained by using the chain rule from that neuron to the next layer (Hellman 1999; Tarasenko et al. 1998 and Ko et al. 2000).

Step 5- Selection of the Best Classifiers

Once all three classifiers were trained, they were tested in the remaining data segments of each patient and confusion matrixes were obtained in order to achieve the over-all performance of the classifiers across each patient.

To evaluate the performance of the classifiers, tests were conducted on unknown data (data not used for training), but from which it was known which electrodes lead to seizure and which did not.

The disagreements between the actual classification and the predicted classification are presented in confusion matrixes as illustrated in table 1.

Table 1. Confusion matrix and related terms

		Detected as	
		Not leading	Leading
Actual	Not leading	TN	FP
	Leading	FN	TP

where TN, FP, FN, and TP stand for True Negative, False Positive, False Negative, and True Positive, respectively. For evaluation purposes, the following measures were further computed: the False Positive rate (FPr) and the False Negative rate (FNr). The False Positive rate (also called False Positive fraction) is the proportion of the false positive counts to the negative instances (all electrodes actually not leading to seizure, i.e. TN + FP). Conversely, the False Negative rate (also called False Negative fraction) is the proportion of the false negative counts to the positive instances (all electrodes actually leading to seizure, i.e. FN + TP). The definitions are given in Eq. 8 and 9.

$$FP_r = \frac{FP}{FP + TN} \tag{8}$$

$$FN_r = \frac{FN}{FN + TP} \tag{9}$$

Once the performance of all classifiers across all patients was computed, they were tabulated and further analyzed in order to make assessments about their performance within and between patients. Results obtained are revealed in the next section in order to assess both the validity of the steps so far described and the merit of each step for identifying suitable linear classifiers.

3. Results

3.1. Detailed Results for Patient #1

To gain a better understanding of how the classifiers for a given patient were generated, this section describes the procedure followed for a specific patient (patient #1), which was then repeated across the remaining patients.

Table 2. Weights of the decision functions for each parameter of patient #1

Function	W1	W2	W3	W4
Correlation Sum	13.444123	-1.969053	-2.520771	-0.278356
Mobility	5.782254	7.892331	-3.078757	-1.812404
Complexity	6.819882	8.265253	-3.536731	-1.962363

Patient #1 is used here because it presented a lot of overlapping.

The three classifiers (correlation sum, mobility and complexity) for patient #1 were first trained using cross-validation on the segment #1.

The optimum set of weights that was found after training is shown in table 2 and was then used to test the classifiers on the remaining data segments.

Applying ROC analysis, the performance of the classifiers obtained for each parameter of patient #1 was used for illustrative purposes following these steps:

A complete intra-patient analysis

Training of each classifier for a base segment and testing on the rest of the segments.

Generation of confusion matrices for each file, as well as calculation of the FP and FN rates for each time window.

As an example, table 3 illustrated above shows the complexity-based classifier for this particular patient performed on each one of the data segments during training (segment #1) and testing (remaining segments).

Table 3. Confusion matrices for all EEG segments of worst case scenario (Patient #1) based on complexity. Values are given for False Negative rate (FNr) and False Positive rate (FPr)

Data Segment		Detected -	Detected +	FNr	*FPr*
1 (base)				14.3	*14.3*
	Actual -	6	1		
	Actual +	1	6		
2				42.9	*14.3*
	Actual -	6	1		
	Actual +	3	4		
3				57.1	*0.0*
	Actual -	7	0		
	Actual +	4	3		
4				14.3	*0.0*
	Actual -	2	0		
	Actual +	1	6		
5				14.3	*71.4*
	Actual -	2	5		
	Actual +	1	6		
6				14.3	*71.4*
	Actual -	2	5		
	Actual +	*1*	*6*		

3.2. Compilation of Results for All Cases

Table 4 shows the results obtained for testing the 24 classifiers (three classifiers for each patient) on randomly selected EEG segments for all patients. The results are expressed in terms of the rate of missed detections (FNr) as well as the rate of incorrect positive detections (FPr).

Table 4. Performance of the three classifiers for all patients

PATIENT	Correlation Sum (%)		Mobility (%)		Complexity (%)	
	FNr	FPr	FNr	FPr	FNr	FPr
Patient 1	40.7	0.0	14.3	12.9	14.3	0.0
Patient 2	37.5	0.0	20.0	0.0	0.0	0.0
Patient 3	0.0	8.2	0.0	0.0	0.0	0.0
Patient 4	33.3	0.0	0.0	0.0	0.0	0.0
Patient 5	0.0	5.0	0.0	0.0	0.0	0.0
Patient 6	28.6	0.0	14.3	0.0	14.3	0.0
Patient 7	42.8	0.0	28.6	0.0	14.3	0.0
Patient 8	42.8	5.0	14.3	0.0	0.0	0.0
AVE	28.2	2.3	11.4	1.6	5.4	0.0
STD	18.1	3.3	10.6	4.6	7.4	0.0

In order to compare how well the different classifiers performed, dot-plots were generated (figure 7) that show the statistics (AVE and STD) of the false detection rates (FNr and FPr) of each classifier across all patients).

In assessing the examples treated before, the complexity-based classifier produced the most consistent and reliable results across all 8 patients included in the study. As it can be observed from figure 7, the lowest AVE and STD across all patients are obtained for this classifier. It was therefore concluded that, for the data given in this study, this parameter was the most suitable one for electrode classification.

The total number of electrodes that presented interictal activity was 75, out of which 30 lead to seizure onset and 45 did lead to an ictal state.

The over-all evaluation of the complexity-based classifier in terms of precision, sensitivity and specificity is as follows:

$$Precision = \frac{TP}{TP + FP} = 94\% \quad (10)$$

$$Sensitivity = \frac{TP}{TP + FN} = 97\% \quad (11)$$

$$Specificity = \frac{TN}{TN + FP} = 96\% \quad (12)$$

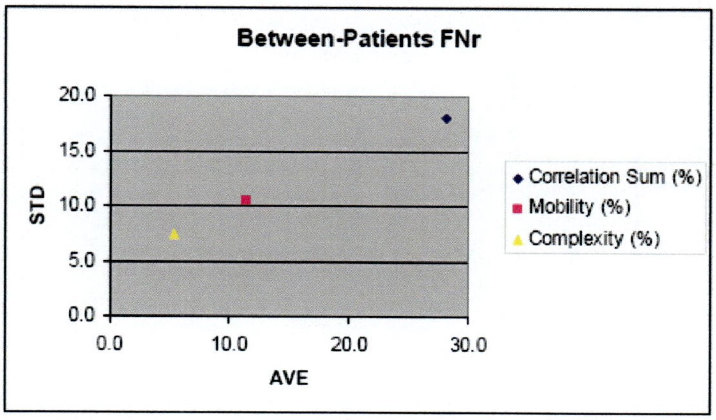

(a)

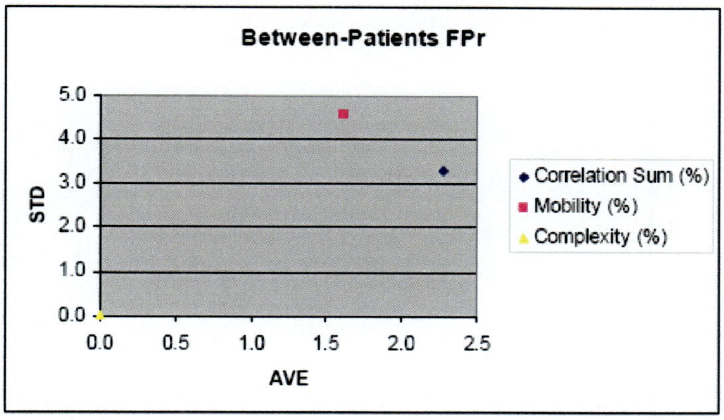

(b)

Figure 7. Dot-plot of the statistics of the performance of each classifier across all patients, based on the FNr (a) and FPr (b).

Examples of results using the complexity-based classifier are given in figures 8-12, with electrodes leading to seizure colored in red (lines or circles) and not leading to seizure colored in blue (lines or plus signs).

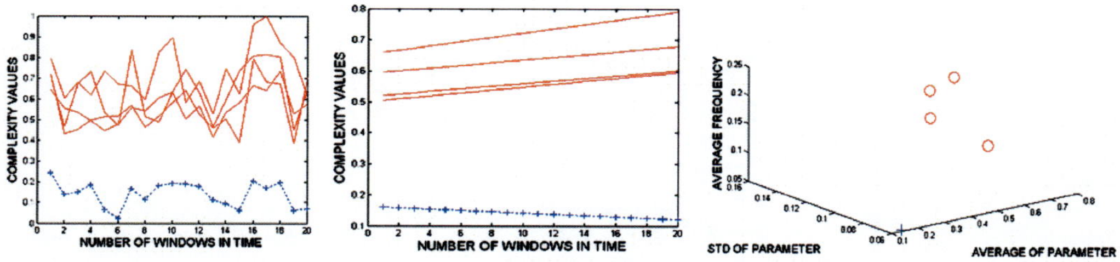

Figure 8. Values of complexity for patient 3.

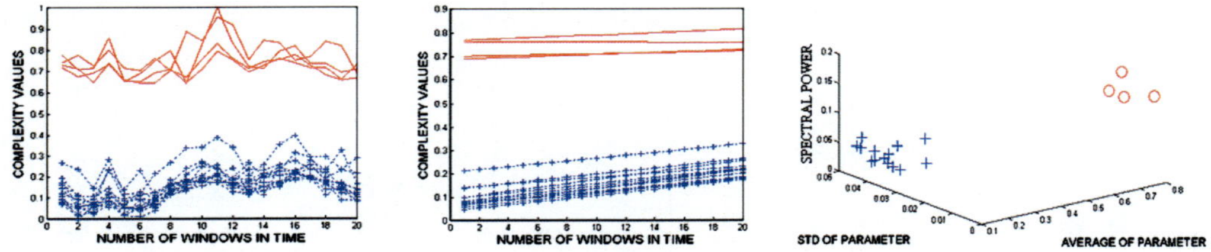

Figure 9. Values of complexity for patient 4.

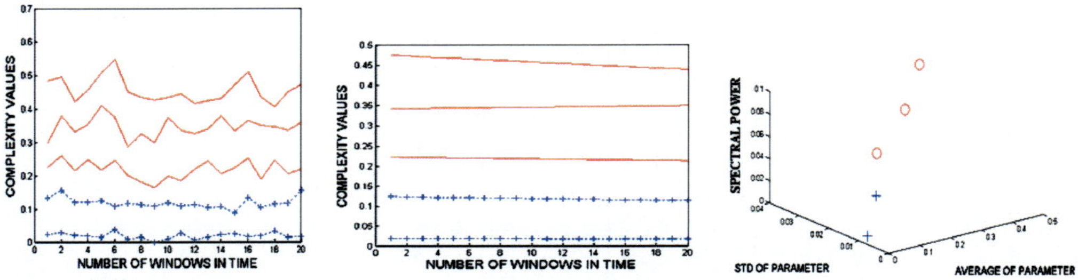

Figure 10. Values of complexity for patient 5.

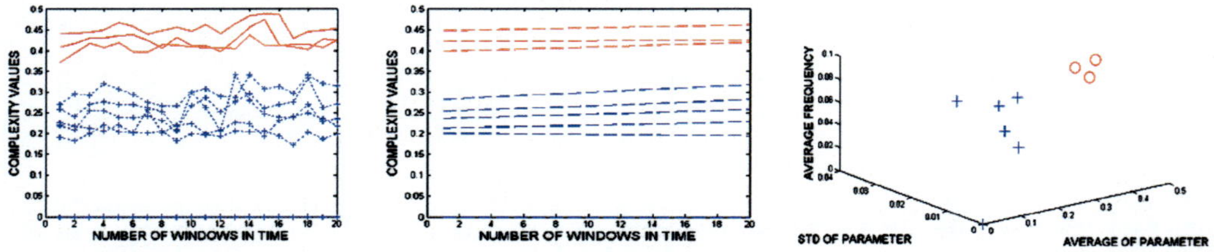

Figure 11. Values of complexity for patient 6.

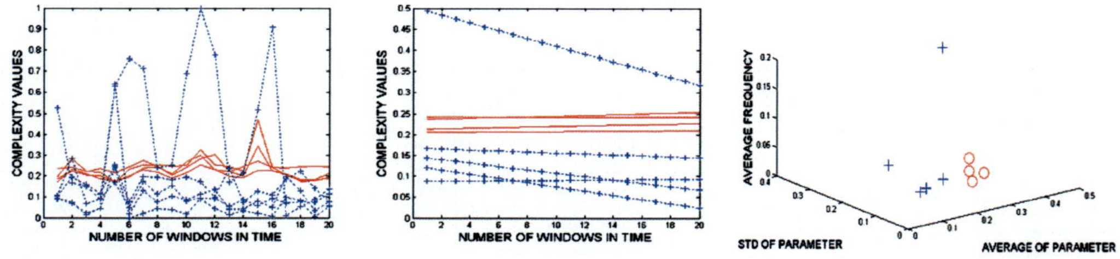

Figure 12. Values of complexity for patient 8.

Note that the three features (μ,σ,Φ) have great potential for classifying electrodes leading to seizure, regardless on what type of classifier was used with respect to the 3 parameters. However, the best separation is achieved for the complexity-based classifier as previously illustrated.

4. Discussion

Key findings can be affirmed as follows: (1) it was found that at any window of time along the EEG signal (independent of time), acceptable classifiers could be obtained using just the complexity values; (2) A search for such decision functions across patients is ineffectual, because experiments reveal that such decision functions are patient dependent; (3) It is extremely important that when one is to search for such decision functions, electrodes should be analyzed only if they are localized in different grids and with interictal spikes not happening simultaneously in all channels.

In assessing the examples treated before, the complexity parameter produces the most consistent and reliable results across all 8 patients included in the study. Nevertheless, a detailed example (figure 13) is provided for a long event consisting of one hour of EEG recording prior to a seizure to see how this parameter changes as we approach an ictal state.

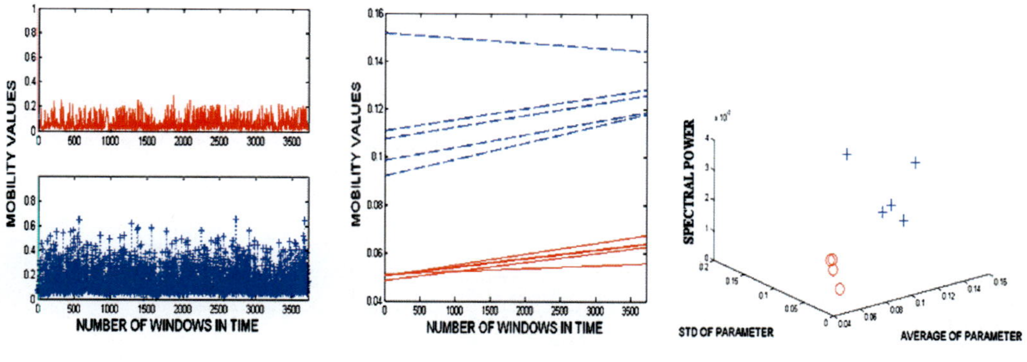

Figure 13. Values of Complexity for a long event (1 hour) for a patient selected at random.

For this particular example, we provided the behavior of the parameter in 2 distinct windows of time for visual appreciation. For each window of time, the behavior of the parameter itself is provided with respect to time as well as through regression line approximations corresponding to that behavior. The respective 3D plots with AVE, STD, and spectral power as x, y, z coordinates are given.

It can be observed, as illustrated in figure 13, in this long event of 1 hour, how the Complexity of the EEG signal can differentiate between the two groups of electrodes. Complexity remains the most reliable feature in this case. The regression lines corresponding to this parameter are separated in two well defined groups. Also correlation sum and mobility show similar distinctions.

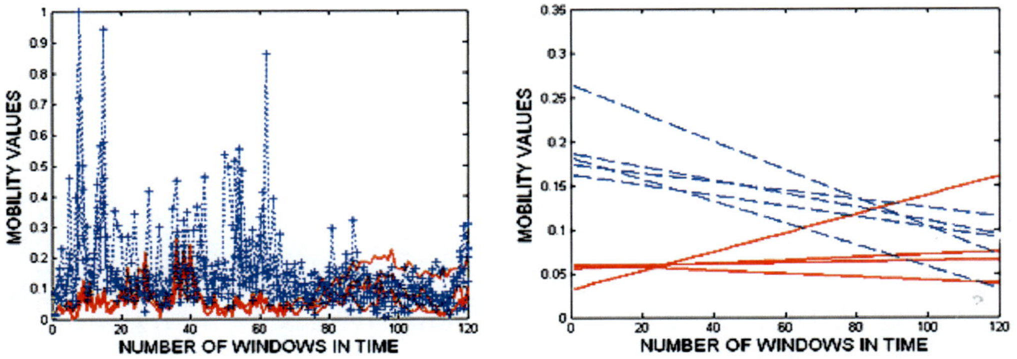

Figure 14. Values of Complexity two minutes before seizure onset for the patient displayed on figure 13. Note how the electrode behavior overlaps shortly before seizure.

As time approaches the onset of the seizure (see figure 14), the trend of the behavior of the measured parameter through time becomes similar for the two classes of electrodes. In other words, just prior to the seizure, the regression lines of the two groups of electrodes converge into one group; there is no clear separation between them. It can be observed in the Complexity plots that 60 seconds prior to the onset of the seizure, the behavior of this parameter becomes the same for all electrodes. The regression line approximations for these signals also show how the two groups (red and blue) converge prior to the onset.

Table 5. Lower ⇓ or higher ⇑ values of the leading to seizure with respect to the not leading to seizure channels

Patient	Mobility (M)	Complexity (C)	Correlation (R)
1	⇑	⇑	⇓
2	⇑	⇑	⇓
3	⇓	⇓	⇑
4	⇑	⇑	⇓
5	⇑	⇑	⇓
6	⇑	⇑	⇓
7	⇓	⇓	⇑
8	⇓	⇑	⇑

Table 5 provides a summary of the results for of all the patients. The arrows indicate for a given parameter whether the values of the red group of electrodes are higher or lower with respect to the blue group of electrodes. As it can be observed, for 5 patients out of 8, the complexity values for those electrodes that lead to an ictal state are higher than the values of those electrodes that do not lead to seizure. Also, the mobility values for these five patients behave in the same manner. Two patients behave in a similar fashion, and their complexity and mobility values are reversed if we compare them with the other five patients.

A closer look at this table reveals the following conditions: If we assign a negative sign (-) to ⇓ and a sign (+) to⇑, then the following relations hold:

$$\begin{aligned} C * R &< 0 \\ M * R &< 0 \\ M * C &> 0 \end{aligned} \tag{13}$$

5. Conclusion

Surgical treatment is being used with increasing frequency for patients with intractable epilepsy. Operative success depends to a large degree on the results of a comprehensive pre-operative patient evaluation, the main purpose of which is to delineate the epileptogenic lesion. The likelihood of the success of surgery is increased when all test results point to a single epileptogenic focus (Eberhard et al. 1990). The unique contribution of this study is that it proves that electrodes can be categorized prior or after the seizures. Thus, focusing the attention on specific electrodes can be very beneficial for epileptogenic focus localization. It will also help to better understand the characteristics of the different interictal epileptiform activities. In all of these performance values of the 3 parameters implemented, it can be said that the results obtained show great promise in delineating electrodes that lead to seizure from those that do not. It is fitting to note that when our results failed to discriminate between these two sets of electrodes, a clinical analysis revealed that those electrodes were indeed situated in the same grid (region) and their interictal spikes were happening simultaneously in all channels. As this study will involve a higher number of patients as they become available, additional results will provide more credence to our findings.

Given the complex nature of EEG recordings, these results, which are supported by clinical experimentation, are most encouraging considering that the patterns applied were computed using data segments of the interictal EEG data irrespective of time and relative position to the onset of a seizure. The integrated algorithm proposed is computationally efficient, fully automated, and designed in a unique way for the extraction of discriminating EEG features. These findings could help in the future to serve as potential predictors of seizure. The use of ictal EEG will likely enhance the precision of the results and add to the merit of this technique.

Through the extraction of parameters from the EEG and their statistical analysis, the influence of time has been completely removed from consideration. With EEG being a time series, it is considered a major accomplishment that these time-independent classifiers perform well in this study.

The results obtained reveal the following findings:

Mobility and complexity had an evident trend in their outcome since both were higher for those electrodes leading to seizure. This indicates that more sharp fluctuations are present in the EEG signals.

There were substantial but characterizing differences in the computed correlation sum parameter. This calculation varies among different patietns and different types of subdural interictal EEG data.

The integration of several parameters (correlation sum, mobility, and complexity) constitutes a unified method for assessing differences in the EEG channels that can lead us to classify in a suitable manner the two groups of electrodes.

It will be futile to search for decision functions that separate the two groups of electrodes across patients because experiments reveal that such decision functions are patient dependent;

It is important to know that when one is to search for such decision functions; all electrodes containing interictal activity should be analyzed only if they are placed in different grids inside the brain and with interictal spikes firing at different times.

In obtaining the aforementioned findings, the following actions played a decisive role:

The selection of key discriminating parameters (correlation sum, mobility, and complexity) used in the implementation.

The selection of unique features to optimize the delineation process of these two types of electrodes, and to get such decision functions.

The development of a back-propagated neural network that automated the decision making process for every patient independent of the others.

The establishment of mathematical functions that elicited the behavior of the key parameters.

Acknowledgements

The authors appreciate the support provided by the National Science Foundation under grants HRD-0317692, CNS-0426125, CNS-0520811, CNS-0540592 and IIS-0308155. The authors are also thankful for the clinical support provided through the Ware Foundation and the joint Neuro-Engineering Program with Miami Children's Hospital.

References

Blume W.T., Holloway G.M., and Wiebe S., Temporal epileptogenesis: localizing value of scalp and subdural interictal and ictal EEG data. *Epilepsia,* 42(4), pp.508-514, April, 2001.

Glover J. R., Raghavan N., Ktonas P.Y., and Frost J. D., Context-based automated detection of epileptogenic sharp transients in the EEG: Elimination of false positives, *IEEE Trans. on Biomedical Engineering,* vol. 36 (5), pp. 519 – 527, 1989.

Greenstein B., and Greenstein A., Color atlas of neuroscience, Neuroanatomy and Neurophysiology, Thieme Stuttgart, New York, 2000.

Gotman B., Practical use of computer-assisted EEG interpretation in epilepsy, *Clinical*

Neurophysiology, vol. 2(3), pp. 251 – 265, 1985.

Martini F. H., Fundamentals of anatomy & physiology, Fifth edition, New Jersey 07458, Prentice Hall, 2001.

Adjouadi M., Cabrerizo M., Ayala M., Jayakar P., Yaylali I., and Barreto A., A new approach to the analysis of epileptogenic data using statistically independent operators, *Journal of Clinical Neurophysiology,* Vol. 22(1), 53-64, January/February 2005.

Adjouadi M., Cabrerizo M., Ayala M., Jayakar P., Yaylali I., and Barreto A., Interictal spike detection using the Walsh Transform, *IEEE Transactions on Biomedical Engineering,* Vol. 51, No. 5, 868-873, May, 2004.

Adjouadi M., Cabrerizo M., Ayala M., Seizing lesions in 3-D, *IEEE Potentials,* Vol. 24, Issue 5, pp. 11-17, December/January, 2006.

Ayala M., Adjouadi M., Yaylali I., and Jayakar P., An optimization approach to recognition of epileptogenic data using neural networks with simplified input layers, *Biomed. Sciences Instrumentation,* Vol. 40, 181-186, 2004.

Cabrerizo M., Adjouadi M., Ayala M., and Sesin A., "3D Epileptic Foci Detection Using an Integrated Neuro-Imaging Approach", *WSEAS Transactions on Information Science and Applications,* Vol. 2 (7), pp. 987-995, August, 2005.

Tito M., Ayala M., Yaylali I., Cabrerizo M., Barreto A., Rishe N., Adjouadi M., "Can EEG Processing Reveal Seizure Prediction Patterns?", Proc. of the IASTED International Conference on Graphics and Visualization in Engineering (GVE 2007), January 3-5, 2007, Clearwater, Florida, USA, ISBN: 978-0-88986-625-6, pp. 47-52.

Popescu S., Trained wavelets used to detect epileptic spikes, Proc. of IEEE-SP Intl. Symposium, Time-Frequency and Time-Scale Analysis, New Jersey, pp. 285–288, 1998.

Gevins A. S., and Remond A., Eds. Methods of analysis of brain electrical and magnetic signals, *Handbook of Electroencephalography and Clinical Neurophysiology,* Vol. 1, Elsevier, Amsterdam 1987.

Birkemeier W. P., Fontaine A. B., Celesia G. G., and Ma M., Pattern recognition techniques for the detection of epileptic transients in EEG, *IEEE Trans on Biomedical Engineering,* vol. 25 (3), pp. 213 – 217, 1978.

Proakis J. G., and Dimitris G. M., Digital signal processing - principles, algorithms and applications, Prentice Hall, Third Edition, 1996.

Gonzalez R. C., Woods R. E., Digital Image Processing, Addison-Wesley Publishing Company, 1993.

Le Van Quyen M., Martinerie J., Navarro V., Baulac M., and Varela F., Characterizing neurodynamic changes before seizure, *Clinical Neurophysiology,* vol. 18(3), pp. 191-208, 2001.

Yaylali I., Kocak H., Jayakar P., Detection of seizures from small samples using non-linear dynamic system theory, *IEEE Trans on Biomedical Engineering,* Vol. 43 (7): 743-751, 1996.

Rosenblatt F. (1958), The Perceptron: A Probabilistic Model for Information Storage and Organization in the Brain, Cornell Aeronautical Laboratory, *Psychological Review,* v65, No. 6, pp. 386-408.

Gurney K. (1997) An Introduction to Neural Networks London: Routledge. ISBN 1-85728-673-1 (hardback) or ISBN 1-85728-503-4 (paperback)

Haykin S. (1999) Neural Networks: A Comprehensive Foundation, Prentice Hall, ISBN 0-13-273350-1

Eberhart R.C., Dobbins R. W. and Hutton L. V., Performance metrics in NeuralNetwork PC Tools, Academic Press, Chapter 7, pp. 161-177, 1990.

Hellmann G., Multifold features determine linear equation for automatic spike detection applying neural networks in interictal EcoG, *Clinical Neurophysiology,* vol. 11 (5), pp. 887-894, May 1999.

Tarassenko L., Khan Y.U., and Holt M.R., Identification of interictal spikes in the EEG using neural network analysis, *IEE Proc. Science, Measurement and Tech.,* 145(6), pp.270–278, 1998.

Ko C.W. and Chung H.W., Automatic spike detection via an artificial neural network using raw EEG data, *Clinical Neurophysiology,* vol. 111(3), pp. 477-481, 2000.

Iasemidis L. D., Barreto A., Gilmore R. L., Uthman B. M., Roper S. A., and Sackellares J.C., Spatiotemporal evolution of dynamical measures precedes onset of mesial temporal lobe seizures, *Epilepsia,* vol. 35, 133-134, 1994.

In: Brain Mapping Research Progress
Editors: Ines C. Girard and Jade S. Andre

ISBN: 978-1-60456-784-7

Chapter VI

Laboratory Memory Tasks and Autobiographical Recollection: Cognitive and Neurofunctional Evidence for Differential Forms of Episodic Memory

Martina Piefke*
Physiological Psychology,
Department of Psychology and Sports Sciences,
University of Bielefeld, Germany

Abstract

The classic model of episodic memory refers to both laboratory tasks requiring the conscious recall or recognition of experimental materials and autobiographical recollection of one's personal past experiences. Recent research in cognitive neuroscience, however, showed evidence that laboratory and autobiographical memory may share aspects of conscious retrieval and reference to the temporal and spatial context at the time of encoding of information, but are different from each other in some important respects. The autobiographical memory domain is characterized by self-referential information processing, subjective emotional evaluation of memories, and the accompanying autonoetic conscious awareness. In contrast, laboratory episodic memory requires the effortful search for impersonal target information and the intentional use of retrieval strategies. Subregions of the prefrontal, medial temporal, and retrosplenial cortices appear to be differentially involved in the neural processing of each type of episodic memory, thus suggesting that they are supported by anatomically and functionally overlapping, but also segregated neural circuits. The empirical data reviewed here support the view that laboratory and autobiographical episodic memory can at least

* Correspondence to: Martina Piefke, Physiological Psychology, Department of Psychology and Sports Sciences, University of Bielefeld, Universitätsstr. 25, 33615 Bielefeld, Germany. Tel.: ++49-521-106-4484. Fax : ++49-521-106-6049. E-mail: martina.piefke@uni-bielefeld.de

in part be distinguished on the cognitive-behavioral and the neurofunctional levels. Accordingly, the review proposes an integrated view of laboratory and autobiographical forms of episodic memory which accounts for an overlap, but also emphasizes the unique features distinguishing the two memory types.

Keywords: fMRI, memory, cognition, self, hippocampus, prefrontal cortex

1. Introduction

The classic episodic memory model introduced by Tulving (1972, 1983) is currently applied to depict both laboratory (i.e., experimental) episodic memory and autobiographical recollection. Experimental episodic memory deals with the conscious recall or recognition of items learned in a laboratory setting while episodic autobiographical recollection provides a direct link into *one's own past*. It allows for the awareness of the time course of one's life history, and is closely interconnected with an individual's sense of self-coherence and self-continuity, as well as emotion processing (Markowitsch, 2003; Piefke et al., 2003). Episodic autobiographical memory builds up the basis of our ability to reconstruct an individual and personally meaningful past (Tulving, 1995; Tulving and Markowitsch, 1998). For both types of episodic memory, the current model requires that the retrieval of information is conscious and includes the spatial and temporal context of information at encoding.

I here review evidence for both commonalities and differences between laboratory and autobiographical episodic memory with regard to behavioral performance and the underlying brain mechanisms. The autobiographical memory domain is uniquely associated with automatic self-referential information processing, subjective emotional evaluation of memory contents, and "mental time travel" (Tulving, 1995). In contrast, the effortful search for impersonal target information and the intentional use of retrieval strategies predominate in laboratory episodic memory. Besides these differences, both memory types are associated with conscious retrieval and include context information (see above). Neuropsychological and functional neuroimaging data support the notion that laboratory and autobiographical episodic memory are at least in part supported by differential brain mechanisms. In particular, there appears to be a functional segregation of regions in the prefrontal, medial temporal, and posterior cingulate cortices related to the neural processing of each memory type (Cabeza et al., 2004; Nyberg et al., 2002; Piefke and Fink, 2005). It is thus conceivable that experimental and autobiographical episodic memories are processed by at least in part functionally and anatomically segregated neural circuits which together constitute a broader episodic memory network.

2. Subdivisions of Long-Term Memory

Tulving (1972) introduced a concept for the partition of human long-term memory which has now become a basic model for the understanding of human memory (Tulving, 1995; Tulving and Markowitsch, 1998): the *multiple memory systems* view. The model proposes two memory systems which act at the implicit, that is, unconscious level of information processing (*procedural memory* and the *priming system*), one memory system acting at the explicit, that is, conscious level of processing (*episodic memory*), and one being involved in both implicit and explicit memory (*semantic memory*). *Figure 1* summarizes this multiple memory systems account of human long-term memory and specifies the kind of information processed by each system.

Episodic and semantic memory are sometimes subsumed under the notion of "declarative memory" (e.g., Squire and Zola, 1996) to describe explicit memory which can be observed in rodents, non-human primates, as well as humans. It is supposed to rely on an intact function of the hippocampal formation. In contrast, non-declarative memory comprises implicit forms of memory which are independent of the hippocampal complex (Squire, 1992; Squire and Zola, 1996; Squire, 1998).

The Multiple Memory Systems View (Tulving, 1995)

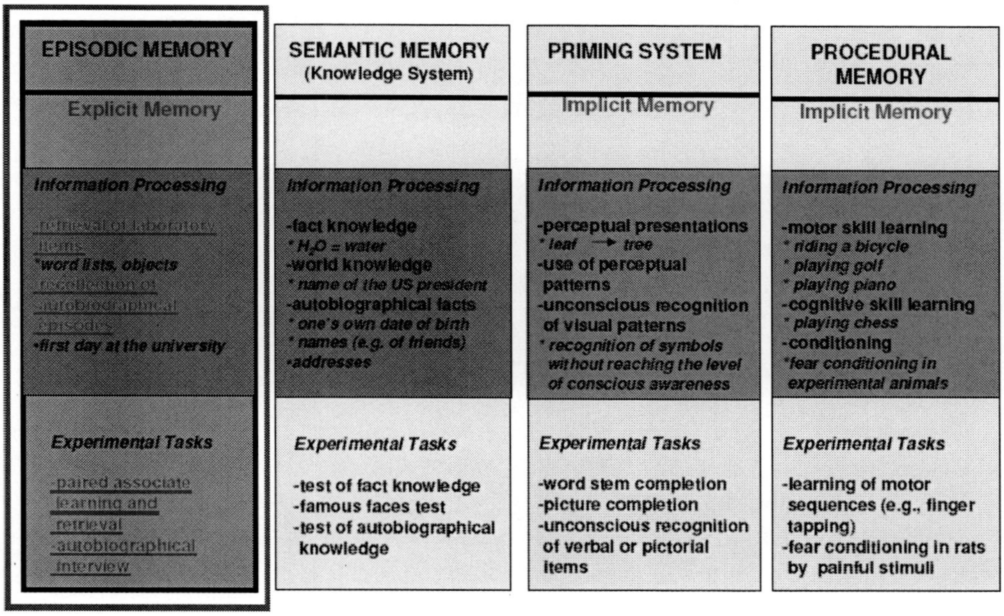

Figure 1. According to the classic multiple memory systems view (Tulving, 1995), human long-term memory comprises at least four memory systems: episodic memory, semantic memory (the knowledge system), the priming system, and procedural memory. The figure specifies the distinct memory types by the categories of information processed by each system and the tasks used to selectively investigate each memory system experimentally. *Both laboratory episodic memory and autobiographical recollection are included the episodic memory system* (highlighted in red). Learning and retrieval of fact knowledge (also autobiographical facts) belong to the domain of semantic memory. Unconscious forms of memory are mediated by the priming system (e.g., perceptual representations) and procedural memory (e.g., skill learning).

Basic and clinical studies on human brain function, however, suggest that episodic and semantic memory represent separate forms of declarative memory. According to the multiple memory systems view (Tulving, 1995), semantic memory does not refer to the context of information encoding. It implies "noetic" awareness, that is, the awareness of retrieving pieces of knowledge (such as "London is the capital of Great Britain") detached from the situational context of information encoding. Episodic memory, in contrast, provides context information and is associated with "autonoetic" awareness. The notion of autonoetic awareness depicts conscious recollection with contextual detail related to time and space of information encoding.

3. The Episodic Memory Account

The initial concept of episodic memory (Tulving, 1972) referred to the free recall and recognition of items within their temporal and spatial context of presentation in a given laboratory setting. It is widely used in behavioral and neuroimaging experiments on human memory (e.g., Burgess et al., 2001; Dalla Barba et al., 1997). However, the concept has also been adapted to studies of conscious memory encoding and retrieval (e.g., of a word list or a series of pictures) without controlling for the inclusion of contextual aspects into the information retrieved (e.g., Henson et al., 2000). Even animal studies of learning and memory in rodents sometimes refer to the episodic memory model (e.g., Meilandt et al., 2004; Remondes and Schuman, 2004), in particular, when tasks are applied which include some kind of declarative spatial, conceptual, or contextual memory (e.g., Morris water maze). Other investigators have retained the broad episodic memory concept, but also developed the model into a framework which allows, at least in part, for the specification of autobiographical recollection (Tulving, 1995; Tulving and Markowitsch, 1998; Piefke et al., 2003). According to this account, laboratory and autobiographical episodic memory share basic similarities which allow for the inclusion of the two forms of memory into one episodic memory model.

The extended use of the episodic memory model calls for a revisit of issues concerning the characteristics of this form of human memory and, in particular, a reconsideration of overlapping and distinct features of autobiographical and laboratory episodic memory.

4. Laboratory and Autobiographical Episodic Memory

4.1. Cognitive Neuropsychology of Episodic Memory

The introduction of "remember-know paradigms" aimed at identifying autonoetic awareness in laboratory experiments of episodic memory (Gardiner and Java, 1993; Knowlton and Squire, 1995; Dalla Barba et al., 1997). Typically, a remember-know paradigm includes a learning phase and a subsequent testing phase requiring the recognition of studied items out of a set of new and learned stimuli. For each item recognized, participants additionally indicate whether they "remember" having seen the item in the study phase including the respective temporo-spatial context information (e.g., that it was displayed in the upper left of the screen), or rather "know" that it was one of the studied items (in the sense of a "feeling of familiarity") but are unable to provide information about the specific context of the item's presentation. In terms of this approach, only "remember-responses" are indicators of autonoetic conscious awareness and thus for episodic memory of an item. The remember-know account claims to show evidence for the coherence of laboratory and autobiographical forms of episodic memory: it refers to the presentation of experimental stimuli in a laboratory context as "mini-events" in the autobiographical sense (Tulving, 1972, 1983). However, laboratory "remember responses" differ from episodic autobiographical recollections at least with respect to the following aspects:

(i) the *time-window* of memory-related information processing which is restricted to the experimental setting in the laboratory type of episodic memory but potentially covers one's entire life history during autobiographical recollection,
(ii) the (often emotional) *re-experience* of an autobiographical event during its recollection which is usually absent in laboratory episodic memory,
(iii) the (emotionally and cognitively determined) *personal significance* of autobiographical recollections which cannot be attributed to laboratory episodic memories,
(iv) the *self-referential perspective* naturally associated with autobiographical recollection but not with laboratory episodic memory tasks,
(v) processes of *mental time travel* associated with autobiographical recollection which are absent or marginal during non-autobiographical episodic memory,
(vi) *reconstructive mechanisms* of autobiographical memory which enable us to reconstruct our personally meaningful past, but are absent (or at least widely reduced) in laboratory episodic memory tasks.

The same is true for the "source memory paradigms" developed some time later (e.g., Cansino et al., 2002). A standard laboratory source memory task requires that a subject learns items (e.g., objects or abstract figures) and their spatial position on the screen (context information). In the following recognition memory test, the participant has to decide whether each shown item was one of the studied items (old/new judgment). If yes, the paradigm requires the localization of the item's position on the screen at encoding. Although source memory paradigms are well applicable for a measure of experimental episodic memory (as are remember-know paradigms), they are no surrogate of a study of episodic autobiographical memory. *Figure 2* illustrates the source memory paradigm used by Cansino et al. (2002).

It is in good accordance with this view that the philosophical perspective of Gallagher (2000) associates autonoetic consciousness with the senses of *self-ownership* (i.e., that I am the one who is undergoing an experience) and *self-agency* (i.e., that I am the source or the initiator of an action). In the non-pathological case, we are therefore sure to have episodic autobiographical memories of our *own* personal past (Fink et al., 1996). Both senses are "naturally" involved in episodic autobiographical memory, but unlikely to emerge during recall of a word list within a laboratory experiment, even if reference to the context at encoding of information is required.

Laboratory tests developed in experimental psychology are the tools used intentionally as simplifications of real life to allow for the controlled assessment of a relevant cognitive process. Although these tests represent valuable approaches that yielded a wealth of knowledge on episodic memory and other brain functions, I would like to argue for the abovementioned reasons that laboratory episodic memory tasks lack crucial aspects of the cognitive and emotional characteristics of autobiographical recollection.

Source Memory Paradigm (Cansino et al. 2002)

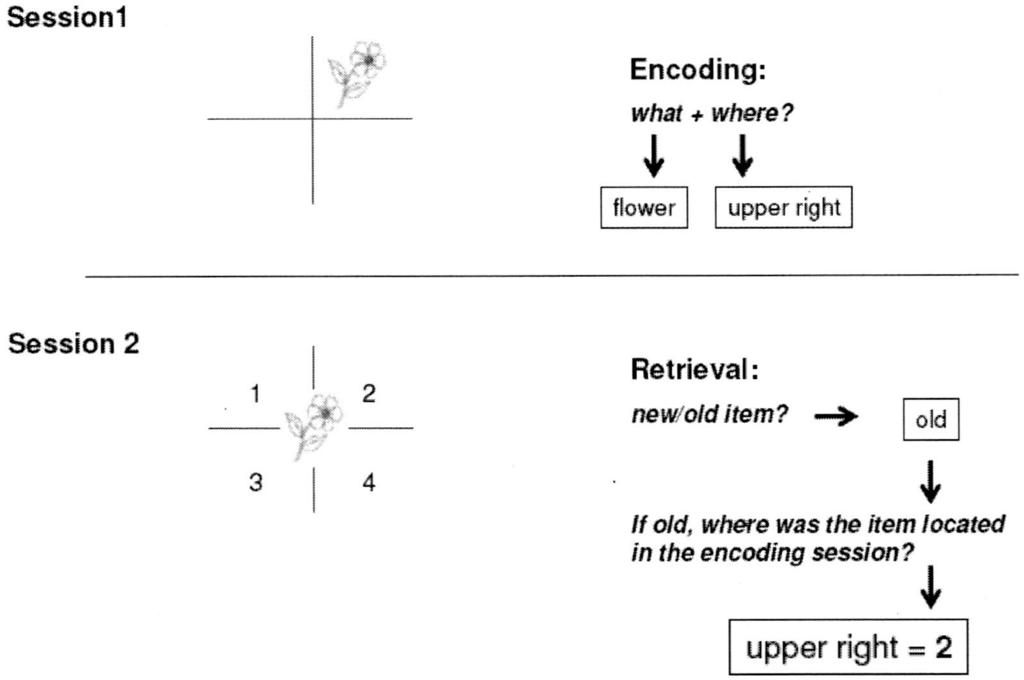

Figure 2. Source memory paradigm which requires the learning (session 1; upper part of the figure) and retrieval (session 2; lower part of the figure) of objects and their position on the screen (four positions are possible). In session 1, participants are asked to learn what is presented and where it is located on the screen (here: flower in the upper right part of the screen). In session two, subjects see the learned objects in their positions and additional new objects located in one of the four positions on the screen. Participants are initially asked to decide whether the item is one of the learned objects or a new one. If it is regarded as one of the learned items, they then have to indicate where it was located in the learning session (here: upper right part of the screen, i.e., quadrant 2). Source memory paradigms allow for the assessment of laboratory episodic memory.

Conway and Pleydell-Pearce (2000) aimed at modeling the specificity of autobiographical memory by the introduction of a "self-memory system" which operates on distinct types of autobiographical information (e.g., knowledge of specific events and lifetime periods). The approach is based on the argument that finally all memories are autobiographical in nature and that "episodic memory" represents a general system which provides sensory and perceptual information on recent events (retention interval: minutes to hours) which has to be integrated into the "autobiographical knowledge base" (Conway, 2001). Therefore, experimental and autobiographical episodic memory cannot be differentiated by this account.

4.2. Brain Correlates of Episodic Memory

Studies of brain damage and neuropsychological performance of amnesic patients suggest that the hippocampus and adjacent medial temporal brain structures, prefrontal, posterior cingulate, and retrosplenial regions all support both laboratory and autobiographical episodic memory. Importantly, however, the studies also indicate that these brain areas may at least in part be differentially involved in the two forms of episodic memory (Aggleton et al., 2000; Bowers et al., 1988; Gaffan et al., 2001; Gainotti et al., 1998; Markowitsch, 1995; Mayes and Downes, 1997; Mayes and Montaldi, 2001; Valenstein et al., 1987). Functional neuroimaging studies of healthy human subjects support these patient data (e.g., Maddock and Buonocore, 1997; Nyberg et al. 2002; Piefke et al., 2003). Moreover, they have shown some evidence for differences in hemispheric lateralization of the two types of episodic memory (Maguire and Frith, 2003a; Piefke et al., 2003; Ranganath et al., 2000).

4.2.1. The Prefrontal Cortex

The "Hemispheric-Encoding-Retrieval-Asymmetry" (HERA) account (Tulving et al., 1994; Habib et al., 2003) assumes that the left prefrontal cortex (PFC) is predominantly involved in episodic encoding, and that right prefrontal regions are mainly recruited during episodic retrieval. According to the model encoding deficits should predominate in patients with episodic memory impairments resulting from left prefrontal lesions, and dysfunctions of episodic retrieval should occur in patients with right prefrontal brain damage. In particular for verbal materials, there is some evidence in support of the HERA account (e.g., Incisa della Rocchetta and Milner, 1993; Stuss et al., 1994; Schacter et al., 1996a). Note, however, that encoding and retrieval deficits can hardly be isolated from each other by studies of laboratory episodic memory in amnesic patients. The application of episodic non-autobiographical memory tests in a laboratory setting is restricted to the investigation of *anterograde memory*, that is, memory of information encoded and retrieved after the occurrence of brain damage. Clues are thus unavailable which may help to decide whether the patient failed to successfully encode the respective information or suffers from a retrieval deficit. In tests of autobiographical recollection, retrograde and anterograde memory deficits can selectively be detected. With regard to anterograde autobiographical memory, however, the problem of the differentiation between encoding and retrieval deficits is the same as in tests of laboratory episodic memory. Given that there is a corresponding lateralization of prefrontal involvement in laboratory and autobiographical episodic memory processing, combined assessment of the experimental and autobiographical forms of episodic memory may nevertheless help to elucidate the validity of the HERA account. Functional neuroimaging studies of normal volunteers cannot directly contribute to the issue since autobiographical encoding may hardly be assessed in a magnetic resonance imaging (MRI) or positron emission tomography (PET) scanner. Moreover, data on prefrontal lateralization during autobiographical memory retrieval are currently rare and inconsistent (Fink et al., 1996; Piefke et al., 2003, 2005). The study of Piefke et al. (2005) suggests that differences in the hemispheric lateralization of autobiographical memory retrieval may also depend on a gender-specific variation in the laterality of brain functions.

No consensus has yet been achieved with regard to the issue of hemispheric lateralization of episodic autobiographical and non-autobiographical memory processes. Recent functional neuroimaging data suggest that laterality effects in the neural activation patterns associated with laboratory tasks of episodic memory encoding and retrieval may depend upon *distinct stimulus characteristics, the complexity of stimulus materials and information to be retrieved, and specific task demands rather than a clear functional hemispheric specialization for memory encoding and retrieval* (as suggested by the HERA account; for a review, see Lee et al., 2003). In fMRI studies of Nolde et al. (1998a, b), laboratory episodic memory tasks with low complexity yielded right prefrontal activations, but the left PFC became activated only with *increasing complexity of retrieval demands* (see also Hunkin et al., 2000). *It is thus conceivable that working memory and executive control processes contribute to the varying laterality of prefrontal activation patterns related to laboratory episodic memory tasks* (Lee et al., 2003; Wager and Smith, 2003). Ranganath et al. (2000) reported a further putative determinant of hemispheric lateralization: in their study, demands of laboratory episodic retrieval of *specific perceptual information* increased neural activity in the left PFC.

In general, these data converge with recent functional neuroimaging studies of autobiographical recollection which provide evidence for a left hemisphere predominance of PFC activations during the retrieval of *complex autobiographical episodes with highly specific perceptual details* (Addis et al., 2004; Maguire and Frith, 2003a, Piefke et al., 2003; but see Fink et al., 1996). The findings suggest that the degree of lateralization of PFC activity associated with both laboratory and autobiographical episodic memory is at least in part determined by a non-linear function of perceptual and cognitive complexity of information processing. With regard to the assumption that there may also exist neurofunctional differences in the brain mechanisms of laboratory and autobiographical episodic memory, it is important to note that laterality effects were mainly *restricted to the PFC in laboratory episodic memory* (Nolde et al., 1998a, b; Ranganath et al., 2000) while *additional medial temporal and parieto-occipital brain regions showed left lateralized activity in autobiographical recollection* (Addis et al., 2004; Maguire and Frith, 2003a; Piefke et al., 2003).

With respect to laboratory episodic memory, evidence has been shown for a high degree of functional segregation within the PFC (for reviews, see Aron et al., 2004; Wager and Smith, 2003). However, the data are inconsistent: right PFC regions have been implicated in "retrieval mode" (Kapur et al., 1995; Nyberg et al., 1995; Tulving, 1983), "retrieval effort" (Schacter et al., 1996b), and "post-retrieval monitoring" (Rugg et al., 1996; Shallice et al., 1994). Fletcher et al. (1998) proposed a dorsolateral/ventrolateral functional segregation within the right PFC, with dorsolateral regions being recruited by increasing monitoring demands and ventrolateral mediating retrieval mode. An alternative view relates differential patterns of PFC involvement in laboratory episodic memory to a neurofunctional differentiation between "retrieval attempt" and "retrieval success" (e.g., Kapur et al., 1995; Nyberg et al., 1995; Rugg et al., 1996; Buckner et al., 1998a, b). The differentiation between memory processes and other cognitive functions that may correspond to ventrolateral and dorsolateral activations, however, has turned out to be difficult. Both regions subserve executive functions such as working memory, cognitive control, and strategic planning (for reviews, see Aron et al., 2004; Wager and Smith, 2003). Any of these processes may be involved in laboratory episodic memory tasks. Accordingly, one cannot easily determine the extent to which PFC activations are directly related to memory functions or rather subserve executive control (e.g., monitoring of retrieved information). In addition to the ventrolateral and dorsolateral PFC, laboratory episodic memory tasks may sometimes recruit orbitofrontal and frontal polar regions. Involvement of these PFC areas in laboratory episodic memory has been related to high context memory demands (Fujii et al., 2004; Nyberg et al., 2002) and emotional aspects (e.g., Smith et al., 2004) of a given task.

The ventrolateral and dorsolateral PFC is also implicated in the executive control of autobiographical episodic recollection (e.g., Maguire et al., 2001a, Piefke et al., 2003; Vanderkerckhove et al., 2005). However, orbitofrontal and medial PFC regions play a predominating role in remembering the personal past. They are involved in self-referential (Vogeley et al., 2001) and social cognition (e.g., theory of mind: Gallagher et al., 2000), as well as emotion and its control (e.g., empathy: Geday et al., 2003; emotional memory: Piefke et al., 2003; Smith et al., 2004). These cognitive and emotional abilities build up major components of autobiographical recollection.

In a review of functional neuroimaging data on corresponding and differential PFC activations associated with laboratory and autobiographical episodic memory, Gilboa (2004) proposed that the right mid-dorsolateral PFC is primarily involved in experimental episodic memor. In contrast, the left ventromedial PFC would predominate in autobiographical recollection. The author interprets the observed prefrontal functional segregation in terms of *distinct modes of post-retrieval verification and monitoring of episodic non-autobiographical and autobiographical memories*. According to this account, autobiographical memories are monitored by a subjective “feeling of rightness” related to a “self-schema” which recruits the left ventromedial PFC. In contrast, experimental episodic memory requires more elaborate monitoring and control strategies to avoid errors such as omissions and repetitions. Therefore, the laboratory type of episodic memory engages the right mid-dorsolateral PFC. It seems conceivable that the monitoring of retrieved information is built upon differential cognitive strategies in laboratory and autobiographical episodic memory. However, it is unlikely that PFC involvement in either type of episodic memory can be reduced to differences in monitoring demands. Distinct aspects concerning the quality of context memory, self-referential information processing, emotional evaluation, and autonoetic conscious awareness which may directly be mediated by functionally segregated prefrontal areas need to be considered, as well.

4.2.2. The Hippocampus

In both animals and humans, the hippocampus plays a key role in declarative memory processing (Markowitsch, 2003; Squire, 1992; Squire and Knowlton, 2000). There is a longstanding debate, however, on the time-window of hippocampal functions in the consolidation, storage, and retrieval of declarative memories. The consolidation theory (Squire, 1992) assumes that memory functions of the hippocampus are time-limited such that older (consolidated) memories which have already been transferred to neocortical storage sites become independent of the hippocampal complex. By contrast, the “multiple trace theory” (MTT; Nadel and Moscovitch, 1997) argues that at least episodic (but not necessarily semantic) memories always depend on the hippocampus. To date, neither model fully accounts for the various forms of amnesia resulting from hippocampal lesions in humans and animals. Differences in the location and the extent of hippocampal lesions, and the application of a wide range of differential tasks in studies of retrograde amnesia may contribute to the inconsistent data reported from studies on memory impairments following damage of the hippocampus (Barr et al., 1990; Bolhuis et al., 1994; Kapur et al., 1992, 1994; Kim and Fanselow, 1992; McDonald and White, 1993; Rempel-Clower, et al., 1996; Scoville and Milner, 1957; Walker, 1957; Zola-Morgan et al., 1986). *Figure 3* depicts the assumptions of the consolidation theory and the MTT, respectively.

Time-Dependent Role of the Hippocampus in Episodic Memory Processing?

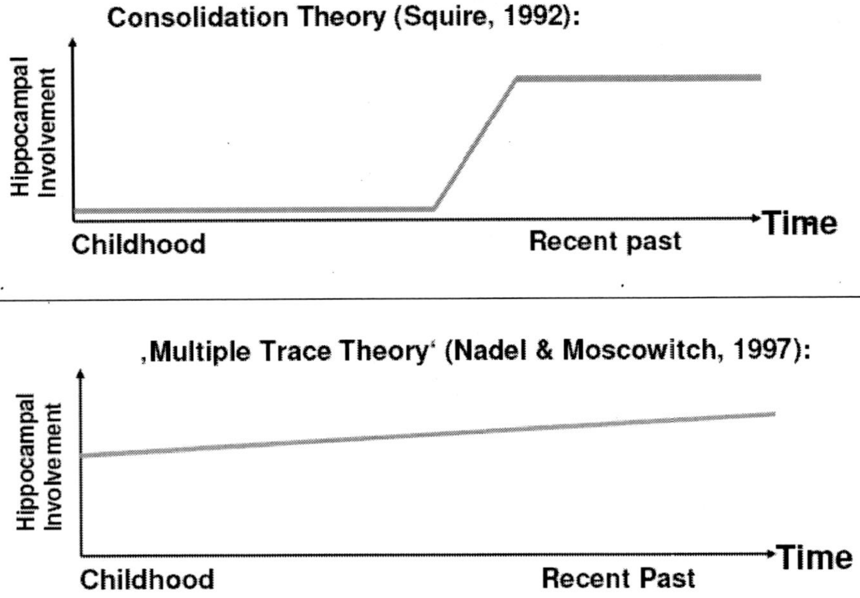

Figure 3. Assumptions of the consolidation theory and the multiple trace theory (MTT) concerning involvement of the hippocampus in episodic memory retrieval. The classic consolidation model (upper part of the figure) presumes a time-limited involvement of the hippocampus in the retrieval of recent episodic memories during the consolidation period. Later, upon long-term storage of information in the neocortex, retrieval processes become independent of the hippocampus. In contrast, the MTT (lower part of the figure) suggests that the hippocampus is always needed for the retrieval of episodic memories, irrespective of the length of the time-period which has passed since the encoding of information. It predicts a flat gradient of hippocampal involvement in retrieval processes as time passes (with remote information requiring less engagement of the hippocampus) which can be due, for example, to the association-related stabilization of information. It is still a matter of debate which of the two theories might better account for the currently available clinical and neuroimaging data on hippocampal memory functions.

When considering the consolidation theory with respect to the assumption of neuropsychological and neurofunctional differences between laboratory and autobiographical episodic memory, it is important to note that the two forms of episodic memory *differ from each other with regard to the time-window defining recent and remote memories*. Laboratory episodic memory tasks normally bear upon time intervals ranging from minutes to hours while the time-window of autobiographical recollection covers one's whole life history.

It remains to be investigated whether temporally graded autobiographical memory loss following hippocampal damage may be paralleled by a corresponding pattern of experimental episodic memory impairment on much shorter time scales. The time-window of experimental declarative memory appears to be sufficient for the assessment of temporally graded retrograde amnesia in animals. In rats with hippocampal lesions induced *after* the learning of target information, temporally graded retrograde amnesia sometimes covered days to weeks (for a review, see Squire, 1992). Reference to the concept of declarative memory in experimental animals, however, does not necessarily contribute to the issue of behavioral and neurofunctional differences between laboratory and autobiographical episodic memory in humans.

Neuropsychological assessment of patients with hippocampal damage suggests that the hippocampus is involved in both laboratory and autobiographical episodic memory (Cohen and Eichenbaum, 1993; Scoville and Milner, 1957; Squire and Zola-Morgan, 1991; Vargha Khadem et al., 1997). Surprisingly, however, functional neuroimaging studies of laboratory episodic memory in healthy volunteers do not consistently reveal hippocampal activations (for a preliminary discussion, see Maguire and Frith, 2003b). In contrast, the hippocampus was activated in most functional neuroimaging investigations of autobiographical recollection (Addis et al., 2004; Fink et al., 1996; Gilboa et al., 2004; Maguire and Frith, 2003b; Maguire et al., 2001a; Niki and Luo, 2002; Piefke et al., 2003). These functional neuroimaging findings suggest that the hippocampus and perhaps adjacent structures of the medial temporal lobe are more sensitive to the characteristics of episodic autobiographical memories (e.g., their complex spatial, temporal, and self-referential contexts, and their emotional significance) than laboratory episodic memory tasks. *It is reasonable to assume that the autobiographical life-time context and the associated processes of mental time travel and self-referential emotional cognition act as modulators of hippocampal memory functions. The degree to which these characteristics of autobiographical memory can be elicited during laboratory episodic memory tasks most likely influences hippocampal involvement in a given experimental task.*

In the autobiographical memory domain, the hippocampus has differentially been implicated in recent (relative to remote) memories by some, but not all functional neuroimaging experiments (Addis et al., 2004; Niki and Luo, 2002; Piefke et al., 2003; but see Maguire et al., 2001a; Ryan et al., 2001; Viard et al., 2007; Cabeza and St. Jacques, 2007). *Figure 4* displays fMRI evidence for differential activations of the hippocampus in the recollection of recent (relative to remote) emotional autobiographical episodes (Piefke et al., 2003).

The finding of differential hippocampal engagement in the recollection of recent (relative to remote) episodic autobiographical information supports the consolidation theory (Squire, 1992; see above). In this regard, the lack of consistent functional neuroimaging evidence for hippocampal activation during laboratory episodic memory tasks is even more intriguing since the processes of encoding and retrieval of "laboratory events" belong to the category of recent memory per se.

Differential Hippocampal Activity Associated with Recent Relative to Remote Emotional Autobiographical Memory Retrieval

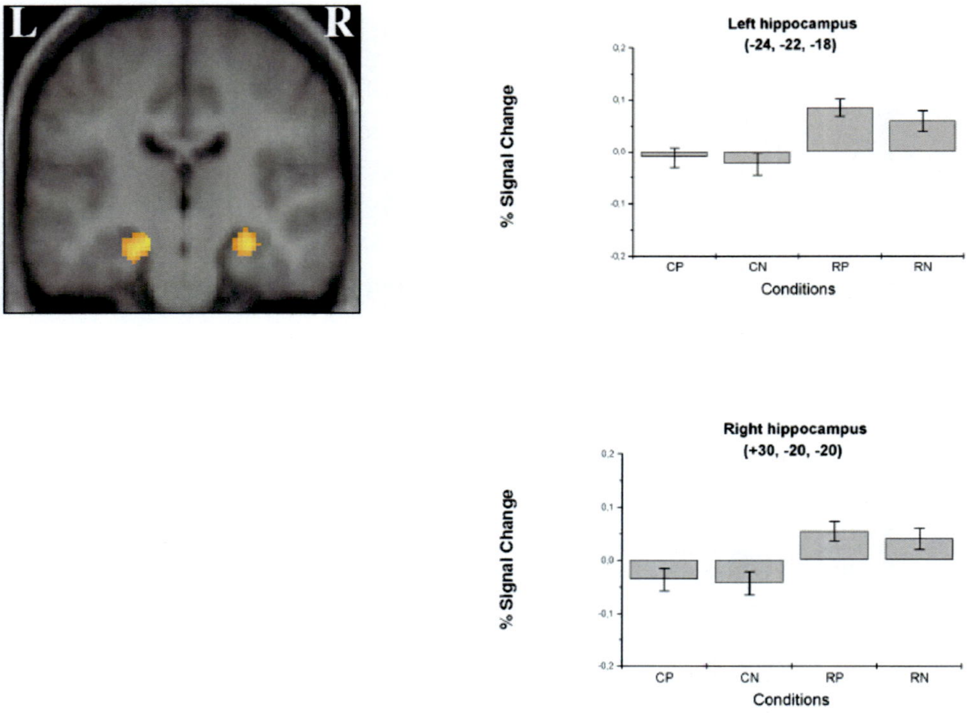

Figure 4. Relative increases in hippocampal activity associated with the recollection of recent compared to remote emotional autobiographical episodes (irrespective of positive or negative valence) of memories reported by Piefke et al. (2003). The histograms display the percentage BOLD signal change for the maxima of significantly increased hippocampal activity as a function of the respective experimental condition. The reverse contrast (remote relative to recent memories) did not yield any statistically significant activations.

R = right; L = left; A = anterior, P = posterior. CP = positive childhood events, CN = negative childhood events, RP = positive recent events, RN = negative recent events.

Functional neuroimaging data suggesting a time-limited hippocampal involvement in recent autobiographical episodic memory is corroborated by the sequential development of memory deficits in patients with Alzheimer's disease (AD) (for a review, see Piefke and Fink, 2005). The loss of recent memories appears during Braak stages III-IV, when conspicuous neurofibrillary changes are mainly restricted to the hippocampal and parahippocampal regions (Braak et al., 1996). Only during later stages of AD, (Braak stages V-VI), as the neurofibrillary changes spread out to the association areas of the neocortex, memories of remote autobiographical events also become impaired. *Figure 5* illustrates the progression of brain pathology and autobiographical memory loss typically associated with AD.

Clinical evidence for AD-related laboratory episodic memory deficits in the anterograde (and thus per se recent) domain (Backman et al., 2001; Eustache et al., 2001; for a review, see Buckner, 2004) may also support of the consolidation theory.

Progression of Brain Pathology in Alzheimer's Disease

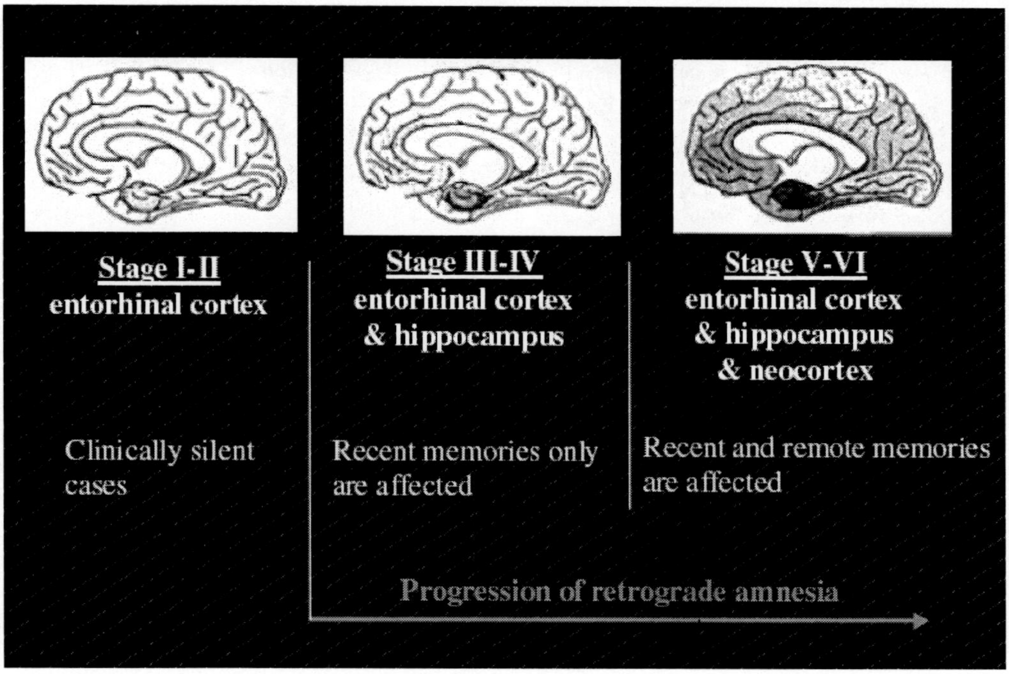

Figure 5. Progression of memory disturbances in patients with Alzheimer's disease (AD) according to Braak et al. (1996). Braak stages I and II depict clinically silent cases where minor changes of the entorhinal cortex can frequently be observed. The sequential development of memory decline is characterized by the early loss of recent memories appearing in the course of Braak stages III-IV during which conspicuous neurofibrillary alterations are typically restricted to hippocampal and entorhinal regions. As the neurofibrillary changes spread out into association areas of the neocortex during the later Braak stages V-VI, remote memory also becomes impaired.

However, other clinical data showing that MTL atrophy in AD patients may result in retrograde amnesia covering both recent and remote episodic autobiographical memories to a similar degree rather support the MTT (see, e.g., Gilboa et al., 2005). Issues concerning the time-window of hippocampal involvement in laboratory and autobiographical memory thus need to be further investigated.

4.2.3. The Posterior Cingulate and Retrosplenial Cortices

The retrosplenial cortex lies adjacent to the retrocommissural hippocampus, a small tissue stripe extending around the posterior end of the corpus callosum. It is interconnected with the entorhinal, the parahippocampal, and the perirhinal cortices and thus closely associated with the hippocampal formation and other structures of the medial temporal lobe subserving memory functions and emotion processing (Insausti et al., 1987). The retrosplenial cortex and its multiple anatomical connections could provide a basis for the typical interplay of emotion and cognition in autobiographical recollections.

Clinical studies reported severe and lasting amnesia for both laboratory and autobiographical materials following selective retrosplenial damage (Bowers et al., 1988; Gainotti et al., 1998; Heilman et al., 1990). Functional neuroimaging studies relate the retrosplenial and posterior cingulate cortices to *emotional* memory in the non-autobiographical (Maddock and Buonocore, 1997; Maratos et al., 2001) and the autobiographical episodic memory domain (Fink et al., 1996; Piefke et al., 2003; Markowitsch et al., 2003). Moreover, the retrosplenial cortex has been related to emotion processing in a more general sense (for a review, see Maddock, 1999).

However, there is also some evidence in support of a specific retrosplenial engagement in autobiographical recollection. Neuropsychological and neuroimaging data converge on the view that autobiographical memory decline associated with normal cognitive aging as well as dementia may be related to pathology of the hippocampal-retrosplenial circuits (for a review, see Piefke and Fink, 2005). Most functional neuroimaging studies on normal volunteers are in good accordance with these clinical data (Fink et al., 1996; Maguire et al., 2001b; Piefke et al. 2003; Shah et al., 2001; Sugiura et al., 2005; but see Maddock, 1999). Piefke et al. (2003) reported increased neural activity in the retrosplenial cortex in combination with bilateral hippocampal activation during the retrieval of recent (relative to remote) emotional autobiographical memories (see also Fink et al., 1996). This finding corroborates the view that the retrosplenial region closely interacts with the hippocampus, and that this interaction may be this interaction may be crucial for the recall of emotionally salient and familiar autobiographical episodes of one's recent past.

Retrosplenial areas have further been implicated in the recognition of personally familiar faces and voices (Shah et al., 2001) as well as objects and places (Sugiura et al., 2005). Although the two latter studies did not directly assess autobiographical recollection, the autobiographically familiar stimulus materials employed in these experiments are likely to have triggered the recall of personal past episodes. Sugiura et al. (2005) argued that the retrosplenial and posterior cingulate cortices are composed of a number of functionally segregated subdivisions. Based on a meta-analysis of functional neuroimaging data on retrosplenial/posterior cingulate involvement in episodic retrieval, they proposed a functional differentiation between the caudal posterior cingulate cortex (cPPC), middorsal PCC (mPCC), posterodorsal PCC (pPCC), and the retrosplenial cortex.

According to this account, the pPCC and the retrosplenial cortex are selectively activated during tasks requiring the retrieval of "real life information", including autobiographical episodes (e.g., Maguire and Frith, 2003b; Piefke et al., 2003), familiar people, and other self-related real world entities (e.g., Leveroni et al., 2000; Kircher et al., 2002; Zysset et al., 2003), and the mental imagery of moving around in a personally familiar environment (Mellet et al., 2000). Activations associated with the retrieval of materials learned in a laboratory context, by contrast, were predominantly located in the mPCC (e.g., Buckner et al., 1996; Henson et al., 1999; Konishi et al., 2000). Finally, the cPCC has been implicated in memory-related navigation in large-scale space (for a review, see Maguire, 2001) and effortful episodic retrieval (Sugiura et al., 2005). The meta-analysis of Sugiura et al. (2005) supports the view suggesting a retrosplenial/posterior cingulate neurofunctional segregation between laboratory and autobiographical episodic memory. *Figure 6* illustrates activation of the retrosplenial area during the recollection of real life information.

Involvement of the Retrosplenial Cortex in the Recollection of Real Life Information

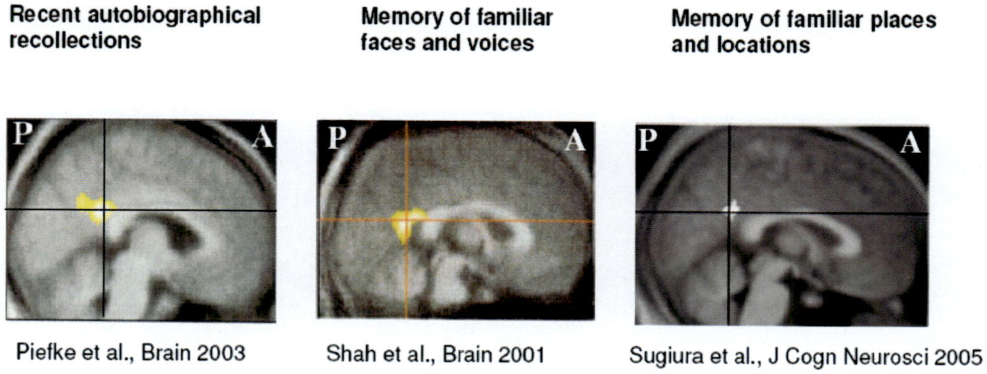

Figure 6. FMRI evidence for retrosplenial activation during the retrieval of real life information. Piefke et al. (2003) demonstrated increased neural activity in the retrosplenial cortex (in combination with bilateral hippocampal activation) during the retrieval of recent (relative to remote) emotional autobiographical memories, suggesting that this brain region is specifically involved in the *recall of emotionally salient and familiar autobiographical episodes of one's recent past* (*a*) (see also Markowitsch et al., 2003). Shah et al. (2001) implicated a corresponding retrosplenial area in the retrieval of personally familiar faces and voices (*b*), and Sugiura et al. (2005) reported activation of the retrosplenial cortex associated with memories of familiar places (*c*). The two latter studies did not directly assess autobiographical recollection. However, the autobiographically familiar stimulus materials used have presumably triggered the recall of personal past episodes.

5. Direct Functional Neuroimaging Comparison of Labortory and Autobiographical Episodic Memory

The studies reviewed above provide evidence that prefrontal, hippocampal and adjacent medial temporal areas, as well as retrosplenial/posterior cingulate brain regions may support both episodic non-autobiographical and autobiographical memory. Parts of these brain structures, however, appear to be differentially engaged in laboratory episodic memory tasks and autobiographical recollection, thus suggesting a *neurofunctional segregation of specific functions involved in each memory type*.

There are some previous neuroimaging experiments which contrasted the brain activations related to autobiographical event memory with those underlying the retrieval of autobiographical facts, public event memory, and the retrieval of general knowledge (Maguire and Mummery, 1999; Maguire and Frith, 2003a, b; Maguire et al., 2001a). However, these do not directly differentiate between laboratory and autobiographical episodic memory: they are based on the distinctions between (i) episodic and semantic memory and (ii) self-referential and impersonal information processing using a 2 x 2 factorial design. Only two functional neuroimaging studies have been published which *directly compared the neural correlates of laboratory episodic memory and autobiographical recollection* using a within-subject design (Cabeza et al., 2004; Nyberg et al., 2002). Nyberg et al. (2002) used a Crovitz cueing technique (Crovitz and Schiffman, 1974) to trigger autobiographical memories across each individual's whole life span and memories of items learned in a recent laboratory context. The types of episodic memories investigated in that study necessarily differed from each other with regard to the main parameters discussed above. These are *memory age* (recent to remote retrograde memory in the autobiographical condition, recent anterograde memory in the laboratory condition), the degree of *self-referential* information processing, the memories' *emotional significance*, the *recollective experience* associated with memory retrieval (which were all high in the autobiographical condition and lacking or at least low in the laboratory condition), and the differential degree and quality of *executive control* (see Gilboa, 2004). Differential neural activations associated with the two memory types were observed in medial and lateral prefrontal as well as parietal brain regions. This finding may indicate the operation of differential brain mechanisms underlying laboratory and autobiographical episodic memory. However, the above confounding between-condition differences have to be taken into consideration when interpreting the data.

Cabeza et al. (2004) a priori defined dimensions determining differences between laboratory and autobiographical episodic memory which were used for the control for confounding variables. Dimensions comprised (i) the proportion of retrieval processes (production and monitoring), (ii) age of memories, (iii) emotional content, (iv) retrieval success, (v) self-referential information processing, (vi) visual/spatial memory, and (vii) recollection. A photo paradigm was used which included photos of (pre-selected) places *taken by the subjects themselves* ("controlled autobiographical condition") and photos of the same places taken by others, but *shown to the subjects in the laboratory* ("laboratory condition"). During the fMRI measurement, participants viewed both types of photos, as well as new ones. They indicated by button press whether each photo had been taken by themselves, shown to them in the laboratory context, or was a new photo. Differential activations related to the controlled autobiographical (relative to the laboratory) condition were observed in the medial prefrontal cortex (an area engaged in self-referential information processing), visual areas and the parahippocampal gyrus (regions involved in visuo-spatial memory), and the hippocampus (a structure implicated in recollective experience). The fMRI data of Cabeza et al. (2004) are in good accordance with the here proposed view of a neurofunctional segregation of laboratory and autobiographical episodic memory in the prefrontal, medial temporal, and retrosplenial/posterior cingulate cortices.

Further investigations are needed, however, in order to evaluate whether the experimental design employed by Cabeza et al. (2004) sufficiently assessed the characteristic attributes of autobiographical memory. Even if the subjects remembered the "real-life" photo-taking episodes during "autobiographical photo recognition", *these episodes remain experimental events*, that is, events which did not occur in the "natural" context of each participant's life history. The attempt to match laboratory and "real life autobiographical" episodic memory for some major dimensions of putative differences between them may have raised the problem that the experimental "real life events" lost some basic attributes of autobiographical episodes. Moreover, the recognition task could well have engaged subjects in the recognition and categorization (own versus others' photo) of photo materials by button presses, but not in the episodic recollection of each respective event. Similar recognition paradigms had been applied in previous functional neuroimaging experiments on autobiographical memory (e.g., Maguire and Frith 2003a, b; Maguire et al., 2001; Ryan et al., 2001). This approach, however, should be treated with caution: one cannot be sure to which degree a neurofunctional measure of recognition memory may give information on *autobiographical recollective re-experience* during memory retrieval.

The photo paradigm employed by Cabeza et al. (2004) meets the requirements of an autobiographical memory study to a higher degree than, for example, fMRI virtual reality (VR) experiments in which VR events were used as a "surrogate" of autobiographical episodes (e.g., Burgess et al., 2001). VR events lack the characteristic features of real life experiences. Rather, they represent experimental events in the sense of an encounter with any kind of stimulus materials which implies visuo-spatial context information. The criteria used by Cabeza et al. (2004) for the identification of differences between autobiographical recollection and laboratory episodic memory are well applicable to the purpose of an up-to-date differentiation between laboratory and autobiographical episodic memory model. Two further aspects could be added: (i) the normal processes and changes of subjective autobiographical reconstruction across time and (ii) the emotional and cognitive evaluation of autobiographical episodes which allow for their integration into a meaningful personal past.

6. Implications of the Present Review

Based on the evidence provided by behavioral, clinical, and neuroimaging studies of laboratory and autobiographical episodic memory reviewed above, I here aim at providing a first step towards a view of episodic memory which accounts for both the commonalities and differences between laboratory and real life autobiographical episodic memory. The classic episodic memory model of the multiple memory systems account (Tulving, 1972, 1983; Tulving and Markowitsch, 1998) represents a well elaborated starting point for a specification of the relationship between laboratory and autobiographical episodic memory. Before the main criterions differentiating laboratory and autobiographical memory will be extracted from the studies reviewed in this article, some important points made by the classic episodic memory model should be summarized. According to the model, common characteristics of laboratory and autobiographical episodic memory concern (i) conscious memory retrieval (but not necessarily conscious encoding, see below) and (ii) reference to the spatial and temporal context of the situation of information encoding. *Laboratory memory tasks which do not explicitly require the conscious processing of spatio-temporal context information during retrieval would therefore not be considered as episodic memory tasks by this account.* In contrast, laboratory tasks relying on remember-know (e.g., Dalla Barba et al., 1997) or source memory paradigms (e.g., Cansino et al., 2002) can be assumed appropriate measures of experimental episodic memory as they require the conscious retrieval of the spatial and/or temporal context of information encoding.

A measure of autobiographical episodic memory can be achieved only by referring to an individual's whole real life context. It always deals with the conscious episodic retrieval of one's own personal past experiences. This point has not always been emphasized by the classic model of episodic memory. The main cognitive-behavioral differences between laboratory and autobiographical episodic memory can be defined along the following criteria:

(1) The requirements of encoding of laboratory and autobiographical episodic information (and the underlying neural mechanisms) differ from each other. Laboratory episodic learning is characterized by an experimentally induced (i.e., artificial) conscious awareness of information processing. This aspect does not need to include the intentional learning of target materials. For example, the semantic categorization of verbal items ("deep encoding") or detection of a particular letter in words or pseudo-words ("shallow encoding") have also been used as episodic memory encoding tasks (e.g., Fletcher et al., 2003; Otten et al., 2001). Autobiographical memory encoding differs from experimental learning in an important respect: the encoding of autobiographical episodes occurs automatically and depending on the subjective relevance of an event such that it does not require any artificial task instruction. To my knowledge, these encoding differences between experimental and autobiographical episodic memory have not explicitly been considered by any neuropsychological or functional neuroimaging study on human memory, yet. In the study of Cabeza et al. (2004), subjects were instructed to learn and intentionally memorize each picture taking episode as an individual event including physical (e.g., light) and psychological (e.g., mental associations) context information. Most likely, the intentional and thus artificial learning of the photo taking events implicates that the "controlled autobiographical events" departed from being autobiographical in nature.

(2) Autonoetic conscious awareness is uniquely associated with autobiographical recollection. Consciousness during laboratory episodic memory retrieval is restricted to an individual's conscious awareness of being engaged in contextual memory retrieval. It needs to be further investigated whether the autonoetic consciousness emerging during autobiographical recollections may at least in part be built upon the processes of automatic encoding of episodic autobiographical information.

(3) The extension of a self-referential context across an individual's whole life history and its association with social-cultural norms during autobiographical information processing may operate as key factors in both the (unconsciously) relevance-oriented automatic encoding of autobiographical episodes and the appearance of autonoetic conscious awareness during autobiographical recollection. The absence of these aspects in laboratory episodic memory tasks most likely requires one's engagement in a conscious and intentional effort to achieve successful encoding and retention of target information.

The neuropsychological and behavioral commonalities and differences of laboratory and autobiographical episodic memory are reflected by a partial integration and segregation of brain mechanisms underlying the two memory types. The prefrontal, temporal, and retrosplenial/posterior cingulate cortices are involved in both laboratory and autobiographical episodic memory, however, with subregions showing a differential engagement in the two memory types. The common aspects include basic neuronal interactions between prefrontal, temporal, and posterior brain regions underlying conjoint conscious item *and* context memory and the monitoring of information retrieval. A segregation of laboratory and autobiographical memory functions occurs at diverse levels of processing. This neurofunctional differentiation can be defined by the following criteria:

(1) The neural mechanisms of the two memory types differ from each other in respect of PFC subregions involved in the executive control of retrieval processes (see also Gilboa, 2004). The dorsolateral and ventrolateral PFC predominate in the support of retrieval effort and post-retrieval monitoring during laboratory episodic memory tasks (e.g., Fletcher et al., 1998). In contrast, the medial PFC is a key player in the self-referential and emotional control of autobiographical recollections (e.g., Cabeza et al., 2004; Piefke et al., 2003). Since the dorsolateral and ventrolateral PFC also mediate strategic aspects of information retrieval, these areas have sometimes also been implicated in autobiographical memory (Gilboa, 2004; Maguire et al., 2001a, Piefke et al., 2003, 2005). Moreover, these PFC regions are involved in the maintenance and manipulation of information in working memory (Cornette et al., 2001; D'Esposito et al., 2000) such that they could act as mediators of the interplay between episodic long-term and working memory processes (Lee et al., 2003; Ranganath et al., 2003). Successful encoding and retrieval of information in laboratory episodic memory tasks particularly depend on strategic "online" manipulation of relevant information. It is thus conceivable that laboratory episodic memory makes higher demands on working memory functions and relies more on lateral PFC regions than autobiographical recollections.

(2) Although the hippocampus is involved in laboratory episodic learning and memory, the degree to which an experimental task approaches the cognitive demands of autobiographical recollections (reference to one's autobiographical life-time context, re-experience of episodes, mental time travel, and self-referential cognition, emotional evaluation) modulates hippocampal and adjacent medial temporal involvement in episodic memory functions (see also Maguire and Frith, 2003b).

(3) The autonoetic conscious awareness which is uniquely associated with autobiographical episodic memory most likely emerges from fine-tuned interactions of circumscribed medial prefrontal, hippocampal, and retrosplenial brain areas. Therefore, it might be the whole cognitive set of autobiographical encoding and retrieval that allows for autonoetic consciousness. The cognitive set of autobiographical recollection is thus likely to differ qualitatively from that of experimental episodic memory. This assumption agrees with recent research on the brain substrates of diverse aspects of consciousness (Egan et al., 2003; Tononi, 2005; Vogt and Laureys, 2005).

Conclusion

The empirical data on laboratory and autobiographical episodic memory reviewed here indicate that the neuropsychological and neurofunctional differences between experimental and autobiographical forms of episodic memory call for an integrative view of the two memory types which considers both their overlapping and differential components. Currently, the laboratory and the autobiographical form of episodic memory may best be modeled as different subsystems of a large-scale neural circuit supporting basic episodic memory functions. To deal with the unresolved issues such as automatic episodic autobiographical memory encoding, the formation of autonoetic conscious awareness during autobiographical recollection, and the role of intentional (in the sense of experimentally induced) cognitive processing in laboratory episodic memory, further cognitive-behavioral and neurofunctional investigations are needed. The suggestions of this review may open the door for the elaboration of novel approaches to both laboratory and autobiographical episodic memory which are qualified for the assessment of such intricate questions.

Acknowledgements

MP is supported by the Hans Lungwitz Foundation, Berlin and the START program of the Rheinisch-Westfälische Hochschule (RWTH) Aachen.

References

Addis, D.R., Moscovitch, M., Crawley, A.P., McAndrews, M.P. (2004). Recollective qualities modulate hippocampal activation during autobiographical memory retrieval. *Hippocampus* 14, 752-762.

Aggleton, J.P., McMackin, D., Carpenter, K., Hornak, J., Kapur, N., Halpin, S., Wiles, C.M., Kamel, H., Brennan, P., Carton, S., Gaffan, D. (2000). Differential cognitive effects of colloid cysts in the third ventricle that spare or compromise the fornix. *Brain* 123, 800-815.

Aron, A.R., Robbins, T.W., Poldrack, R.A. (2004). Inhibition and the right inferior frontal cortex. *Trends Cogn Sci* 8, 170-177.

Backman, L., Small, B.J., Fratiglioni, L. (2001). Stability of the preclinical episodic memory deficit in Alzheimer's disease. *Brain* 124, 96-102.

Barr, W.B., Goldberg, E., Wasserstein, J., Novelly, R.A. (1990). Retrograde amnesia following unilateral temporal lobectomy. *Neuropsychologia* 28, 243-256.

Bolhuis, J.J., Stewart, C.A., Forrest, E.M. (1994). Retrograde amnesia and memory reactivation in rats with ibotenate lesions to the hippocampus or subiculum. *Q. J. Exp. Psychol. B* 47, 129-150.

Bowers, D., Verfaellie, M., Valenstein, E., Heilman, K.M. (1988). Impaired acquisition of temporal information in retrosplenial amnesia. *Brain Cogn* 8, 47-66.

Braak, H., Braak, E., Yilmazer, D., de Vos, R.A., Jansen, E.N., Bohl, J. (1996). Pattern of brain destruction in Parkinson's and Alzheimer's diseases. *J. Neural. Transm.* 103, 455-490.

Buckner, R.L. (2004). Memory and executive function in aging and AD: multiple factors that cause decline and reserve factors that compensate. *Neuron.* 44, 195-208.

Buckner, R.L., Raichle, M.E., Miezin, F.M., Petersen, S.E. (1996). Functional anatomic studies of memory for auditory words and visual pictures. *J. Neurosci.* 16, 6219-6235.

Buckner, R.L., Koutstaal, W., Schacter, D.L., Wagner, A.D., Rosen, B.R. (1998a). Functional-anatomic study of episodic retrieval using fMRI: I. Retrieval effort versus retrieval success. *Neuroimage* 7, 151-162.

Buckner, R.L., Koutstaal, W., Schacter, D.L., Dale, A.M., Rotte, M., Rosen, B.R. (1998b). Functional-anatomic study of episodic retrieval. II. Selective averaging of event-related fMRI trials to test the retrieval success hypothesis. *Neuroimage* 7, 163-175.

Burgess, N., Maguire, E.A, Spiers, H.J., O'Keefe, J. (2001). A temporoparietal and prefrontal for retrieving the spatial context of lifelike events. *Neuroimage* 14, 439-453.

Cabeza, R., St. Jacques, P. (2007). Functional neuroimaging of autobiographical memory. *Trends Cogn. Sci.*, epub ahead of print.

Cabeza, R., Prince, S.E., Daselaar, S.M., Greenberg, D.L., Budde, M., Dolcos, F., Labar, K.S., Rubin, D.C. (2004). Brain activity during episodic retrieval of autobiographical and laboratory events. *J. Cogn. Neurosci.* 16, 1583-1594.

Cansino, S., Maquet, P., Dolan, R.J., Rugg, M.D. (2002). Brain activity underlying encoding and retrieval of source memory. *Cereb. Cortex* 12, 1048-1056.

Cohen, N.J., Eichenbaum, H. (1993). *Memory, amnesia, and the hippocampal system.* Cambridge, MA: MIT Press.

Conway, M.A. (2001). Sensory-perceptual episodic memory and its context: autobiographical memory. *Philos Trans R Soc Lond B. Biol. Sci.* 356, 1375-1384.

Conway, M.A., Pleydell-Pearce C.W. (2000). The construction of autobiographical memories in the self-memory system. *Psychol. Rev.* 107, 261-288.

Cornette, L., Dupont, P., Salmon, E., Orban, G.A. (2001). The neural substrate of orientation working memory. *J. Cogn. Neurosci.* 13, 813-828.

Crovitz, H.F., Schiffman, H. (1974). Frequency of episodic memories as a function of age. *Bull. Psychon. Soc.* 5, 517-518.

Dalla Barba, G., Mantovan, M.C., Ferruzza, E., Denes, G. (1997). Remembering and knowing the past: a case study of isolated retrograde amnesia. *Cortex* 33, 143-154.

D'Esposito, M., Postle, B.R., Rypma, B. (2000). Prefrontal cortical contributions to working memory: evidence from event-related fMRI studies. *Brain Res.* 133, 3-11.

Egan, G., Silk, T., Zamarripa, F., Williams, J., Federico, P., Cunnington, R., Carabott, L., Blair-West, J., Shade, R., McKinley, M., Farrell, M., Lancaster, J., Jackson, G., Fox, P., Denton, D. (2003). Neural correlates of the emergence of consciousness of thirst. *Proc. Natl. Acad. Sci. USA* 100, 15241-15246.

Eustache, F., Desgranges, B., Giffard, B., de la Sayette, V., Baron, J.C. (2001). Entorhinal cortex disruption causes memory deficit in early Alzheimer's disease as shown by PET. *Neuroreport* 12, 683-685.

Fink, G.R., Markowitsch, H.J., Reinkemeier, M., Bruckbauer, T., Kessler, J., Heiss, W.D. (1996). Cerebral representation of one's own past: neural networks involved in autobiographical memory. *J Neurosci* 16, 4275-4282.

Fletcher, P.C., Shallice, T., Frith, C.D., Frackowiak, R.S., Dolan, R.J. (1998). The functional roles of prefrontal cortex in episodic memory. II. Retrieval. *Brain* 121, 1249-1256.

Fletcher, P.C., Stephenson, C.M., Carpenter, T.A., Donovan, T., Bullmore, E.T. (2003). Regional brain activations predicting subsequent memory success: an event-related fMRI study of the influence of encoding tasks. *Cortex* 39, 1009-1026.

Fujii, T., Suzuki, M., Okuda, J., Ohtake, H., Tanji, K. Yamaguchi, K., Itoh, M., Yamadori, A. (2004). Neural correlates of contex memory with real-world events. *Neuroimage* 21, 1596-1603.

Gaffan, D., Parker, A., Easton, A. (2001). Dense amnesia in the monkey after transection of fornix, amygdala, and anterior temporal stem. *Neuropsychologia* 39, 51-70.

Gainotti, G., Almonti, S., DiBetta, A.M., Silveri, M.C. (1998). Retrograde amnesia in a patient with retrosplenial tumour. *Neurocase* 4, 519-526.

Gallagher, H.L., Happe, F., Brunswick, N., Fletcher, P.C., Frith, U., Frith, C.D. (2000). Reading the mind in cartoons and stories: an fMRI study of "theory of mind" in verbal and nonverbal tasks. *Neuropsychologia* 38, 11-21.

Gallagher, I.I. (2000). Philosophical conceptions of the self: implications for cognitive science. *Trends Cogn. Sci.* 4, 14-21.

Gardiner, J.M., Java, R.I. (1993). Recognizing and remembering In: A.F. Collins, S.E. Gathercole, M.A. Conway, P.E. Morris (Eds.), *Theories of Memory* (pp. 163-188). Hove (UK): Erlbaum.

Geday J., Gjedde, A., Boldsen, A.S., Kupers, R. (2003). Emotional valence modulates activity in the posterior fusiform gyrus and inferior medial prefrontal cortex in social perception. *Neuroimage* 18, 675-684.

Gilboa, A. (2004). Autobiographical and episodic memory - one and the same? Evidence from prefrontal activation in neuroimaging studies. *Neuropsychologia* 42, 1336-1349.

Gilboa, A., Winocur, G., Grady, C.L., Hevenor, S.J., Moscovitch, M. (2004). Remembering our past: functional neuroanatomy of recollection of recent and very remote personal events. *Cereb. Cortex* 14, 1214-1225.

Gilboa, A., Ramirez, J., Köhler, S., Westmacott, R., Black, S.E., Moscovitch, M. (2005). Retrieval of autobiographical in Alzheimer's disease: relation to volumes of medial temporal lobe and other structures. *Hippocampus* 15, 535-550.

Habib, R., Nyberg, L., Tulving, E. (2003). Hemispheric asymmetries of memory: the HERA model revisited. *Trends Cogn Sci* 7, 241-245.

Heilman KM, Bowers D, Watson RT, Day A, Valenstein E, Hammond E, Duara R. (1990). Frontal hypermetabolism and thalamic hypometabolism in a patient with abnormal orienting and retrosplenial amnesia. *Neuropsychologia* 28, 161-169.

Henson, R.N., Rugg, M.D., Shallice, T., Josephs, O., Dolan, R.J. (1999). Recollection and familiarity in recognition memory: an event-related functional magnetic resonance imaging study. *J. Neurosci.* 19, 3962-3972.

Henson, R.N.A., Rugg, M., Shallice, T., Dolan, R.J. (2000). Confidence in recognition memory for words: dissociating right prefrontal roles in episodic retrieval. *J. Cogn. Neurosci.* 12, 913-923.

Hunkin, N.M., Mayes, A.R., Williams, S.C.R., Gregory, L.J., Nunn, J.A., Nicholas, A,K., Brammer, M.J., Bullmore, E.T. (2000). Does frontal lobe activation during retrieval reflect complexity of retrieved information? *Neuroreport* 11, 557-561.

Incisa della Rocchetta, A., Milner, B. (1993). Strategic search and retrieval inhibition: the role of the frontal lobes. *Neuropsychologia* 31, 503-524.

Insausti, R., Amaral, D.G., Cowan, W.M. (1987). The entorhinal cortex of the monkey II: Cortical afferents. *J. Comp. Neurol.* 264, 356-395.

Kapur, N., Ellison, D., Smith, M.P. McLellan, D.L., Burrows, E.H. (1992). Focal retrograde amnesia following bilateral temporal lobe pathology. A neuropsychological and magnetic resonance study. *Brain* 115, 73-85.

Kapur, N., Ellison, D., Parkin, A.J., Hunkin, N.M., Burrows, E., Sampson, S.A., Morrison, E.A. (1994). Bilateral temporal lobe pathology with sparing of medial temporal lobe structures: lesion profile and pattern of memory disorder. *Neuropsychologia* 32, 23-38.

Kapur, S., Craik, F.I., Jones, C., Brown, G.M., Houle, S., Tulving, E. (1995). Functional role of the prefrontal cortex in retrieval of memories: a PET study. *Neuroreport* 6, 1880-1884.

Kim, J.J., Fanselow, M.S. (1992). Modality-specific retrograde amnesia for fear. *Science* 256, 675-677.

Kircher, T.T.J., Brammer, M., Bullmore, E., Simmons, A., Bartels, M., David, A.S. (2002). The neural correlates of intentional and incidental self processing. *Neuropsychologia* 40, 683-692.

Knowlton, B.J., Squire, L.R. (1995). Remembering and knowing: two different expressions of declarative memory. *J. Exp. Psychol. Learn Mem. Cogn.* 21, 699-710.

Konishi, S., Wheeler, M.E., Donaldson, D.I., Buckner, R.L. (2000). Neural correlates of episodic retrieval success. *Neuroimage* 12, 276-286.

Lee, A.C.H., Robbins, T.W., Owen, A.M. (2003). Episodic memory meets working memory in the frontal lobe: functional neuroimaging studies of encoding and retrieval. *Crit. Rev. Neurobiol.* 14, 165-197.

Leveroni, C.L., Seidenberg, M., Mayer, A.R., Mead, L.A., Binder, J.R., Rao, S.M. (2002). Neural systems underlying the recognition of familiar and newly learned faces. *J. Neurosci.* 20, 878-886.

Maddock, R.J. (1999). The retrosplenial cortex and emotion: new insights from functional neuroimaging of the human brain. *Trends Neurosci.* 22, 310-316.

Maddock, R.J., Buonocore, M.H. (1997). Activation of left posterior cingulate gyrus by the auditory presentation of threat-related words: an fMRI study. *Psychiatry Res.* 75, 1-14.

Maguire, E.A. (2001). The retrosplenial contribution to human navigation: a review of lesion and neuroimaging findings. *Scand. J. Psychol.* 42, 225-228.

Maguire, E.A., Mummery, C.J. (1999). Differential modulation of a common memory retrieval network revealed by positron emission tomography. *Hippocampus* 9, 54-61.

Maguire, E.A., Frith, C.D. (2003a). Lateral asymmetry in the hippocampal responses to the remoteness of autobiographical memories. *J. Neurosci.* 23, 5302-5307.

Maguire, E.A., Frith, C.D. (2003b). Aging affects the engagement of the hippocampus during autobiographical memory retrieval. *Brain* 126, 1511-1523.

Maguire, E.A., Henson, R.N., Mummery, C.J., Frith, C.D. (2001a). Activity in the prefrontal cortex, not hippocampus, varies parametrically with increasing remoteness of autobiographical memories. *Neuroreport* 12, 441-444.

Maguire, E.A., Vargha-Khadem, F., Mishkin, M. (2001b). The effects of bilateral hippocampal damage on fMRI regional activations and interactions during memory retrieval. *Brain* 124, 1156-1170.

Maratos, E.J., Dolan, R.J., Morris, J.S., Henson, R.N., Rugg, M.D. (2001). Neural activity associated with episodic memory for emotional context. *Neuropsychologia* 39, 910-920.

Markowitsch, H.J. (1995). Which brain regions are critically involved in the retrieval of old episodic memories? *Brain Res. Brain Res. Rev.* 21, 117-127.

Markowitsch, H.J. (2003) The functional anatomy of learning and memory. In: P. Halligan, U. Kischka, G. Beaumont (Eds.), *Handbook of Clinical Neuropsychology* (pp. 724-740). Oxford (UK): Oxford University Press.

Markowitsch, H.J., Vanderkerkhove, M.M., Lanfermann, H., Russ, M.O. (2003). Engagement of lateral and medial prefontal areas in the ecphory of sad and happy autobiographical memories. *Cortex* 3, 643-665.

Mayes, A.R., Downes, J.J. (1997). What do theories of the functional deficit(s) underlying amnesia have to explain? *Memory* 5, 3-47.

Mayes, A.R., Montaldi, D. (2001). Exploring the neural bases of episodic and semantic memory: the role of structural and functional neuroimaging. *Neurosci. Biobehav. Rev.* 25, 555-573.

McDonald, R.J., White, N.M. (1993). A triple dissociation of memory systems: hippocampus, amygdala, and dorsal striatum. *Behav. Neurosci.* 107, 3-22.

Meilandt, W.J., Barea-Rodriguez, E., Harvey, S.A., Martinez, J.L. (2004). Role of hippocampal CA3 mu-opioid receptors in spatial learning and memory. *J. Neurosci.* 24, 2953-2062.

Mellet, E., Briscogne, S., Tzourio-Mazoyer, N., Ghaem, O., Petit, L., Zago, L., Etard, O., Berthoz, A., Mazoyer, B., Denis, M. (2000). Neural correlates of topographic mental exploration: the impact of route versus survey perspective learning. *Neuroimage* 12, 588-600.

Nadel, L., Moscovitch, M. (1997). Memory consolidation, retrograde amnesia, and the hippocampal complex. *Curr. Opin. Neurobiol.* 7, 217-227.

Niki, K., Luo, J. (2002). An fMRI study on the time-limited role of the medial temporal lobe in long-term topographical autobiographic memory. *J. Cogn. Neurosci.* 14, 500-507.

Nolde, S.F., Johnson, M.K., Raye, C.L. (1998a). Left prefrontal activation during episodic remembering: an event-related fMRI study. *Neuroreport* 9, 3509-3514.

Nolde, S.F., Johnson, M.K., Raye, C.L. (1998b). The role of prefrontal cortex during tests of episodic memory. *Trends Cogn. Sci.* 2, 399-406.

Nyberg, L., Tulving, E., Habib, R., Nilsson, L.G., Kapur, S., Houle, S., Cabeza, R., McIntosh, A.R. (1995). Functional brain maps of retrieval mode and recovery of episodic information. *Neuroreport* 7, 9-10.

Nyberg, L., Forkstam, C, Petersson, K.M., Cabeza, R., Ingvar, M. (2002). Brain imaging of human memory systems: between-systems similarities and within-systems differences. *Brain Res. Cogn. Brain Res.* 13, 281-192.

Otten, L.J., Henson, R.N., Rugg, M.D. (2001). Depth of processing effects on neural correlates of memory encoding: relationship between findings from across- and within-task comparisons. *Brain* 124, 399-412.

Piefke, M., Weiss, P., Zilles, K., Markowitsch, H.J., Fink, G.R. (2003). Differential Remoteness and emotional tone modulate the neural correlates of autobiographical memory. *Brain* 126, 650-668.

Piefke, M., Weiss, P., Markowitsch, H.J., Fink, G.R. (2005). Gender differences in the functional neuroanatomy of emotional episodic autobiographical memory. *Hum. Brain Mapp.* 24, 313-324.

Piefke, M., Fink, G.R. (2005). Recollections of one's own past: the effects of aging and gender on the neural mechanisms of episodic autobiographical memory. *Anat. Embryol.* 210, 497-512.

Ranganath, C., Johnson, M.K., D'Esposito, M. (2000). Left anterior prefrontal activation increases with demands to recall specific perceptual information. *J. Neurosci.* 20, 1-5.

Ranganath, C., Johnson, M.K., D'Esposito, M. (2003). Prefrontal activity associated with working memory and episodic long-term memory. *Neuropsychologia* 41, 378-389.

Remondes, M., Schuman, E.M. (2004). Role for a cortical input to hippocampal area CA1 in the consolidation of long-term memory. *Nature* 43, 699-703.

Rempel-Clower, N.L., Zola, S.M., Squire, L.R., Amaral, D.G. (1996). Three cases of enduring memory impairment after bilateral damage limited to the hippocampal formation. *J. Neurosci.* 16, 5233-5255.

Rugg, M.D., Fletcher, P.C., Frith, C.D., Frackowiak, R.S.J., Dolan, R.J. (1996). Differential activation of the prefrontal cortex in successful and unsuccessful memory retrieval. *Brain* 119, 2073-2083.

Ryan, L., Nadel, L., Keil, K., Putnam, K., Schnyer, D., Trouard, T., Moscovich, M. (2001). Hippocampal complex and retrieval of recent and very remote autobiographical memories: evidence from functional magnetic resonance imaging in neurologically intact people. *Hippocampus* 11, 707-714.

Schacter, D.L., Curran, T., Galluccio, L., Milberg, W.P., Bates, J.F. (1996a). False recognition and the right frontal lobe: a case study. *Neuropsychologia* 34, 793-808.

Schacter, D.L., Alpert, N.M., Savage, C.R., Rauch, S.L., Albert M.S. (1996b). Conscious recollection and the human hippocampal formation: evidence from positron emission tomography. *Proc. Natl. Acad. Sci. USA* 93, 321-325.

Scoville, W.B., Milner, B. (1957). Loss of recent memory after bilateral hippocampal lesions. *J. Neurol. Neurosurg. Psychiatry* 20, 11-20.

Shah, N.J., Marshall, J.C., Zafiris, O., Schwab, A., Zilles, K., Markowitsch, H.J., Fink, G.R. (2001). The neural correlates of person familiarity: A functional magnetic resonance imaging study with clinical implications. *Brain* 124, 804-815.

Shallice, T., Fletcher, P., Frith, C.D., Grasby, P., Frackowiak, R.S., Dolan, R.J. (1994). Brain regions associated with acquisition and retrieval of verbal episodic memory. *Nature* 368, 633-635.

Smith, A.P., Henson, R.N., Dolan, R.J., Rugg, M.D. (2004). FMRI correlates of the episodic retrieval of emotional contexts. *Neuroimage* 22, 868-878.

Squire, L.R. (1992). Memory and the hippocampus: a synthesis from findings with rats, monkeys, and humans. *Psychol. Rev.* 99, 195-231.

Squire, L.R. (1998). Memory systems. *CR Acad. Sci. III* 321, 153-156.

Squire, L.R., Knowlton, B.J. (2000). The medial temporal lobe, the hippocampus, and memory systems of the brain. In: M.S. Gazzaniga (Ed.), *The New Cognitive Neurosciences* (pp. 765-779). Cambridge, MA: MIT.

Squire, L.R., Zola-Morgan, S. (1991). The medial temporal lobe memory system. *Science* 253, 1380-1386.

Squire, L.R., Zola, S.M. (1996). Structure and function of declarative and nondeclarative memory systems. *Proc. Natl. Acad. Sci. USA* 93, 13515-13522.

Stuss, D.T., Alexander, M.P., Palumbo, C.L., Buckle, L., Sayer, L., Pogue, J. (1994). Organizational strategies of patients with unilateral or bilateral frontal lobe injury in word list learning tasks. *Neuropsychology* 8, 355-373.

Sugiura, M., Shah, N.J., Zilles, K., Fink, G.R. (2005). Cortical representations of personally-familiar objects and places: functional organization of the human posterior cingulate cortex. *J. Cogn. Neurosci.* 17, 183-198.

Tononi, G. (2005). Consciousness, information integration, and the brain. *Progr. Brain Res.* 150, 109-126.

Tulving, E., (1972). Episodic and semantic memory. In: E. Tulving, W. Donaldson (Eds.), *Organization of Memory* (pp. 381-403). New York: Academic Press.

Tulving, E. (1983). Elements of Episodic Memory. Oxford: Claredon Press.

Tulving, E. (1995). Organization of memory: Quo vadis? In: M.S. Gazzaniga (Ed.), *The Cognitive Neurosciences* (pp. 839-847). Cambridge, MA: MIT Press.

Tulving, E., Markowitsch, H.J. (1998). Episodic and declarative memory: Role of the hippocampus. *Hippocampus* 8, 198-204.

Tulving, E., Kapur, S., Craik, F.I.M., Moscovitch, M., Houle, S. (1994). Hemispheric encoding/retrieval asymmetry in episodic memory: Positron emission tomography findings. *Proc. Natl. Acad. Sci.* 91, 2016-2020.

Valenstein, E., Bowers, D., Verfaellie, M., Heilman, K M., Day, A., Watson, R.T. (1987). Retrosplenial amnesia. *Brain* 110, 1631-1646.

Vanderkerckhove, M.M., Markowitsch, H.J., Mertens, M., Woermann, F.G. (2005). Bi-hemispheric engagement in the retrieval of autobiographical episodes. *Behav. Neurol.* 16, 20-210.

Vargha-Khadem, F., Gadian, D.G., Watkins, K.E., Connelly, A., Van Paesschen, W., Mishkin, M. (1997). Differential effects of early hippocampal pathology on episodic and semantic memory. *Science* 277, 376-380.

Viard, A., Piolino, P., Desgranges, B., Chetelat, G., Lebreton, K., Landeau, B., Young, A., de la Sayette, V., Eustache, F. (2007). Hippocampal activation for autobiographical memories over the entire lifetime in healthy aged subjects. An fMRI study. *Cereb. Cortex*, epub ahead of print.

Vogeley, K., Bussfeld, P., Newen, A., Herrmann, S., Happe, F., Falkai, P., Maier, W., Shah, N.J., Fink, G.R., Zilles, K. (2001). Mind reading: neural mechanisms of theory of mind and self-perspective. *Neuroimage* 14, 170-181.

Vogt, B.A., Laureys, S. (2005). Posterior cingulate, precuneal, and retrosplenial cortices: cytology and components of the neural network correlates of consciousness. *Prog. Brain Res.* 150, 205-217.

Wager, T.D., Smith, E.E. (2003). Neuroimaging studies of working memory: a meta-analysis. *Cogn Affect Behav Neurosci* 3, 255-274.

Walker, A.E. (1957). Recent memory impairment in unilateral temporal lesions. *Arch. Neurol. Psychiatry* 78, 543-552.

Zola-Morgan, S., Squire, L.R., Amaral, D.G. (1986). Human amnesia and the medial temporal region: enduring memory impairment following a bilateral lesion to field CA1 of the hippocampus. *J. Neurosci.* 6, 2959-2967.

Zysset, S., Huber, O., Samson, A., Ferstl, E.C., von Cramon, D.Y. (2003). Functional specialization within the anterior medial prefrontal cortex: a functional magnetic resonance imaging study with human subjects. *Neurosci. Lett.* 335, 183-186.

In: Brain Mapping Research Progress
Editors: Ines C. Girard and Jade S. Andre

ISBN: 978-1-60456-784-7

Chapter VII

Brain Electric Source Imaging by an Iterative Correlation Matrix Based Multiple Signal Classification Approach

Dezhong Yao*
Perception-Motor Interaction Laboratory, School of Life Science and Technology,
University of Electronic Science and Technology of China,
Chengdu 610054, PR China

Abstract

How to localize the neural electric activities effectively and precisely from the scalp EEG recordings is a critical issue for clinical neurology and cognitive neuroscience. In the 1980s and 1990s, suggested approaches included the dipole localization, cortical imaging, scalp Laplacian and 3D tomography. The 3D tomography may be realized by a direct linear inversion, or an indirect algorithm such as the subspace projection scanning method named MUltiple SIgnal Classification (MUSIC). However, the classical MUSIC algorithm is limited for its assumption of random noise. In this work, we propose to use a delay-correlation matrix instead of the previous zero-delay-correlation matrix in the signal-subspace estimate of the MUSIC algorithm to get a better performance over a spatial coherent but temporal random noisy disturbance. Then an Iterative application of the Delay-correlation MUSIC (IDM) is emphasized to derive a reasonable reconstruction of the multi-sources. The present simulation and empirical data experiment show that final promising results are obtained.

Keywords: Electroencephalography; inverse algorithm; delay correlation; multiple signal classification (MUSIC); subspace correlation; computer simulation; evoked potential; iteration

---

* E-mail: dyao@uestc.edu.cn, www.neuro.uestc.edu.cn

Introduction

Noninvasive measurements of human brain functions have been attracting much interest. Such measurements often use various kinds of sensory stimuli, especially when measuring higher-order cognitive functions or identifying brain dysfunction. Among the different modalities that provide functional brain images, electroencephalogram (EEG) has a distinct characteristic that it can provide a temporal resolution less than 1 ms at a much less cost than the Positron Emission Topography (PET) or functional Magnetic Resonance Imaging (fMRI) and magnetoencephalography (MEG).

Recently, a considerable amount of effort has been made in the development of EEG–based source imaging and multi-sources localization techniques. Representative approaches in source-imaging include the low resolution electromagnetic topography (LORETA) [Pascual-Marqui et al., 1994; Yao et al., 1998; Yao et al, 2001b; Xu et al, 2007], scalp Laplacian [Yao, 2002a, 2002b] and the cortical imaging techniques [Sidman et al., 1992; Gevins et al., 1993; Srebro, 1993; Nunez et al., 1994; Yao et al., 1995, 1996, 2004a, 2004b].

Multi-sources localization from scalp-recorded EEGs provides quantitative three-dimensional information regarding electrical activities inside the brain, and it can be formulated in terms of finding a least-squares fit of a set of current dipoles with the observed data. A fundamental problem is that the least-squares cost function is highly non-convex with respect to the locations of the dipoles. Consequently, inverse methods such as gradient–based optimization or nonlinear simplex searches often become trapped in local minimums, yielding significant localization errors [Miltner et al., 1994; Supek et al., 1997a; Huang et al., 1998]. One of the attempt to overcome the difficulty of the least-squares fit is the application of the MUltiple SIgnal Classification (MUSIC) algorithm into EEG/MEG inverse problem [Schmidt, 1986; Mosher et al., 1992]. The canonical MUSIC-based EEG inverse algorithm localizes the multi-sources with a procedure in which a single dipole is scanned through a grid confined to a three-dimensional (3-D) head volume conductor. At each point on this grid, the forward model (transfer matrix) of a dipole at this grid point is projected against a signal subspace that has been estimated with the EEG/MEG data. The locations on this grid where the source model gives the best projections onto the signal subspace correspond to the dipole locations [Mosher et al., 1992]. The scanning manipulation instead of the non-linear multi-sources search makes it very attractive to the peers [Supek et al., 1997b]. However, the Canonical MUSIC (CM) algorithm suffers from two limitations (Yao et al., 1999): 1) the data are corrupted by additive spatial white noise; 2) the algorithm is based on the assumption that the data are generated by a set of asynchronous dipolar sources. To breakthrough these limitations, a few improvements have been made in recent years (Yao et al. 2000, 2001a). The nonwhite noise problem has been investigated under an assumption that the covariance of the background noise is known or it can be estimated [Soong et al., 1995; Sekihara et al., 1997, 1998], and a Recursive MUSIC (RM) was proposed to proceed synchronous activities [Mosher et al., 1998]. In the RM, the recorded EEGs are considered to be a sum of contributions from a fixed number of spatio-temporal independent topographies (IT), each IT being considered to be a source comprising one or more fixed dipoles which collectively have a single time-course.

In this work, a Delay MUSIC (DM) (Yao et al. 2000) based on a non-zero delay-correlation matrix instead of the CM on a zero-delay-correlation matrix is proposed as a novel algorithm for extracting the multi-sources from data corrupted by spatial coherent noise. And an Iterative/alternative idea is emphasized in the application of the DM (IDM) (Yao et al. 2001a) to get a promising result in practice.

IDM Algorithm

DM Algorithm

The EEGs may be formulated as the following mathematical model:

$$y(t) = A(L)x(t) + e(t), t = 1,...., N \tag{1}$$

where, $y(t) \in R^{M\times1}$ are the scalp recording potentials, M is the number of electrodes, $x(t) \in R^{L\times1}$ are the multi-sources inside the brain, and L is the number of sources, $e(t) \in R^{M\times1}$ are the noise which stem from environmental noise and random spontaneous electrical activities. A(L) is the transfer matrix accomplishing the transfer from the sources to the scalp electrodes, which is decided by the head model.

We may express the delay-correlation matrix of the scalp recordings as (Yao et al., 2000)

$$R(\beta) = < y(t)y^T(t+\beta) > = AP(\beta)A^T + W(\beta) \tag{2}$$

where $P(\beta) = < x(t)x^T(t+\beta) >, W(\beta) = < e(t)e^T(t+\beta) >$, T represents matrix transfer. β ranges from zero (CM) to other desired non-zero value (DM).

Suppose the following three notes hold for our problems:

Note 1: M>L , so rank(A)=L.

Note 2: Suppose the data is the evoked potential(EP) or evoked field(EF), and the main noise is the spontaneous EEG/MEG, then the delay correlation of the signal (EP/EF) will be much better than that of the noise. So β may be chosen approximately as the minimum delay corresponding to the zero-level delay correlation of the noise, hence equation (2) simplifies to

$$R = APA^T, W(\beta) = 0 \tag{3}$$

Note 3: The sources may be independent of each other, then we derive rank(P)=L, $rank(APA^T) = L$ [Mosher et al., 1992; Supek et al., 1997b; Yao et al., 1999]. If some of the multi-dipoles are synchronous, each synchronous set should be grouped as an "integrated source", i.e., an " independent topographies(IT)" model, then rank(P)=L_1<L,

$rank(APA^T) = L_1 < L$ [Mosher et al., 1998]. If some of the multi-dipoles are partly synchronous, we get rank(P)=L_2<=L, $rank(APA^T) = L_2 <= L$. Obviously, the first two are particular cases of the partly synchronous source model.

We may decompose the correlation matrix R as

$$R = U\Sigma V^T \tag{4}$$

where $\Sigma = diag[\lambda_1,...,\lambda_M]$, λ_i is the eigenvalues of the correlation matrix R, and $\lambda_i > 0, i = 1,..., L_s; \lambda_i \approx 0, i = L_s + 1,..., M$. The orthogonal matrix U and V are formed by the associated eigenvectors. Based on the eignevalues, the orthogonal matrix U or V may be decomposed into two parts, for example $U = [S \mid G] = [u_1,..,u_{L_s} \quad u_{L_s+1},...,u_M]$. The spans of the columns of matrix $S = [u_1,..,u_{L_s}]$ and matrix $G = [u_{Ls+1},...,u_M]$ are respectively called the signal subspace and the noise subspace. In theory, Ls should be one of the L, L_1 or L_2.

If the dipoles are independent of each other, we may calculate the Subspace Correlation(SC) between the subspaces spanned by the matrix S and transfer matrix A_i corresponding to a dipole at a grid point. The distribution of the SC or its function over a discrete grid of the solution space will show us the source locations [Mosher et al., 1992]. If the dipoles can be separated into a few independent synchronous set, i.e. a few IT models, the RM may be used, where the SC is between the subspaces spanned by the matrix S and transfer matrix A_{IT} [Mosher et al., 1998]. For the partly synchronous sources model, the following IDM may be used, where the SC is between the subspaces spanned by the matrix S and transfer matrix A_g, and the A_g is the transfer matrix of the partly synchronous sources configuration. In the IDM, not only the synchronous dipoles collectively with a single time-course but also the dipoles with a few partly synchronous time-courses are "grouped" as an " integrated source".

The subspace correlations(SC) are defined as

$$\{c_1, c_2,...\} = subcorr\{A_*, S\} \tag{5}$$

where the A_* may either be the A_i or A_{IT} or A_g. $\{c_1,...c_r\}$ are the ordered set of the SC, $1>=c_1>=...>=c_r>=0$, between the two subspaces spanned by the matrix A_* and matrix S.

The steps of computing the subspace correlations may be found in references [Golub et al., 1984; Mosher et al., 1998]. In practice, which to choose in the set $\{c_1,...c_r\}$ as the imaging metric still remains as a problem. Our opinion is stated in the following IDM algorithm (Yao et al., 2001a).

IDM Algorithm

IDM denotes an Iterative application of the Delay-correlation MUSIC algorithm. The steps are as follows:

(1) The delay-correlation matrix of the measured spatio-temporal data is calculated by $R = E\{yy^T(\beta)\}$, where β is decided by a prior judgement about the delay correlation of the signal and the noise or by a trial and error. If the noise is assumed to be white time-course noise, β =1.

(2) Singular Value Decomposition(SVD) of the matrix R performs as $R = U\Sigma V^T$, and the signal subspace is assumed being spanned by the eigenvectors correspond to the nonzero eigenvalues, and the number of the nonzero-level eigenvalues is called the Signal Subspace Dimensionality(SSD).

(3) Create a relatively dense grid of dipolar source locations in the solution space. In this work, a grid ranging from z=0.0 to z=0.80 with grid size 0.1 are created in the brain volume conductor (the solution space) whose surface radius is 1.0 and the total grid number is 1509.

(4) For index starts at 1.

(5) Let $G = [A_{*(1)}, A_{*(2)},..., A_{*(index-1)}]$ be the transfer matrix of the sources extracted out of the previous loops (It is a null matrix for the first loop).

(6) For index, concatenate the transfer matrix $A_{g(index)}$ (the A_i and A_{IT} are considered to be special cases of the A_g) to the present extracted model, $W = [G, A_{g(index)}]$. Calculate the subspace correlations(SC), $\{c_1, c_2, ...\} = subcorr\{W, S\}$.

(7) If c_{l-1} has been unit 1.0 (supposing l=1 and $c_{l-1}= c_0=1.0$ for the first loop), check the maximum of the c_l in the ordered set of the SC and the distribution map of the c_l or its function over the discrete grid of the solution space. If the maximum is closely enough to unit 1.0, and the map "clearly and simplely" shows local activities, they may be explained as effective activities. If the SC c_l has been used as the imging metric in the previous loops, i.e. the l is the same as that in these previous loops, the new identified activities is interpreted as (partly) synchronous activities with the sources which are extracted by the SC c_l in the previous loops; If the SC c_l has not been used in the previous loops, for example, the c_l in the first loop, the new identified local activities is interpreted as independent sources. If the c_l =1.0, let l=l+1. Finally let index=index+1, and back to step 5). If the map is blurred, there may be two reasons, one of which is that the source model of the A_g is simpler than the actual model, hence we should try a more complex model such as two dipolar sources instead of one dipolar source or three dipolar sources instead of two dipolar sources, etc. In such case, we should keep the index without change, and back to step 5) to start a new calculation with the new transfer matrix A_g. The other reason is that the next dipoles are asynchronous with the extracted sources. In such event, c_l to c_l mainly represent the SC of the previous extracted sources, then we should check the next SC c_{l+1}. If the maximum of the c_{l+1} is closely enough to unit 1.0, and the map of

the c_{l+1} or its function "clearly and simplely" shows local activities, the local activities is explained as new "independent sources", then let index=index+1, l=l+1, and back to step 5). If the actual "new independent sources" is an "integrated sources" with a more complex sources configuration, we should keep the index without change, and back to step 5) and increase the complexity of the transfer matrix A_g to start a new calculation. If both c_l and c_{l+1} can not give us any more reasonable source information through a trial and error, proceed to step 8). Apparently, l is a number without relation to the index and the source number. It is the number of the correlation coefficients of the SC that are equal to 1.0 or closely enough to 1.0.

(8) stop;

Obviously, the practice of the IDM is an interactive process between the man's assumption and the scanning results. In such sense, the "iterative" in the IDM is a more general concept than the "recursive" in the RM [Mosher et al., 1998]. The detail interactive process will be illustrated clearly in the following simulation and empirical data tests.

Besides, to get a reasonable reconstruction of the actual sources, there are a few problems to be considered in practice. First, the SSD should be carefully chosen. In theory, it is the number of independent sources, but, for a noisy data especially for a data corrupted by spatial coherent noise as shown in the following numeric tests, it had better to be chosen as a larger number than the actual independent signal number. In our practice, it is decided by the distribution of the singular values and assumed being the number of the non-zero level singular values, i.e. SSD=L_s, which is always equal to or larger than the L or L_1 or L_2.

The second is about the optimization of the sources assemblage with more than one dipolar source. The scanning of all the combinatories is a multidimensional search similar to the non-linear least-squares algorithm, and a random subset of the possible combinations is used in the RM[Mosher et al., 1998]. In this work, a similar subset search is utilized, however, the obtained scanning results are emphasized to be used as a prior information for choosing the next subset and searching region.

Finally, we'd like to point out the difference of the definitions of G in the IDM and RM. The whole transfer matrix of the sources extracted in the previous loops is concatenated to the current G in the IDM, it means that only the locations of the extracted sources are used as prior information in searching the next source(s) location. However, in the RD, both the dipole locations and orientations of the extracted sources are used as prior information in searching the next source(s), accordingly, where G is defined as $G=[a_{i(1)},a_{i(2)},..,a_{i(index-1)}]$, with $a_{i(k)}=A_{i(k)}\hat{u}_k$, $\hat{u}_k$ is the obtained unit dipole-orientation vector [Mosher et al.,1998]. In our numeric tests, we find that the reconstruction of location is more robust than that of orientation, and a wrong orientation of a extracted dipole may result in an ill reconstruction of the next source. So in our IDM algorithm, the orientations of the extracted dipoles are allowed of further adjustment with the new sources together. Another difference between the RM and IDM is that, in the RM, the extracted model is assumed to be fixed, and if the first one is wrong, the later will be influenced [Koles, 1998], while in the IDM, we may fix the later extracted sources and optimize the former sources again, therefore a more general "iterative" idea is involved in the IDM through the interaction between man's guess and the recursive application of the DM.

Computer Simulation

Simulation Method

Volume Conductor Model and Electrode Configuration

The concentric three-spheres head model is used to represent the head volume conductor [Rush et al., 1969]. The radii of the brain, the skull, and the scalp spheres are taken as 0.87,0.92 and 1.0, respectively. The conductivity of the scalp and the brain is taken as 1.0, and that of the skull as 0.0125. The number of the scalp electrode is 120, and the configuration is derived from the Neuro SCAN electrode configuration projecting on the best-fit and normalized spherical surface of the group averaged head model over 10 subjects. About the Cartesian coordinate system of the Neuro SCAN electrode configuration, the midpoint between the left and right preauricular points is defined as the coordinate origin. The axis directed away from the origin toward the left preauricular point is defined as the +y axis, and that from the origin to the nasion is the +x axis. The +z axis is defined as the axis that is perpendicular to both these axes and directed from the origin to the vertex.

Signal Model

The time-course is supposed to be a Gaussian function modulated by a sine function, the waveform is controlled by adjusting the parameters [Yao et al., 1999]. The function is

$$f(t) = \exp(-(2\pi f_m (t - t_0)/\gamma)^2)\cos(2\pi f_m (t - t_0) + v) \qquad (6)$$

Supposing dt=2ms,v=π/2, γ=3 and π=3.14159, the other parameters of source 1 used in the following simulation are f_m =5Hz, t_0=10*dt, and that of source 2 are f_m =15Hz, t_0=20*dt and that of source 3 are fm=10Hz, t_0=30*dt. The correlation coefficient between the source 1 and source 2 is –0.2925, and that between source 1 and source 3 is –0.0494. The total sample point is 150. In Figure 1 the three time-courses are shown.

Noise and Noise-Signal Ratio (NSR)

The time-course of the noise is white Gaussian. The spatial white (incoherent) noise denotes that the noise for each channel is generated independently, and the spatial color (coherent) noise means that the noise is same for all the 120 channels. The noise-signal ratio(NSR) is defined as the ratio of the squared Frobenius norm of the noise matrix to the squared Frobenius norm of the noiseless signal matrix.

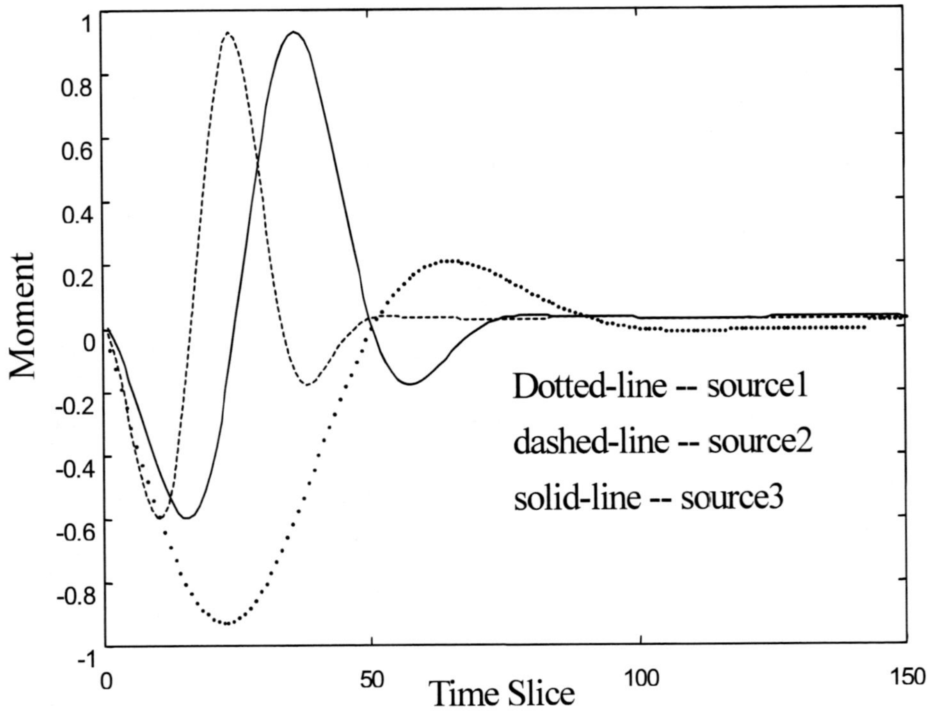

Figure 1. Time-courses of the simulated electrical generators.

Normalized Blurring Index (NBI)

A NBI of a function distribution is defined as to indicate the relative blurring level [Yao et al, 2001b; 1999), which is written as

$$NBI_i = \sqrt{\sum_k \|\vec{r}_k - \vec{r}_i\|^2 X^2(k) / \sum_k X^2(k)} \Big/ \sqrt{\sum_k \|\vec{r}_k - \vec{r}_i\|^2 / \sum_k 1} \tag{7}$$

where the order i denotes a grid point where the NBI is to be estimated and k denotes a grid point within a subregion of the point i, for example, within a subsphere originated at point i with radius equal to or smaller than 0.2. The $\vec{r}_i$ stands for the displacement of the grid point i. Apparently, if the distribution function X(k) is uniform in the subregion, the NBI will approach unit 1.0, and if the distribution is similar to a Dirc function $\delta(k-i)$, the NBI will approach to zero. Obviously, a smaller NBI is preferred in EEG inverse problem. Here the imaging metric X is defined as $X = 1./\sqrt{1.001 - c_l^2}$ in simulation study and $X = 1./(1.001 - c_l^2)$ for empirical data test, where the 0.001 is introduced to remove the singular point when c_l=1.0. The c_l is the SC explained in the last section.

Simulation Results

The CM algorithm has been tested by a few authors [Supek et al., 1997; Yao et al., 2002]. Here the simulation will emphasize on the following items.

Effect of the SSD and the Delay

The signal-subspace estimate is the crux of the MUSIC-based algorithm. After the data acquisition, the remaining problems will be the selections of the delay parameter β and SSD. The signal subspace is spanned by eigenvectors associated with the non-noise level eigenvalues where the number of the non-noise level eigenvalues is believed to be the signal number [Schmidt, 1986]. However, due to the limited data length, low signal/noise ratio, the breakpoint between the noise level and non-noise level eignevalues is blurred, and because the (partly) synchronous sources and distributed source nature instead of the dipolar source model, it is difficult to determine the SSD in EEG inverse practice [Mosher et al.,1992; Greenblatt, 1993; Knosche, 1997]. In the following simulation, β=0(CM) and β=1(DM), SSD=2~6 are taken.

Supposing two radial asynchronous dipoles are located at (-0.3 -0.4 0.7) and (0.3 -0.4 0.7), whose time-courses are source 1 and source 2. The minimum delays are 1, 31 and 8 corresponding to the white time-course noise, source 1 and source 2, respectively, so β=1 is selected in the practice of the DM.

Table 1. Singular value distribution

	1	2	3	4	5	6
CM 0%	1.181794	0.546704	0	0	0	0
CM 10%nc	1.182127	0.545491	0.00477	0.000465	0.000438	0.000433
CM 10%c	1.183096	0.546621	0.012800	0	0	0
CM 80%nc	1.200860	0.551688	0.030564	0.029774	0.028000	0.027747
CM 80%c	1.550651	0.830970	0.411151	0	0	0
DM 0%	1.187160	0.539090	0	0	0	0
DM 10%nc	1.187320	0.537738	0.000313	0.000287	0.000280	0.000277
DM 10%c	1.186150	0.536900	0.000889	0	0	0
DM 80%nc	1.195314	0.533601	0.020022	0.018361	0.017963	0.017751
DM 80%c	1.172151	0.517173	0.059794	0	0	0

CM-Canonical MUSIC, DM –Delay MUSIC ; c- spatial coherent noise; nc – spatial non-coherent noise.

Table 1 shows the first six singular values of the delay-correlation matrix when different noise is added to the signal. Based on Table 1, actual rank 2 is revealed in results of the CM in cases of white spatial noises and in cases of spatial color noises with small NSR, and in results of the DM in all cases. Figure 2 shows the NBI of the reconstructed imaging maps, which is calculated around the known actual source locations, and the result is the average of the results on the two source locations. On the Figure, only the results of SSD=2 and 6 are shown, because the results from SSD=3 to 6 are similar to one another. Figure 3 shows the source imaging maps plotted according to the metric $X = 1./\sqrt{1.001 - c_1^{\ 2}}$ when SSD=2, 3 and 6, where only the maps on slice with z=0.7 are shown for saving space.They are reconstructed by the CM and DM when different noise in type and content is added.

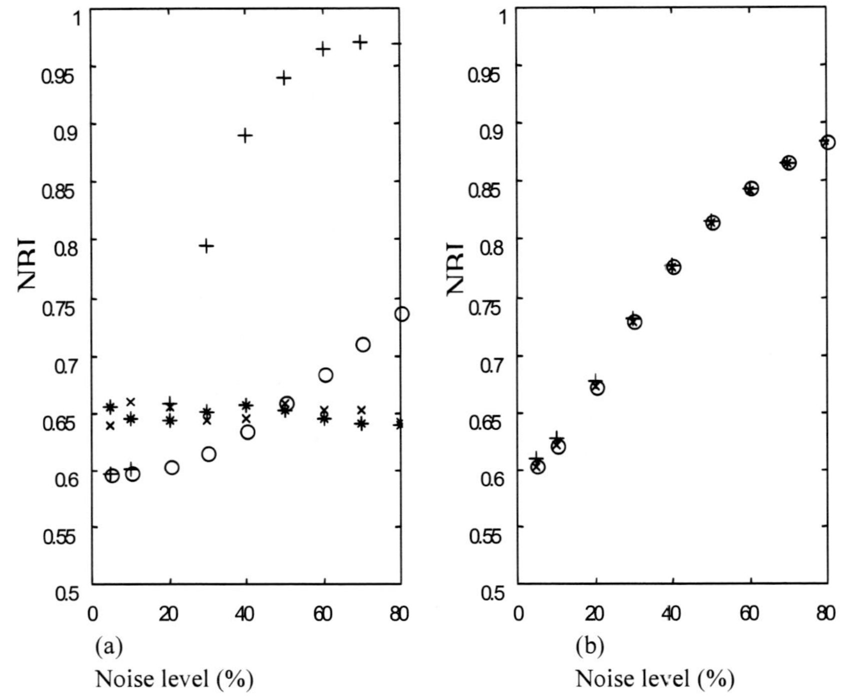

Figure 2. Normalized blurring index(NBI). The left figure corresponds to spatial coherent (color) noise, and the right figure corresponds to spatial incoherent (white) noise. O—DM, SSD=2; x—DM , SSD=6; + --NM, SSD=2; * --NM , SSD=6.

For spatial coherent noise, as shown by the point-curves (o,x) in Figure 2(a) and Figure 3(1,5,9,13,17), the DM conducts a very robust reconstruction no matter the rank is chosen equal to (2) or larger than (3,6) the true rank (2). The CM with the true rank 2 is sensitive to the NSR level as shown by the point-curve (+) in Figure 2(a) and Figure 3(3,7,11). When the NSR is equal to or larger than 50%, one source is missed (Figure 3(7,11)). However, if a larger rank (3,6) than the true rank (2) is chosen, the results of the CM are almost the same as that of the DM (the point-curve (*) in Figure 2(a) and Figure 3(15,19)).

For spatial incoherent noise, the performance of the CM and DM is similar to each other no matter the rank is equal to (2) or larger than (3,6) the true rank (2) (Figure 2(b), Figure 3(2,6,10,14,18) and Figure 3(4,8,12,16,20)). The differences among the Figure 3(2,6,10,14,18; 4,8,12,16,20) are due to the random spatial coherence of the white time-course noise. The random spatial coherence is almost equivalent to both the DM and CM, and this fact is shown by the wide singular value distribution of both the DM and CM (Table 1, *%nc). Besides, for the spatial incoherent noise, the imaging maps (Figure 3) shown again that nearly identical results are obtained with true or over-selected rank [Mosher et al., 1998; Supek et al., 1997b] and the larger the NSR is, the worse the map is [Yao et al., 2002].

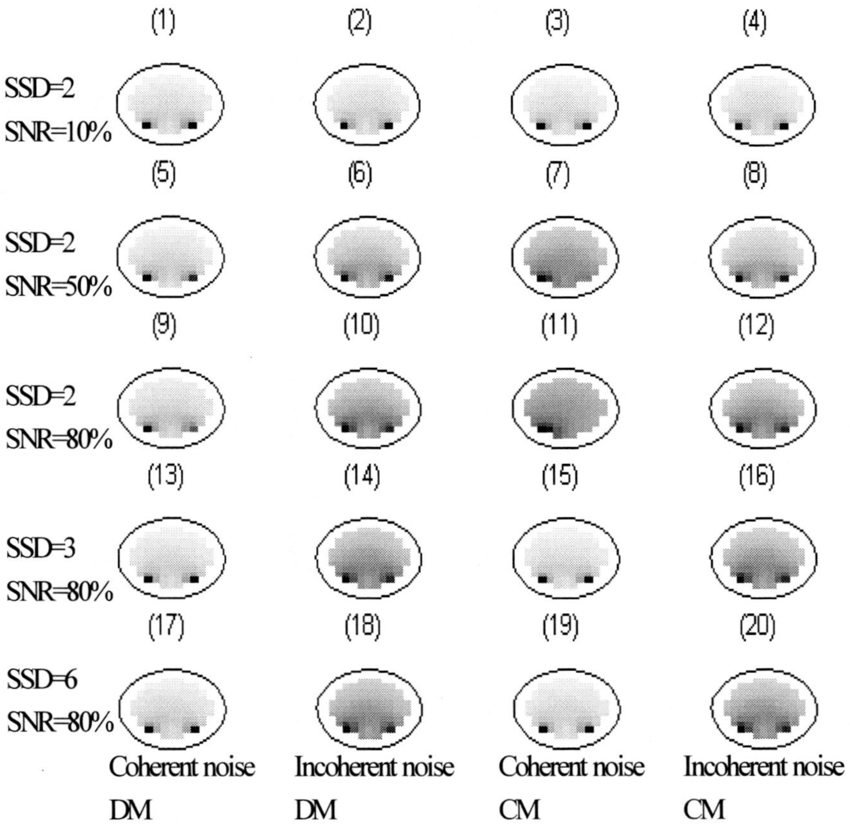

Figure 3. Maps of the metric $X = 1./(1.001 - c_1^{\ 2})$. The results are for slice with z=0.7 under different noise level, noise type (coherent/incoherent) and different SSD and method (CM/DM).

For the spatial coherent noise, due to its white time-course nature, it is depressed by the delay correlation no matter the content of the noise, and so the DM shows a very robust reconstruction when different NSR and SSD are involved. The bad performance, Figure 3(7,11), of the CM with true rank (2) is due to that the spatial coherent noise acts as a " signal" in the zero-delay-correlation matrix. In fact, rank 3 is implicated by the singular values (Table 1, CM 80%c). It means that the signal subspace should be spanned by its first three eigenvectors because these three eigenvectors can not be further divided into two groups with the first two pertaining to the "signal" and the third to the "coherent noise ". The similar performance between the CM with rank SSD=3 to 6 and DM may be due to that the extended signal subspace guarantees that the whole signal-subspace information is included. So on one hand, we can prove the subspace correlation between the actual source transfer matrix and the signal subspace. On the other hand, the noise subspace spanned by eigenvectors over-included by a larger SSD than the true rank does not correlate with an actual transfer matrix. It means that an over-selected eigenvectors do not change much of the correlation between the transfer matrix of a dipole at a grid point and the signal subspace.

Concretely, for the spatial coherent noise used here, though it acts like a "signal" in the zero-delay correlation as shown by the singular values of the " CM 80%c" in Table 1, it is not a dipole field, and it can not be extracted by the dipole scanning. Therefore, though a larger rank (3 to 6) is chosen, the resultant source number still is 2 (Figure 3). Finally, if the spatial coherent noise is not same in each channel, it can be considered as a combination of a spatial coherent noise and incoherent noise, and the results will be an intermediate state [Yao et al., 2002].

In summary, when the noise is spatially incoherent and the SSD is equal to or larger than the true rank, the performance of the CM and DM is similar to each other. If the noise is spatially coherent, the DM is very effective when a proper β is selected, the result of the CM pertaining to over-selected rank is better than that to true rank. So the DM and the CM with an over-selected SSD are more effective in repressing the spatial coherent noise than the CM with true rank. These results suggest that for data corrupted by unknown noise type, the DM is prefer to the CM, and an over-selected SSD is not a compromise [Mosher et al., 1998] but a necessary choice. Nevertheless, it can results in some false activities that the random subspace correlation (SC) between the transfer matrix of some grid-points and the "signal subspace" originated from an over selected SSD, so we do not commend that the larger the rank is, the better the result is. We choose the SSD based on the singular value distribution, and we believe that a trial and error is necessary in the choice of a proper SSD in some practices.

IDM Identifies Synchronous Activities

Supposing that there are three sources. One radial dipole locates at (0.0 0.0 0.6) with the source 1 time-course. The other two synchronous radial sources locate at (-0.3 –0.3 0.6) and (0.3 0.3 0.6) with the same source 3 time-course. The noise is the spatial coherent noise with NSR=80%. $\beta=1$ is used in the IDM because of the white time-course of the noise. The first six singular values are 1.153057, 0.066178, 0.010905, 0.0, 0.0, 0.0, they imply SSD=1~3. We choose SSD=3, and starting scanning with $W=A_i$, we get Figure 4(a). The maximum is $c_1=1.0$, which is located at the (0.0 0.0 0.6). Then after scanning the second dipole with $W=(A_{i(0.0,\ 0.0,\ 0.6)}(\text{extracted}), A_i)$, we get figure 4(b), and its corresponding second maximum $c_2=0.974$ is at (0.1 0.2 0.0). Though the 0.974 is larger than the recommended criterion 0.95[Mosher et al., 1998], the map of the metric X is quite blurred which implicitly means the second dipole is not an independent dipole, so we start a two-dipoles scanning with $W=(A_{i(0.0,\ 0.0,\ 0.6)}(\text{extracted}), A_i\ (\text{fixed}), A_i)$. We try to find some prior information from Figure 4(b). It is clear that there is a seriously deep blurred region and then is a "two sources" projection on slices z=0.6 and z=0.7. These facts implicitly tell us that the seriously blurred region should be an "equivalent source region" of two or more dipoles. And the actual dipoles may be within a sub-region around slices z=0.6 and z=0.7. We choose the maximum point on slices z=0.6 and 0.7 as the A_i(fixed), which is at (0.1 0.0 0.6) with $c_2=0.9536$, and we define a smaller scanning region which is composed by slices from z=0.5 to z=0.8. After a two-dipoles scanning with $W=(A_{i(0.0,\ 0.0,\ 0.6)}(\text{extracted}), A_i\ (\text{fixed}), A_i)$, we choose the grid point where the maximum c_2 located at as the new A_i(fixed).

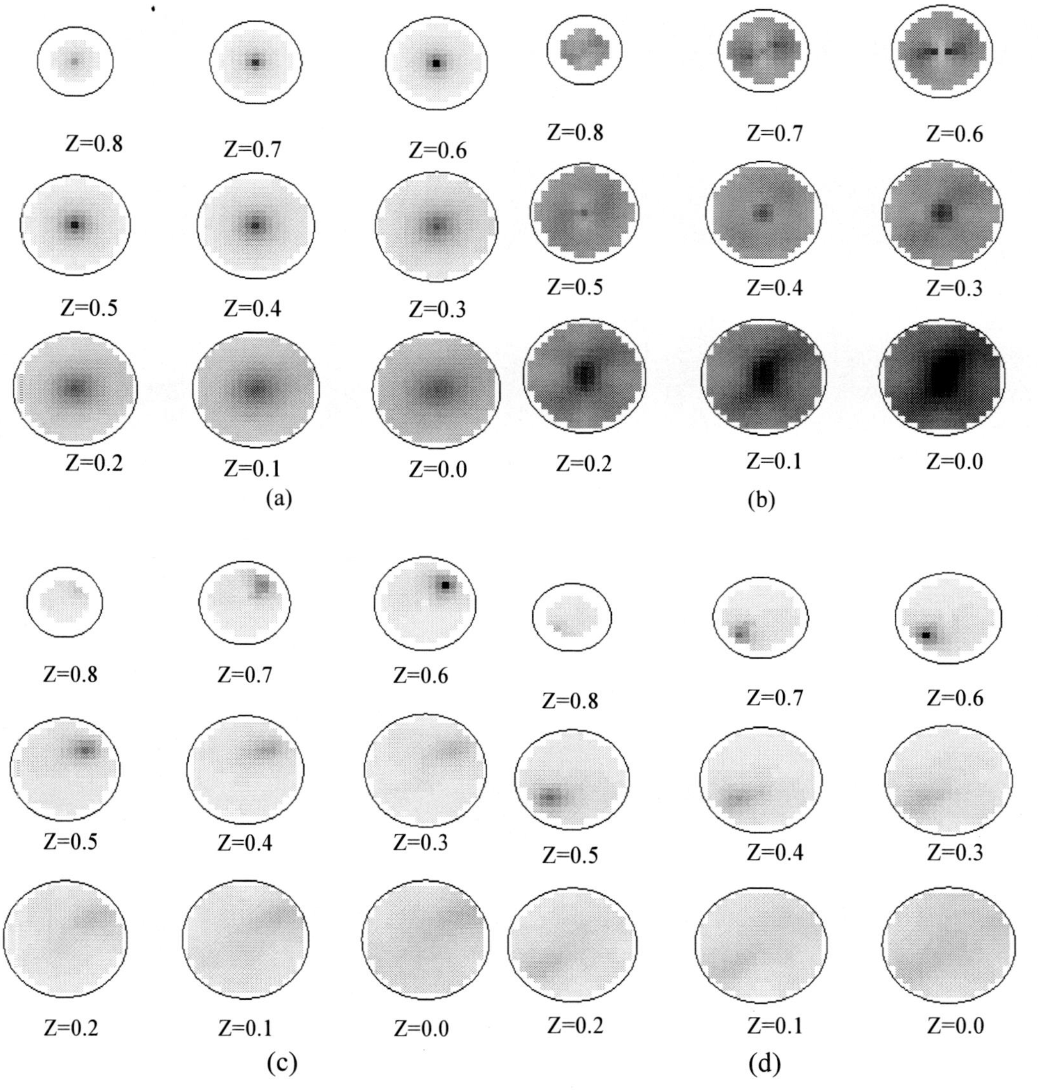

Figure 4. Maps of the metric X. Each map is a distribution of the imaging metric on a transverse plane, and the corresponding z-axis value is shown under the map. (a) Map of the $X = 1./\sqrt{1.001 - c_1^{\ 2}}$ in an one-dipole scanning; (b) map of the $X = 1./\sqrt{1.001 - c_2^{\ 2}}$ in a scanning after a dipole is assumed at (0.0 0.0 0.6); (c) map of the $X = 1./\sqrt{1.001 - c_2^{\ 2}}$ in a two-dipoles scanning after a dipole is assumed at (0.0 0.0 0.6) and one of the two-dipoles is fixed at (-0.3 –0.3 0.6); (d) map of the $X = 1./\sqrt{1.001 - c_2^{\ 2}}$ in a two-dipoles scanning after a dipole is assumed at (0.0 0.0 0.6) and one of the two-dipoles is fixed at (0.3 0.3 0.6).

Repeating this process, finally, we find that a two-dipoles scanning with W=($A_{i(0.0,\ 0.0,\ 0.6)}$(extracted), $A_{i(0.3\ 0.3\ 0.6)}$(fixed), A_i) results in maximum c_2=1.0 at (-0.3 –0.3 0.6) (Figure 4(d)); and a two-dipoles scanning with W=($A_{i(0.0,\ 0.0,\ 0.6)}$(extracted), $A_{i(-0.3\ -0.3\ 0.6)}$(fixed), A_i) results in maximum c_2=1.0 at (0.3 0.3 0.6) (Figure 4(c)). The maps, Figure 4(c) and Figure

4(d), are "simple and clear" and distinctly different from the Figure 4(b). And that the maximum points on Figure 4(a,c,d) are consistent with the actual source locations.

Empirical Data Test

Evoked by a check-board flashed to the right visual field on the horizontal line, the visual ERP data are collected. The check-board used as stimuli is shown in Figure 5. Volunteers sit in a sofa 60cm from the monitor, and fix his eyes on a cross at the center of the monitor. The visual angle is from 1.5° to 4.5°. The inter-stimulus intervals (ISIs) are from 250-550ms. The data used here is the grand average data over 10 healthy right-handed subjects with a mean age of 24. Subjects had normal or rectified-to-normal visual acuity. Due to an unreasonable singular waveform, the channel 86 is rejected.

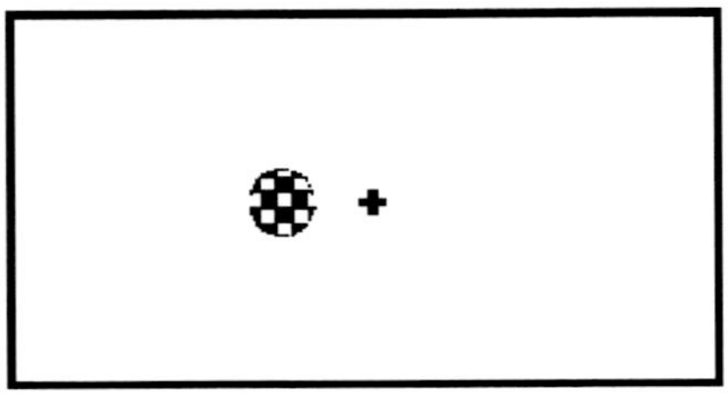

Figure 5. Visual stimulus pattern.

We are interested in source locations of the early visual electrical activities (t<160ms). Fig.6 shows scalp animations from post-stimuli 52ms to 140ms. It indicates three activities. They may be the C_1 before 80 ms on the visual cortex, and the P_1 after 60ms on left visual cortex and right visual cortex subsequently [Clark et al., 1995].

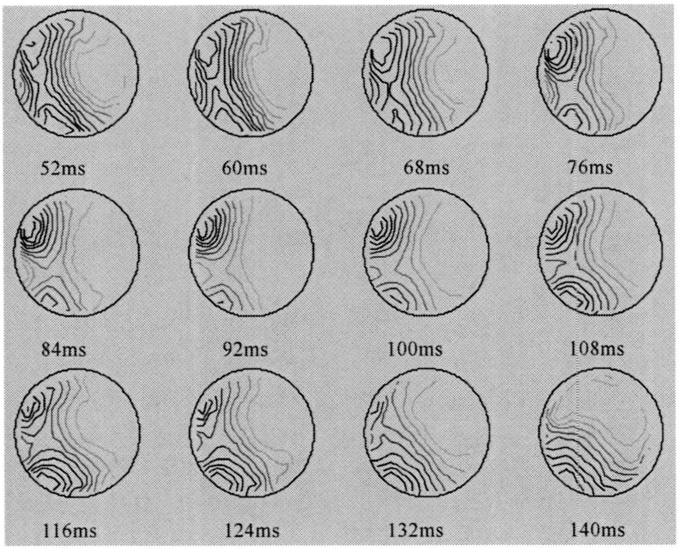

Figure 6. Successive scalp mapping from 52ms to 140ms poststimuli.

The first ten singular values of the delay-correlation matrix are 18.329, 10.3244, 0.40978, 0.2254, 0.18257, 0.09792, 0.05919, 0.03265, 0.02990, 0.02591. They hint two main signals and some small activities or distributed spontaneous activities in the data. Because there is not a clear breakpoint of the singular value distribution, we over-select SSD=5 and β=1.

We start scanning with W=A_i, and get the first maximum c_1=0.9903 located at the (-0.1 –0.1 0.6). However, the map, Figure 7(a), of the metric $X = 1./(1.001 - c_1^{\ 2})$ shows that there are two active regions. The other is centered on (-0.5 0.3 0.5) with c_1=0.9884. We note that these two active regions are the imaging result of the DM, and the active on the right visual cortex hinted by the animation, Figure 6, is lost. It means that the DM localizes fewer sources than the actual sources just as the CM does when synchronous sources existed [Supek et al., 1997; Mosher et al., 1998]. So an iterative search is necessary to improve the result of either the CM or the DM. Now, we choose the active on the left visual cortex centered on (-0.5 0.3 0.5) as the A_i(fixed), and do a scanning with W=($A_{i(-0.5,\ 0.3,\ 0.5)}$(fixed), A_i), we get the map of the metric $X = 1./(1.001 - c_1^{\ 2})$ (Figure 7(b)), which clearly shows an active on the right visual cortex centered on (-0.5 -0.5 0.5) with maximum c_1=0.9937, and we get a map of the metric $X = 1./(1.001 - c_2^{\ 2})$ (Figure 7(c)) with maximum c_2=0.9895 centered on (-0.1 0.0 0.6) — a point close the point (-0.1 –0.1 0.6). In order to affirm these three active regions, we choose the (-0.5 -0.5 0.5) as the A_i(fixed) , and get two activities centered on (-0.5 0.3 0.5) with c_1=0.9937 and on (-0.1 0.0 0.6) with c_1=0.9948 on the map of the metric $X = 1./(1.001 - c_1^{\ 2})$. And if the (-0.1 0.0 0.6) are chosen as the A_i(fixed), we get the maximum c_1=0.9949 at (-0.5 -0.5 0.5) and maximum c_2=0.9895 at (-0.5 0.3 0.5). These results repetitively affirm the three active regions centered on (-0.1 0.0 0.6), (-0.5 0.3 0.5) and (-0.5 -0.5 0.5). Their radii are 0.61, 0.77 and 0.87 in the unit sphere head model. These results are qualitatively consistent with the known early visual electrical generators, i.e. the early C_1, P_1 (left) and P_1 (right) [Clark et al., 1995]. However, the depth 1-0.61=0.39 of the C_1 is much deeper than the supposed region 17 and the depth 1-0.87=0.13 of the P_1 activity on the right visual cortex is shallower than the cortical surface. Such shortfalls may be due to the distributed nature of the actual sources, which is different from the dipole model used in the MUSIC scanning.

About the relations among the three activities, the activity centered on (-0.5 0.3 0.5) should be (partly) synchronous with the activity centered on (-0.5 -0.5 0.5), because when we choose one of them as the A_i(fixed), and do a scanning with W=(A_i(fixed), A_i), the other always appear on map of the c_1. It means that these two actives together respond to the SC c_1. The active centered on (-0.5 -0.5 0.5) should be (partly) synchronous with the active centered on (-0.1 0.0 0.6) due to the same reason. However, the actives centered on (-0.3 0.3 0.5) and (-0.1 0.0 0.6) should be asynchronous because both of them appear on the map of the metric X related to c_1 in the primary one dipole scanning (Figure 7(a)), and both them appear on the map of X related to c_1 when (-0.5 -0.5 0.5) is chosen as the A_i(fixed) . And because when one of them is chosen as the A_i(fixed), the other always appears on the map of the metric X related to c_2 . Based on these phenomena, the actives may be started in region centered on (-0.1 0.0 0.6). And then an (almost) independent active appears on the left visual cortex centered on (-0.5 0.3 0.5) (the stimuli is on the right visual field). At last, a secondary active appears on the right visual cortex centered on (-0.5 -0.5 0.5), and it may be a secondary evoked activity by the activities centered on (-0.5 0.3 0.5) and (-0.1 0.0 0.6).

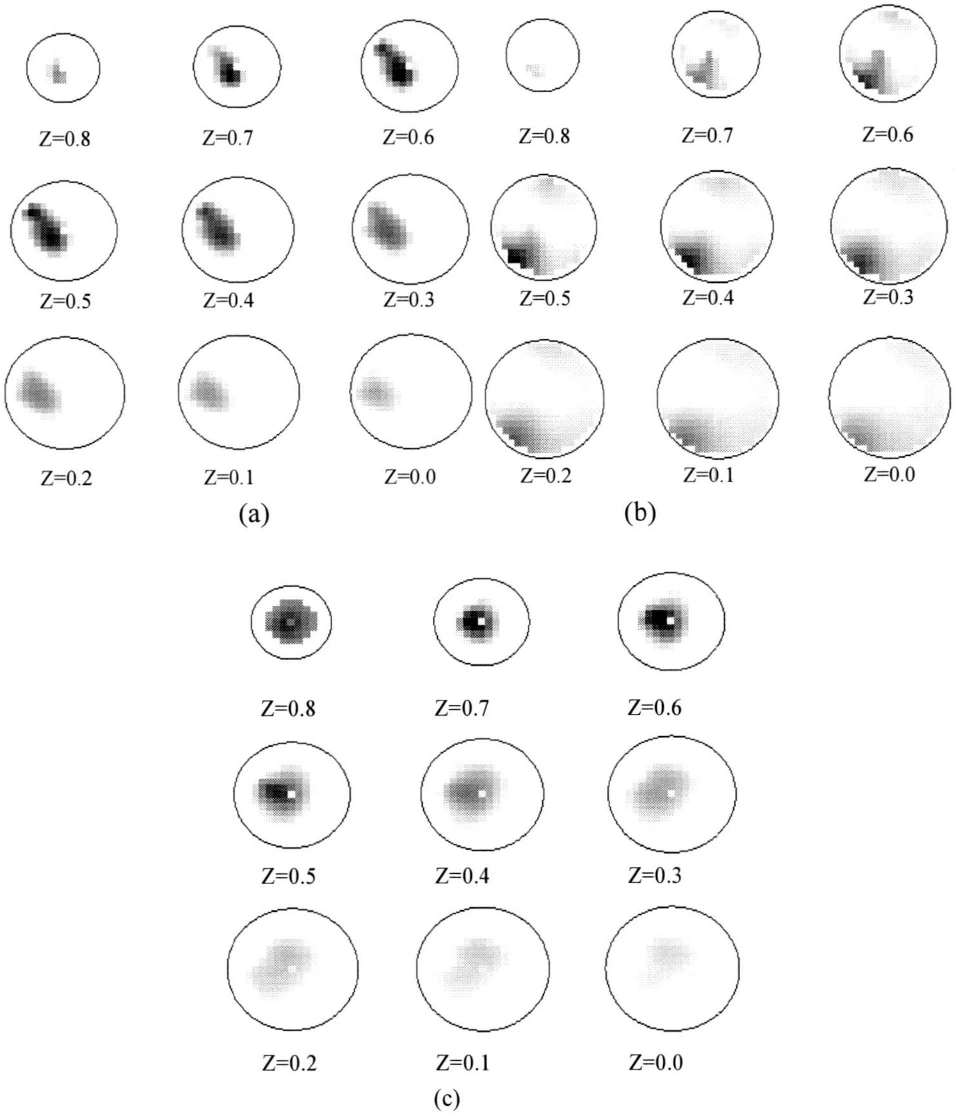

Figure 7. Maps of the metric X. Map of the $X = 1./(1.001 - c_1^2)$ in an one-dipole scanning; (b) map of the $X = 1./(1.001 - c_1^2)$ in a scanning after a dipole is assumed at (-0.5 0.3 0.5); (c) map of the $X = 1./(1.001 - c_2^2)$ in a scanning after a dipole is assumed at (-0.5 0.3 0.5).

Finally, the above result can be further improved if a finer grid and a realistic head model are involved. And due to the (partly) synchronous activities among the three source regions, a nonlinear multidimensional search is useful to further improve the location parameters of the three actives. However, since the nonlinear search algorithm is a problem under study, it is not included in this work.

Conclusion and Discussion

Based on the CM and the recently developed recursive framework, a new algorithm denoted as IDM is provided to localize the brain electrical activities. The non-zero delay correlation is introduced to replace the zero-delay correlation in the estimate of the signal subspace of the MUSIC-based algorithm. Numeric simulation shows a better performance of the new algorithm than that of the CM in repressing the spatial coherent noise. Numeric simulation also shows that a relative larger signal-subspace rank is preferred to the true rank, especially when the data are corrupted by spatial coherent or partly coherent noise. Besides, an iterative process is emphasized in the practice of the algorithm, and the iterative process is also an interactive process between man's guess and the practice of the DM. The results show that the IDM is a new choice in the EEG inverse problem.

The difference between the DM and the other pre-whitening methods is that the DM only requires the delay correlation is dramatically different between the signals and the noise [Yao et al., 2000], and the other methods require to estimate the noise covariance [Sekihara et al., 1997]. Reviewing the procedure to implement the IDM, the undesired subjective judgement is required in the selection of the SSD, and in the selection of a starting point of a muti-sources scanning, and some interactive guesses are required in the practice of the IDM. Meanwhile, for the coherent source imaging, there are some other methods are proposed in recent years, such as the frequency domain method [Gross et al., 2001], the fourth order cumulant matrix decomposition subspace method [Yao, 2000] and the multivariate correlation coefficient decomposition [Zhang et al, 2006], they are meaningful to evaluate these methods in the near future especially by empirical data.

Though an objective procedure has been the goal of the field for a long time, subjective participation still plays an important role in the current practice of EEG inverse problem like the BESA software [Scherg, 1990; Miltner et al. 1994]. Based on the state-of-the-art of the field, the non-unique of the EEG inverse problem has not been and may never be solved, we believe a positive barge is necessary for almost all the current dipole localization algorithms [Miltner et al., 1994; Supek et al., 1997a; Huang et al., 1998].

Acknowledgment

This work was supported by NSFC #30525030, #60571019 and 60736029. The authors would like to thank the previous master students Min Zeng , Fansheng Meng, Xiao Hu, Yingchun Zhou for their contributions in programs and discussions, and Prof Lin Chen, Silu Fan and Dr Xinyu Ao for providing the ERP data.

References

Cadzow JA (1998). A high-resolution direction –of- arrival algorithm for narrow-band coherent and incoherent sources. *IEEE Trans. ASSP* 36: 965-979.

Cadzow JA (1990). Multiple source location –the signal subspace approach. *IEEE Trans ASSP* 38:1110-1125.

Clark VP, Fan S, and Hillyard S (1995). Identification of early visual evoked potential generators by retinotopic and topographic analysis. *Human brain mapping* 2:170-187.

Gevins AS, Le J, Martin, NK, et al (1994). High resolution EEG: 124-channel recording, spatial de-blurring and MRI integration methods. *Electroenceph. Clin. Neurophysiol* , 90:337-358.

Golub GH and Van Loan CF (1984). *Matrix Computations.* 2nd ed. Baltimore, MD: Johns Hopkins Uni. Press.

Huang M, Aine CJ, Supek S, Best E, Ranken D, Flynn ER (1998). Multi-start downhill simplex method for spatio-temporal source localization in magnetoencephalography. *Electroenceph. Clin. Neurophysiol.* 108:32-44.

Greenblatt RE (1993). Probabilistic reconstruction of multiple sources in the bioelectromagnetic inverse problem. *Inverse Problem* 9:271-284.

Gross J,Kujala J, Hämäläinen M, Timmermann L, Schnitzler A, Salmelin R (2001). Dynamic imaging of coherent sources: study in gneural interactions in the human brain. *PNAS*, 98(2): 694-699.

Knosche T (1997). *Solutions of the neuroelectromagnetic inverse problem-- an evaluation study.* Ph.D thesis of Universiteit Twente.

Koles ZJ (1998). Trends in EEG source localization. *Electroenceph. Clin. Neueophysiol.* 106:127-137.

Miltner W, Braun C, Johnson R Jr, Simpson GV, Ruchkin DS (1994). A test of brain electrical source analysis (BESA): a simulation study. *Electroenceph. Clin. Neurophysiol.* 91: 295-310.

Mosher JC, Lewis PS, Leahy RM (1992). Multiple dipole modeling and localization from spatio-temporal MEG data. *IEEE Trans. BME* 39:541-557.

Mosher JC, Leahy RM (1998). Recursive MUSIC: A framework for EEG and MEG source localization. *IEEE Trans. BME* 45(11): 1342-1354.

Nunez PL, Silibertein RB, Cdush PJ, Wijesinghe RS, Westdrop AF et al (1994). A theoretical and experimental study of high resolution EEG based on surface Laplacian and cortical imaging. *Electroenceph. Clin. Neurophysiol.* 90:40-57.

Pascual-Marqui, RD, Michel, CM and Lehmann D (1994). Low resolution electromagnetic tomography: a new method for localizing electrical activity in the brain. *Int. J. Psychophysiol* 18:49-65.

Rush S, Driscoll DA (1969). EEG electrode sensitivity – An application of reciprocity. *IEEE Trans. BME* 16:15-22.

Scherg M (1990). Fundamentals of dipole source analysis. In: Grandori F, Hoke M, Roman GL (eds): *Auditory Evoked Magnetic Fields and Electrical Potentials.* Basel: Karper, 40-69.

Schmidt RO (1986). Multiple emitter location and signal parameter estimation. *IEEE Trans AP* 34:276-280.

Sekilhara K, Poeppel D, Marantz A et al (1997). Noise covariance incorporated MEG-MUSIC algorithm: A method for multiple-dipole estimation tolerant of the influence of background brain activity. *IEEE Trans. BME* 44(9):839-847.

Sekilhara K, Poeppel D, Marantz A, et al (1998). MEG covariance difference analysis: a method to extract target source activities by using task and control measurements. *IEEE Trans. BME* 45(1):87-97.

Sidman R, Vincent D, Smith D, et al (1992). Experimental tests of the cortical imaging techniques- applications to the response to median nerve stimulation and the localization of epileptiform discharges. *IEEE Trans. BME* 39:437-444.

Soong ACK and Koles AJ (1995). Principal-component localization of the sources of the background EEG. *IEEE Trans. BME* 42(1): 59-67.

Srebro R, Oguz RM, Hughlett K et al (1993). Estimating regional brain activity from evoked potential field on the scalp. *IEEE Trans. BME* 40:509-516.

Supek S, Aine CJ (1997). Spatio-temporal modeling of neuromagnetic data: I. Multi-source location versus time-course estimation accuracy. *Human Brain Mapping* 5: 139-153.

Supek S, Aine CJ (1997). Spatio-temporal modeling of neuromagnetic data: II. Multi-source resolvability of a MUSIC-based location estimator. *Human Brain Mapping* 5: 154-167.

Xu P, Tian Y, Chen HF, Yao D(2007). Lp norm iterative sparse solution for EEG source localization. *IEEE Trans Biomed Eng*, 54(3): 400-409.

Yao D (1995). Imaging of EEG by spherical harmonic analysis. *Journal of Electronics* (In Chinese) 17(5): 456-462.

Yao D (1996). The equivalent source technique and cortical imaging. *Electroenceph. and clin. Neurophysiol.* 98:478-483.

Yao D He B (1998). The Laplacian weighted minimum norm estimate of three dimensional equivalent charge distribution in the brain. *Proceedings of the 20th IEEE EMBS*, Hongkong.

Yao D, Fu S, Rao N, Zhou Y, Fan S, Chen L(1999). A computer simulation study of MUSIC algorithm for EEG inverse problem. *Chinese Journal of Biomedical Engineering* (In Chinese), 21(1): 53-58, 83.

Yao D (2000). Electroencephalography inverse problem by subspace decomposition of the fourth-order cumulant matrix. *Sheng Wu Yi Xue Gong Cheng Xue Za Zhi* (In Chinese), 17(2):174-8.

Yao D, Rao N, Fu S, Hu X(2000). A delay sub-space decomposition algorithm of electroencephalography sources localization. *Acta Electronica Sinica* (In Chinese), 28(4): 135-138.

Yao D, Zhou Y, Fan S, Chen L, Ao X(2001a). Multi-dimensional delay-correlation MUSIC: a new method to extract multi-sources of EEGs. *Acta Electronica Sinica* (In Chinese), 29(4): 522-525.

Yao D and He B(2001b). A Self-Coherence Enhancement Algorithm and its Application to Enhancing 3D Source Estimation from EEGs. *Annals of Biomedical Engineering*, 29(11):1019-1027.

Yao D (2002a). The theoretical relation of Scalp Laplacian and scalp current density. *Phys. Med.Biol.*, 47:2179-2185.

Yao D(2002b). High-resolution EEG mapping: a radial-basis function based approach to scalp Laplacian estimate. *Clin. Neurophysiol.*, 113(6): 956-967.

Yao D, Wang L, Nielsen KD, Arendt-Nielsen L,Chen CAN(2004a). Cortical Mapping of EEG Alpha Power Using a Charge Layer Model. *Brain Topogr*. 17(2):65-71.

Yao D, Yin Z, Tang X, Arendt-Nielsen L and Chen CAN(2004b). High-resolution Electroencephalogram mapping: scalp charge layer. *Phys. Med. Biol.*, 49: 5073-5086.

Zhang J, Yao D, Cui Y(2006). Multivariate Correlation Coefficient Decomposition and Its Application to Map the Coherent Sources in Human Brain. *Chinese Journal of Biomedical Engineering* (In Chinese), 25(1): 6-9.

In: Brain Mapping Research Progress
Editors: Ines C. Girard and Jade S. Andre

ISBN: 978-1-60456-784-7

Chapter VIII

Mapping of Brain Operational Architectonics

Andrew A. Fingelkurts* and Alexander A. Fingelkurts
BM-SCIENCE Brain & Mind Technologies Research Centre, Espoo, Finland

Abstract

Recent neuroscience is lacking of consistent theory and methods for understanding the mechanisms through which the brain orchestrate the symphony of perceptions, thoughts and actions. The aim of this Chapter is to contribute to a better understanding of such mechanisms by establishing methodological foundations of the Operational Architectonics framework of brain and mind functioning. The theory we offer provides a framework for mapping and understanding important aspects of the brain mechanisms that constitute perception, cognition, and eventually consciousness.

Keywords: EEG/MEG, Operational Synchrony, Structural Synchrony, Functional Connectivity, Neuronal Assemblies, Brain Operations, Mind, Temporal Structure, Binding, Perception, Cognition, Consciousness, Dynamical, Symbolic, Neurocomputational Approach, Isomorphism

"We may be able one day to use brain waves as indicators of the beginning and end of a mental process..."

Robert S. Woodworth (1938)

* Correspondence concerning this article should be addressed to Dr. Andrew A. Fingelkurts BM-SCIENCE Brain & Mind Technologies Research Centre, PO Box 77, FI-02601, Espoo, Finland. E-mail: fingelkurts@bm-science.com. Url: http://www.bm-science.com/team/fingelkurts.html

Introduction

Attempts to understand systematically the brain and mind and their operations go back at least to the Ancient Greeks, when philosophers such as Plato and Aristotle tried to explain the nature of human knowledge. However, until recently such understanding is simplistic and is still a source of puzzlement. And it is so despite the fact that over last few decades there has been an explosive development of new theories regarding the brain and mind functioning and powerful techniques that allow studying it. Contemporary scientific knowledge about the brain is as follows: Simplifying, the brain is essentially a network of neurons (and glia) interconnected with synapses. Particular neurons are connected to inputs from which they receive information from the outside world. If these neurons receive a sufficiently strong signal, they fire, thereby affecting more neurons, and so on. It is supposed that neurons represent features in the input and that connections between neurons encode relational context among those features (Choe, 2002). Eventually, an output signal, acting on the outside world is generated. However, in such interpretation, the static and passive role is assigned to the brain.

In reality brain does not simply represent the environment in a different format (Erdi, 2000; Buzaki, 2004). It rather generates its own mental representations and behavior, thus been a functional active entity (Alexandrov, 1999; Freeman, 2000; Cariani, 2001)[1]. In another words, the living brain is in a state of permanent flux, been continuously in a change accordingly with its environment (external and internal). It senses the environments, anticipates what actions are appropriate (Freeman, 2000; Erdi, 2000), and acts accordingly through the sequence of operations (Alexandrov, 1999). Here the operations of perception, coordination-anticipation, and action in the organism become the measurements, predictive computations, and actions (Cariani, 2001). By probing its environment, brain extracts from the changing array of stimuli the regularities and covariances that assert the stability of the external world (Paillard, 1991). Such regularities are printed in the neural circuitry of cortical modules through the stabilization of co-activated synapses (see discussion in Phillips et al. 1984). An internal representation of a stable predictable environmental framework (system of mental states or images) thereby emerges, which gives coherence and unity to the spatial relationships that link the organism to its external world. In such a way, brain, been a complex system, achieves a degree of epistemic autonomy relative to its surrounds (see also Cariani, 1994; Erdi, 2000).

It is obvious, that both brain and mind functioning have a *temporal structure* (Pöppel, 1988; Glicksohn, 2001). The time range for complex brain-mind operation is related to the multiple time scales. These temporal scales are (1) information processing in the brain (milliseconds), (2) perception of events in the real outside world (seconds and minutes), (3) processing of these events, and (4) realistic behavior with cognitive tasks (hours and days). In

---

[1] It is not necessary or even desirable to postulate conscious experience or awareness as a basis for active perception. To illustrate this point we've borrowed example from Freeman (2000; pp. 208): "...in the study of conditioned reflexes an observer does not need to know, and with animals cannot know, whether the subjects are aware of the stimulus, only whether a contingent response occurs in conjunction with patterns of neural activity in the brain that are accessible to observation."

general, the brain has to perform in a parallel manner many successive operations in order to achieve a successful result (Bak and Chialvo, 2001).

The fundamental concept of *operation* is common to an organizational structure of brain and mind. Both the material organization that characterizes brain and the informational order that characterizes mind therefore necessarily involve such events as operations at their cores. Here the *operation* is stand for the *process* or series of acts that are limited in time (Krippendorff, 2002). More generally operation is the state of being in effect. This provides a basis for discussion of the relative complexity of operations, where there is a more complex operation/operational act that subsumes the simpler ones (for a more detail conceptualization, see Fingelkurts and Fingelkurts, 2003). In this sense, a simplified description of the operation of a neuron is that it processes the electric currents which arrive on its dendrites and transmits the resulting electrical current to other connected neurons using its axon. Such "blind" neurophysiological operation, at the same time, is the elemental physical operation of the brain (Tabl. 1). Such operations have a fully neurophysiological ontology and they are completely NONconscious phenomena, which according to Searle (1992) have no mental/subjective ontology whatsoever. More complex physical operations of the brain emerge from the collective activity of many neurons – *neuronal assembly*[2]. It is well established, that single neurons (highly distributed along the cortex) can quickly become associated (or dis-associated) by synchronization of their activity and giving rise to functional transient assemblies (Kogan and Choraian, 1977; von der Malsburg, 1999). Anatomical connections are not necessarily important prerequisite for such synchronization; it is rather a stimulus (external – physical or internal – mental) and/or a task that is important and is the causal source of synchrony (see Ryder and Favorov, 2001). Each of these functional assemblies maintains discrete complex brain operations some of which may have already mental/subjective ontology in addition to their neurophysiological ontology (Tabl. 1): They process different attributes of object or environmental scene, thus being simple cognitive operations (Valera et al., 2001; Fingelkurts and Fingelkurts, 2003). The joint functionally connected activity of many neuronal assemblies produces already complex cognitive/mental operations[3] (Tabl. 1; see also McIntosh, 1999, 2000). Each neuronal assembly makes a specific contribution to the performance of complex cognitive operation, and the contribution is determined by the position which a particular neural assembly occupies within the richly connected, parallel, and distributed brain system (see Petersen and Fiez, 1993). The temporal synchronization of many operations of local neuronal assemblies together (*Operational Synchrony,* OS) gives rise to a new level of brain abstractness – metastable[4] brain states (for

[2] A neuronal assembly may be defined as a group of neurons that cooperate to perform a specific computation (operation) required for a specific task (Nunez, 2000).

[3] Using the orchestra metaphor of Raichle (1999, p.44), it is so as "specific members of a large orchestra perform together in a precise fashion to produce a symphony, a group of localized brain areas performing elementary operations work together to exhibit an observable human behavior."

[4] The specific interpretation of metastability in the context of a specific theoretical model of the coordination dynamics of brain and behavior was developed by Kelso (1991, 1995). According to his theory metastability arises because of a specific symmetry breaking in the coordination dynamics. In our reinterpretation metastability arises in the brain because intrinsic differences in activity between the local neuronal assemblies are sufficiently large and they do their own job, while still retaining a tendency to be coordinated together in accordance with cognition and/or behavior (for the review, see Fingelkurts and Fingelkurts, 2001, 2003, 2004).

the review, see Fingelkurts and Fingelkurts, 2004). It is suggested that these metastable brain states or functional *Operational Modules* (OM), as we name them, underlie complex brain functions and/or mind complex operations (cognitive percepts and mental states that have representational nature)[5]. The sequence of these metastable OMs, thus, represents[6] the stream of thoughts (Fingelkurts and Fingelkurts, 2001). It is only at this level of integration we may hope relate brain and mind through *functional isomorphism* principle (see Fingelkurts and Fingelkurts, 2004).

Different parts of this very general picture of brain-mind functioning have been obtained from a large body of behavioral, cognitive, and physiological studies. For example, brain-behavior experiments (Fuchs et al. 1992; Fuchs et al. 2000; Kelso et al. 1992) have demonstrated that neural activity picked up by the magnetoencephalogram (MEG) and electroencephalogram (EEG) shows spatiotemporal transitions when the operation of behavior (movement pattern) switches. This research indicates that the ongoing brain activity is directly related to the behavioral coordination dynamics (Jirsa et al., 1998). The biological advantages of coordination transitions are obvious: They provide a mechanism for flexibility, allowing the system (brain) alternative ways to coordinate itself under changing environmental or task conditions. Thus, behavior implies dynamical sequence of patterns. Such view is in accord with the concept developed by Alexandrov (1999) and introduced by Anokhin (1973; 1978). According to this theory of functional systems, behavior is indeed a continuum of discrete behavioral acts performed by an individual during life. Any behavioral act consists of a number of appropriate operations (Shvyrkov, 1990). The following behavioral act in a sequence is realized only when the previous act is achieved and evaluated. The evaluation process is a necessary part of the organizational architecture of the following behavioral act and is usually rapid, thus, being transitional. During such transitive periods the redundant degrees of freedom of the whole system are eliminated and the decision of what should be done and how to achieve the adaptive result is made (Alexandrov, 1999).

Table 1. The hierarchy of brain-mind operations

OPERATION	One neuron	One neuronal assembly	Several neuronal assemblies	Many Neuronal assemblies
Brain level	simple	complex	more complex	very complex
Cognitive level	—	simple	complex	very complex

From a daily phenomenological experience we are aware also of a discrete sequence of cognitive events, where conscious percepts, mental images and thoughts are constant within a snapshot of variable duration (Mangan, 1993a; Galin, 2000; Bickle et al, 2000). In science,

[5] These states could be divided into two categories: unconscious mental phenomena and conscious mental phenomena (for a detail, see Searle, 1992).

[6] As has been stated by Antonio and Hanna Damasio (1999), such representations are not "pictorial" objects in the brain as was traditionally thought; instead they are the records of the neural activity that takes place in the brain during particular brain operation. Such records define perceived or imagined object and/or event. Generally each of these records can also activate related ones.

the idea of discrete cognition and consciousness was firstly considered by William James (1890). Stroud (1955) was the first who start to use the notion "*perceptual moment*". However, the notion of a "*time quantum*" was initially suggested by von Baer (1864) and important investigations in this vein have been further made by Geissler (1987; 1997). Later, Efron (1970) suggested that conscious cognition is temporally discontinuous and parsed into sensory sampling intervals or "*perceptual frames*." Based on behavioral studies it was shown that there exists a certain minimal interstimulus interval for which two successive events are consistently perceived as simultaneous: one can think of them as occurring within a single *discrete epoch* (Hirsh and Sherrick, 1961; Kristofferson, 1967; Andrews et al., 1996).

In recent years this vein of research has been extended to electrophysiology. Exactly cortical brain oscillations have been found to be closely related to temporal perceptual window (Varela et al., 1981; Gho & Varela, 1988). John (1990) proposed a mechanism, where a cascade of momentary perceptual frames converges on cortical areas to establish a steady-state perturbation (*spatiotemporal signature*) from baseline activity (John, 2002). This mechanism has received substantial support from EEG studies, including research by Lehmann and colleagues (Lehmann, 1971; Lehmann et al., 1987). They have demonstrated that the dynamic of the brain EEG field is represented by the intervals of quasistability or "*microstates*" and by *sudden transitions* between them (Strik and Lehmann, 1993; Pascual-Marqui et al., 1995). Furthermore, they have shown that these microstates have been associated with different modes of spontaneous thoughts (Koenig and Lehmann, 1996) and with spontaneous visual imagery or abstract thoughts (Lehmann et al., 1998).

Different Approaches to Study Brain-Mind Operation

Many theories in brain research try to capture the complex functioning of brain-mind. Amongst general approaches to study how the brain and mind function, there are currently three major types: the *dynamical* approach, the *symbolic* approach, and the neural information processing (*neurocomputational*) approach. While symbolic and dynamical approaches are quite disjoint, considerable overlap exists between each of these and the neurocomputational view (see Cariani, 2001).

Dynamical Approach

The dynamical approach for cognition and brain activity has been adopted in believing that systems of differential or difference equations are the most appropriate tool for modeling brain behavior (Van Gelder, 1995). According to this approach cognition is explained as a multidimensional space of all possible thoughts and behaviors that is traversed by a path of thinking followed by an agent under certain environmental and internal pressures, all of which are captured by sets of differential equations (Van Gelder and Port, 1995). For dynamicists, the brain is considered as a large and complex continuous-time physical system that is described in terms of the dynamics of neural excitation and inhibition (Freeman and Barrie, 1993). The behavior of large number of microscopic neural elements creates discrete basins of attraction for the system that can be switched (Haken, 1999; Tsuda, 2001). These contingently-stable dynamical macro-states form the substrates for mental and behavioral states (John, 2002). Thus, cognitive processes are not rule-governed sequences of discrete symbolic states, but continuous, evolving total states of dynamic systems determined by continuous, simultaneous and mutually determining states of the systems' components (Freeman, 2000). Representation in a dynamic system is essentially information-theoretic; though the bearers of information are not symbols, but state variables or parameters (Beer, 2000). There are several classes of models used within dynamical approach. One class is represented by the models of deterministic chaos (twist-flip maps and the Lorenz, Rössler, and Chua attractors). However, these models are low dimensional, stationary, autonomous, and essentially noise-free, so they inadequately model the brain, which fail to conform to any of these conditions (Freeman et al., 2001). The same is true for the attempts to measure correlation dimensions, Lyapunov exponents, and related numeric features of brain subsystems. These measures have failed to yield normative results and became less considered for brain modeling (Rapp, 1993). Another large class of models is represented by reaction-diffusion equations (chemical morphogenesis; Turing, 1952, and irreversible thermodynamics; Prigogine, 1980) that make "order from disorder". These models also fail, especially when they model the interactions within neural networks and populations (Freeman et al., 2001). Furthermore, it was shown that terminal chaos (Zak, 1993) is impaired in its utility for representing chaotic systems (Freeman et al., 1997). Models based on hydrodynamics and turbulence are unsatisfactory also; there is nothing equivalent to viscosity or to molar convection in neurodynamics (Freeman et al., 2001). The best available models are those from synergetics, which described microscopic particles as being "enslaved" by a macroscopic "order parameter" (Haken, 1991). Generally, dynamic system theories are not be able in any way to explain (1) discrete higher-order thoughts and images, (2) the qualitative or phenomenal character of experience, and (3) how cognitive systems can be both representational and computational (Eliasmith, 1996).

The Symbolic Approach

In the neural and cognitive sciences, the symbol-based approach has been adopted by research traditions whose subject matter lends itself to orderly, rule-governed successions of discrete functional states: The physical systems symbol hypothesis (Newell and Simon, 1976), language symbolic processing (Fodor, 1987; Fodor and Pylyshyn, 1988), symbolic artificial intelligence (Honavar, 1994). Symbol-based approach have proposed that the mind contains such mental representations as logical propositions, rules, concepts, images, and analogies, and that it uses mental operations such as deduction, search, matching, rotating, and retrieval. According to Fodor and Pylyshyn, in normal cognitive agents, there exist intrinsic connections between some thoughts and others. Thoughts (symbols) come in clumps. This putative fact is the *systematicity* of cognitive representations. The *compositionality* of representations says something about the nature of the thoughts that are intrinsically connected. It indicates the nature of the clumps of mental thoughts (symbols): The thoughts in the clumps are semantically related. For example, the thoughts in the clumps have common terms and predicates. Thus, the thoughts 'John loves Mary' and 'Mary loves John' are compositional sets of representations since they both represent 'John,' 'loving,' and 'Mary.' Perception here is seen in terms of microcomputations by discrete feature-detection elements, while mental operations are conceptualized in terms of computations on discrete, functional symbolic states that are thought to be largely autonomous of the underlying neural microdynamics. However, symbolic approaches (1) does a poor job of explaining graceful degradation of function, holistic representation of data, spontaneous generalization, appreciation of context, and many other features of human intelligence and cognition, (2) have ignored problems related to how new symbolic primitives can be created (Piatelli-Palmarini 1980; Schyns et al., 1998).

The Neurocomputational Approach

The neurocomputational approach includes a variety of neurophysiological and neurocomputational perspectives that seek to understand the neural coding – the identification of which aspects of neural activity convey information (Cariani, 1994; Mountcastle 1967; Perkell and Bullock 1968; Rieke et al. 1997; Uttal 1973; Arbib 1989; Churchland and Sejnowski 1992; Marr 1991; McCulloch 1965; Freeman et al., 2001). One of these perspectives is the connectionist model. It seems, that such models are particularly well matched to what we know about the brain. Indeed, the brain is a neural net, formed from massively many units (neurons) and their connections (synapses). Furthermore, several properties of neural network models suggest that connectionism may offer an especially faithful picture of the nature of mind. Neural networks exhibit robust flexibility in the face of the challenges posed by the real world. Noisy input or destruction of units causes graceful degradation of function. In such cases the net's response is still appropriate, though somewhat less accurate. In contrast, noise and loss of circuitry in classical computers typically result in catastrophic failure. Neural networks are also particularly well adapted for problems that require the resolution of many conflicting constraints in parallel. Despite these intriguing features, there are some weaknesses in connectionist models that bear mentioning. First, most neural network research abstracts away from many interesting and possibly important features of the brain and mind. Second, the claim that human brains and minds work by computation is an empirical conjecture and might be wrong. For example, Dreyfus (1992) and Searle (1992) have claimed that computational approach (1) neglects the important role of emotions, (2) ignores the importance of consciousness, (3) disregards the significant role of physical environments, and (4) neglects the fact that the mind is a dynamical system, not a computational one.

The debate between these three approaches is still intense and there is a fast growing literature built around the many issues raised by it. It is clear that neither approach described above is satisfactory in isolation; none of them exploit in an explicit way the actual physical/brain and subjective/mental operations the human brain-mind possesses in the course of organism behavior. The entire brain functioning is described in a somewhat one-side manner. There is, for example, no physiological explanation for abrupt changes in brain-mind states over time, and there is no means for deriving the time needed for brain-mind operations. When inevitable in such cases "paradoxes" appear, where human brain does not behave as the theory predicts, the standard response of the researchers is to alter the initial axioms of theories. This is apparently implausible and requires significant simplification. However, the operational organization of brain-mind functioning (as has been described in the Introduction section) may be an essential framework for cognitive neuroscience. Thus, there is a need for further explanatory theories to be introduced, which would be alternative and superior to either of described above.

Operational Architectonics Postulates

We have suggested the *Operational Architectonics* (OA) framework[7] (Fingelkurts and Fingelkurts, 2001; 2003) of brain-mind functioning, which is a metatheory and is a plausible illustration of the explanatory advantages of integrated view that adopts an approach which supposes from the outset that brain and mental processes essentially evolve over real time (a dynamical approach), have distinct microstates (a symbolic approach), which are the result of communication between neuronal assemblies (a computational approach). This framework explores the temporal structure of information flow and interarea interactions within the network of functional neuronal assemblies by examining topographic sharp transition processes in the scalp EEG (or MEG), on the millisecond scale. Thus, the OA theory may be a sufficient framework that accounts for data covered. by three traditional approaches described above, but which explanatory capacities go beyond those of traditional theories in a number of respects. The OA framework, by contrast to other theories, sets out with the explicit aim to describe, measure and model the brain and mind operations involved in the complex human behavior which is governed by the individual's brain. According to the OA framework, the notion of operation[8] is central for perception, attention, intention, memory, action, and eventually consciousness (Fingelkurts and Fingelkurts, 2003).

In constructing OA, we have drawn on many ideas from other theoreticians especially, of course, those emphasizing the intimate relationship between brain and mind operations. For instance, we share the general perspective of Chalmers (1995) and Varela (Thompson and Varela, 2001) that brain/physics and mind/phenomenology are functionally linked and that it is only their coordination that allows for adaptive behavior. We further adopt the metastability notion put forward by Kelso (1991; 1995), Friston (1997; 2000), and Kaplan (1998), that is circumstantial for the interaction among the elementary neuronal systems in order to generate adaptive behavior within changing and not fully predictable environments. And we also follow Singer (1994; 2001) in assuming that representations of perceptual contents and action plans are content-specific composites of codes presumably stored in a distributed fashion, whereby synchronization of brain activities, going on in different brain areas, is a mechanism for the integration of local circuits within the large-scale anatomical structure and was claimed to be crucial for mental representations (Phillips and Singer, 1997). From a dynamical systems viewpoint, the best way to assess this large-scale level of synchronization is through EEG and/or MEG measures (Nunez, 2000; John, 2002; Freeman, 2003; Basar, 2004). The main three principles utilized by OA concept are (1) the neuronal assembly notion suggested by Hebb (1949) and developed by von der Malsburg (Malsburg,

---

[7] This framework takes its direct origin and is rooted in the work of Kaplan and colleagues (Kaplan, 1995, 1998; Kaplan et al., 1997; Kaplan & Shishkin, 2000; Kaplan et al., 2001).

[8] There is, admittedly, a strong, fallible, assumption that the system is divided into components performing different elementary operations (Bechtel, 2002). Petersen and Fiez (1993), for example, stress that neuroimaging should be seeking to identify elementary operations, not tasks.

1999; Triesch and von der Malsburg, 2001), (2) the large-scale description of information processing in the brain (Nunez, 2000; John, 2002; Freeman, 2003; Basar, 2004), (3) the importance of human consciousness; the work by Chalmers (1995; 2002), Baars (1988; 1997), Edelman and Tononi (2000), Crick and Koch (2003), and Revonsuo (2000; 2001). Below we will discuss each of these principles in detail.

Transient Neural Assemblies

It is now well appreciated that integration of distributed brain activity involve the activities of large number of neurons (deCharms and Zador, 2000). However, there are basically two ways how to describe the mass behavior of neurons (see Hatsopoulos et al., 1998; deCharms, 1998): (1) as by pooling together large number of essentially *independent* neuronal signals (The Independent-Coding Hypothesis), or (2) through the essential *coordination* of neuronal elements into a single signal, as in a symphony (The Coordinated-Coding Hypothesis). According to the independent coding framework each cortical neuron represents a separate signal. Although many neurons may be involved in coding a particular object, the key postulate of the independent-coding hypothesis is that all of the information that can be obtained from any one neuron can be derived from that individual neuron alone, without reference to the activities of others (Georgopoulos, 1990; Schwartz, 1994a,b). It has been proposed that such independent signals may be overlapping, noisy, or redundant and may need to be pooled or averaged over large populations to become clear, but the signal carried by each neuron is carried independently (see deCharms and Zador, 2000).

The coordinated-coding hypothesis, on the contrary, suggests that the dynamic patterns of cooperative activity of neurons cannot be predicted from knowledge of the activity patterns of any single class of neurons, or individual neurons (Mountcastle, 1998). According to this hypothesis the coordinated information could be extracted from the relations between multiple neurons in a population, whereby these relations are reflected in the neural synchrony (Gray et al., 1989; Singer and Gray, 1995). Indeed, it has been shown that changes in such synchrony (a) are stimulus frequency specific, (b) follow the time course of ongoing stimuli, and (c) are systematically mapped across the cortical surface (deCharms and Merzenich, 1996). Here the emphasis is put on the functional brain units or assemblies (von der Malsburg, 1999) executing the basic elemental operations of informational processing (Finger, 1994; McIntosh, 1999; Varela et al., 2001; Crick and Koch, 2003).

Before moving further, we need to be clear about how elementary the operations in question might be (Bechtel, 2002). In a broad sense, basic physics defines elementary operations of all phenomena in nature in terms of quantum mechanics. However, this is typically not necessarily the right level at which we are searching the basic operations that comprise the explanation of a cognitive phenomenon. To illustrate this point we have borrowed example from the Bechtel (2002; p. 233): "To explain how a car generates locomotion we do not jump immediately to quantum mechanics. Rather, we appeal to parts at one level of decomposition down from the whole car – the engine, drive shaft, axles, etc. Each of them makes a contribution which we can understand in light of the goal of generating locomotion – transforming chemical energy to mechanical energy, etc." Similarly, if we are interested in a quest to find the brain operations that comprise the elemental cognitive operations, we should define the appropriate level of brain description.

The individual neurons are seen as imperfect and unreliable pulse generators, partly due to thermal fluctuations in the membranes of their trigger zones, and partly due to their biochemical nature (Freeman, 2000). Moreover, most of the activity of single neurons is expected to be determined by the activity of their peers and only the small part of such activity is determined by the features of the environment (Buzaki, 2004). It has been also stated that individual neuronal activity is only weakly correlated with cognition and behavior. Indeed, the response properties of individual neurons tend to vary only little in awake, sleeping, and anesthetized brains, meaning that the tuned responses of individual neurons are alone not sufficient to support cognition and consciousness in particular (Singer, 2001). Revonsuo in his analytic paper also comes to the same conclusion: "...it appears that the records of single-cell firing rates are not explanatorily adequate for the discovery of the phenomenal level, for we have no idea how the firing rate of a neuron is supposed to contribute to the subject's phenomenology and, consequently, we have no clue how to reconstruct any aspect of the subject's phenomenology from the firing rate data alone." (Revonsuo, 2001; p. 12). When we record activity from the single cells, we observe brain activity at a very low level of organization – we trace the elemental brain *physical* operations – and such observations never allow the visualization of the phenomenon (cognition or mind) we are interested in (for a detail discussion, see Revonsuo, 2001). Thus, the level of the activity of individual neurons (elemental brain physical operations) is most likely an inappropriate level of brain organization for realization of cognition and mind. However, there must be some level of organization in the brain that literally resembles or is *isomorphic* to cognition, that is to say cognition (or mind) itself. So, the appropriate level of brain description should in some way allow reconstruction of the structure (or at least some aspects of it) and/or content of phenomenal level of organization experienced by the subject.

The elemental cognitive brain operations (perception, object feature representation, recognition, and so on) appear to require some kind of "devices" that bridge distances and allow for the fast between-neuron exchange of information. In another words, information represented in some class of neurons has to be bound[9] (Fig. 1 A). Neuronal assemblies are perfectly suited to fit this purpose[10]. Nowadays, in the result of the paradigm change, it seems clear that the coordinated-coding framework, or a theory of neural assemblies plays more and more central role in cognitive sciences (Basar, 2004). Here, the activity of any individual neuron is informational only insofar as it contributes to the overall statistics of the assembly of which it is a member (John, 2002). For example, hippocampal pyramidal cells during rest and sleep produce strongly coherent ensemble bursts believed to be critical in transferring information to the neocortex. Although robust at the assembly level, no amount of sequential

[9] The communication of neurons within the assembly is achieved through the synchronous operations executed by each neuron. Such synchronization occurs among the neurons which tune preferentially to a particular features of their sensory environments and are predictably related to other such features (Phillips and Singer, 1997). It is supposed that this process relay on self-organization (Erdi and Barna, 1984; Singer, 2001) where the crucial role is played by dendrites (Ryder and Favorov, 2001).

[10] Neuronal assemblies allow also overcoming the unavoidable unreliability of individual neurons (see above). By having numerous elements in parallel, a consensus can be found by averaging among them in order to extract a clean signal – this solution is very well known by engineers (Freeman, 2000).

single-cell recording could reveal such cooperative patterns (Buzsaki et al., 1992). Thus, it has been claimed that the cell assembly theory (which describes the *intermediate-level organization* of the brain) seems the only plausible concept that bridges the gap between neural and mental dynamics[11] (Palm, 1990; Eichenbaum, 1993; Pulvermueller et al., 1994; Mountcastle, 1998; von der Malsburg, 1999; Varela et al., 2001; Basar, 2004). According to this theory, higher brain functions (cognition) are based on processing units called cell assemblies (Pulvermueller et al., 1994; Crick and Koch, 2003). Such neuronal assemblies, thus, is thought to serve as the functional elements of brain mental activity – elemental *cognitive* operations[12] (Fingelkurts and Fingelkurts, 2003; see also Basar, 2004). If cell assemblies are the basic units of cognition, they must become active when cognitive processes take place. It is known from animal experiments that synchrony (is taken as an indicator of reverberating activity in cell assemblies, see Merzenich and deCharms, 1996) of neuronal activity reflects gestalt criteria, for example the fact that two objects move together (Singer 1995; Singer and Gray 1995). Further support for the role of neuronal assemblies in cognitive processing comes from studies of electrocortical responses to different memory stages (Fingelkurts et al., 2003a). Moreover, gestalt-like figures such as Kanizsa's triangle have led to stronger EEG responses when compared to physically similar stimuli that are not perceived as a coherent gestalt (Tallon et al., 1995; Tallon-Baudry et al., 1996). It is well documented that the simplest inputs such as single words lead to activation of broad patterns in brain scans. There is no way to accept that the input of a single word would activate such a large fraction of the neurons unless the group activation process is the normal response of the brain (Epstein, 1999). Even more, there is known fact that seeing only the first few letters of a word can create a whole word in our minds; it also shows that a neuronal assembly can be normally activated by those first inputs (Epstein, 1999). It has been even suggested that if cognitive processing does not take place, neuronal assemblies do not become active[13] (Pulvermueller et al., 1994).

---

[11] Only observing statistically representative groups of the neurons can reveal such emergent phenomena as cognition.

[12] This view is alternative to both localizationist and holistic approaches (Pulvermueller, 1999). Localizationists would assume that small cortical areas are fully capable of performing complex cognitive operations. A localizationist would, for instance, propose that a small brain area is the locus of word comprehension (Broca 1861; Lichtheim 1885; Wernicke 1874). According to this view, each complex cognitive operation is restricted to one area – that is, no other areas are assumed to contribute to this specific process. In contrast, a holistic approach would imply that the entire cortex exhibits equipotentiality with regard to all cognitive operations and that all cortical areas can contribute to sufficiently complex mental processes (for discussion see an overview, Deacon 1989). The neuronal assembly theory is in sharp contrast to both of these views (Pulvermueller, 1999). Cell assemblies with defined cortical topographies are assumed to form the neurobiological representations of elemental cognitive operations, whereby complex cognitive operations are represented by the joint activity of many neuronal assemblies at another time scale (Fingelkurts and Fingelkurts, 2003). To illustrate this, lets consider the following example: The elemental cognitive operation lasts some short period *T*. Then at times shorter than *T* one should speak about cognitive (or brain) microstate, whereas at times greater than *T* one observes a succession of microstates (or a state history). The combination of local microstates together will form cognitive (or brain) macrostate that will last some time *Ti* and will have its own history at times greater than *Ti*.

[13] More precisely, cell assemblies may be stimulated and, therefore, become slightly active, but no full activation, no ignition, should take place.

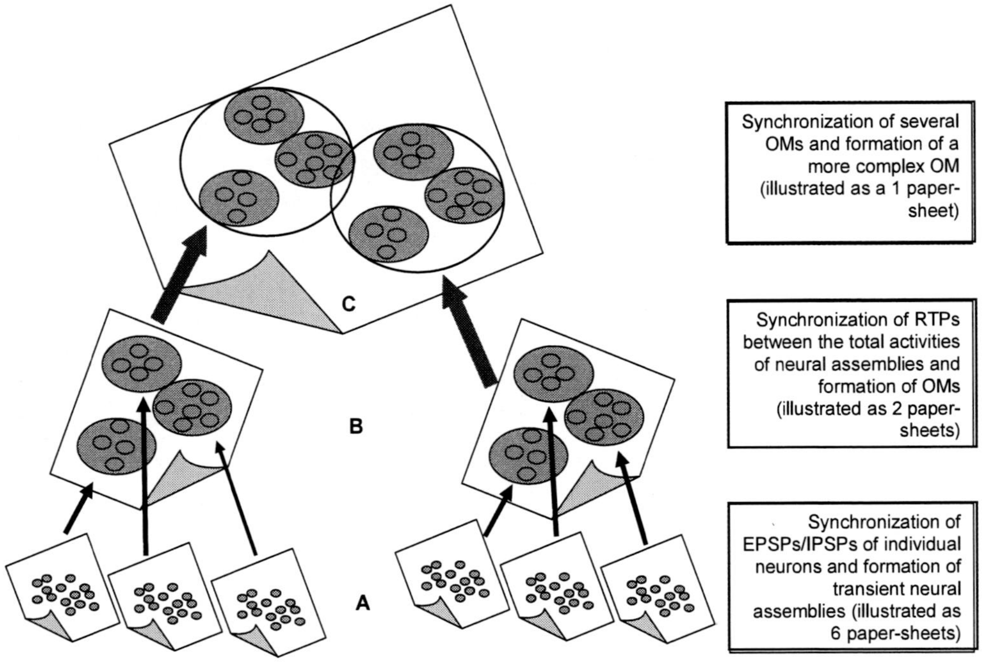

Figure 1. Schematic illustration of operational architectonics of brain functioning. *A*, Microscopic level of individual neurons. *B*, Mesoscopic level of transient neuronal assemblies. *C*, Macroscopic level of operational modules (OMs). *EPSP/IPSP*, excitatory/inhibitory postsynaptic potential. *RTP*, rapid transition periods in electromagnetic field. Figure is modified from Fingelkurts et al., 2005, Progress in Neuropsychopharmacology & Biological Psychiatry ©.

Hebbian Neuronal Assemblies

Early attempts to build the neuronal assembly theory can be traced back to Donald Hebb, who in 1949 proposed that the coactivation of connected cells would result in a modification of weights so that when the presynaptic cell fires, the probability of the postsynaptic cell firing is increased[14] (Hebb, 1949). This implying that group of neurons that have the tendency to fire together will become strengthened as an assembly. Such principle is known as "the principle of cooperativity". Another principle was suggested later – it is "the correlation learning": Connection strength is not only modified by coincident activity, it also changes if only one of two connected neurons is active while the other one is inactive (Pulvermueller, 1999). These two principles have to have two important functional consequences: (1) If a sufficiently large number of the assembly neurons are stimulated by the input (either through sensory input or by internal image), activity will spread to additional assembly members and, finally, the entire assembly will be active. This explosion-like process has been called ignition of the assembly (Braitenberg 1978). (2) After an assembly has ignited, activity will not stop immediately (because of fatigue or regulation processes),

[14] This view corresponds with one of the basic ideas of the Russian neurophysiological school: In the first third of previous century Vvedensky (1906) and Ukhtomsky (1935) proposed that connections between nervous structures are promoted through the correspondence in their frequency characteristics, that is, in equalizing their excitation cycle rate. This is known as the "functional lability" parameter (Ivanitsky and Nikolaev, 1999).

but the strong connections within the assembly will allow activity for some time (Pulvermueller, 1999). Hebb's postulates have been extended into various forms of correlation-based rules and intensively used in many learning networks and in the analysis of activity-driven refinement of developing circuits[15] (Sejnowski and Tesauro, 1989; Brown et al., 1990; see also review by Bi and Poo, 2001).

Even though the explanatory power of neuronal assembly theory is very high and it is the right level of brain organization for the cognition, there is a major problem with using Hebbian cell assemblies to explain perceptual and cognitive processes. For one thing, they are too slow and rely on learning by repetition at a low-level (single neurons) organization of the brain. However, a great part of our cognition and perceptions are fast, unique, and singular in a veritable sense (Bauer and Dicke, 1997). For example, we can perceive individual objects that we see only once, and never again, within a fraction of a second. The coherency of perceptual and cognitive states is achieved rapidly and effortlessly (Edelman and Tononi, 2000). It is obvious that neuronal representations of such objects and related cognitive processes cannot be based on slow anatomical cell assemblies (Bauer and Dicke, 1997). Instead, *functional transient neuronal assemblies* may be appropriate for the purpose since they are fast and do not necessarily depend on the anatomical connections[16] (von der Malsburg, 1999; see also Fingelkurts et al., 2005a).

The other general problem with Hebbian neuronal assemblies is that they have no flexible means of constructing higher-level operations by combining more elementary operations (Fodor and Pylyshin, 1988). It is known as "the binding problem" (von der Malsburg, 1981). To illustrate this, lets consider the following classical example: Imagine that two objects need to be activated/represented in the same mental state in order to be compared. Such coactivation would inevitably lead to what has been named "superposition catastrophe", whereby two neuronal assemblies according to the classical concept will merge into one, and there will be no possibility to express the information needed to subdivide the composite state into its components (von der Malsburg, 1999). So far, the only reliable solution lies in the fast transient neuronal assemblies which (being the discrete functional units[17]) are capable of combinatorial mechanisms through the temporal synchrony of their total activities (Fig. 1 B). As a result they may form the complex units which have explicit structure on the basis of which elements of this structure can be compared, recognized, decomposed, and further combined to build new or even more complex structures (Fig. 1 C;

---

[15] An exciting application of modified Hebbian rules is in a new type of neural network models – the "pulsed neural networks" (Maass and Bishop, 1999) that use precise timing of individual spikes to encode information. Such temporal coding may enable construction of more versatile and powerful networks because it provides larger coding capacity and easier handling of temporal information (Bi and Poo, 2001).

[16] The assembly of neurons which are connected by functional connectivity has been also called "dynamical cell assembly" (Fujii et al., 1996). The important point to note is that neurons composing a dynamical neural assembly need not be fixed; that is to say, a set of neurons joining the assembly may alter in time (Watanabe et al., 2001).

[17] Cell-assembly size is currently estimated to lie between several hundred and about a million neurons (Palm, 1982; 1993). It is relevant to point out here that the boundary between neuronal assemblies is necessary fuzzy. And it is not a problem, since there will be some neurons with high correlations and others whose correlation with these "core neurons" are smaller (Pulvermueller, 1999). In other words, some neurons will always become active together when a certain input pattern is provided, others may only be recruited in some cases, depending, for example, on the neuronal sets activated in the past (Milner, 1957).

see also Fingelkurts and Fingelkurts, 2003). This is the neural architecture that has the capacity for flexible learning and self-organization (for the review, see Fingelkurts and Fingelkurts, 2004).

Transient Functional Neuronal Assemblies

Katchalsky (1974) was the first who start to study the self-organized behavior of fast cell assemblies. The distributed interactions among neurons that arise in neuronal cell assemblies "enslave" the mass of cortical neurons (Haken, 1999). More precisely, with convergence, each receiving neuron sums the dendritic currents triggered by neurons broadly scattered over the transmitting cortex[18] (Freeman, 1992). The only activity that survives this spatial integration is that which has the same instantaneous frequency and phase over the spatial extent of the integration[19], whereas the stimulus-locked activity that is not spatially coherent is washed away (Freeman, 2000). The activity that has this property is the common carrier wave generated by the cortical interaction, which conveys the amplitude modulation patterns. The consequence is that the raw sense data, which can be regarded as a representation of each particular stimulus, is "deleted" by the brain as noise, and the self-organized amplitude modulation pattern is accepted as the signal, that is, the meaning for the individual of the class of the particular stimulus (Freeman, 2000). By tuning or choosing delays and connection weights, functional neural assemblies can be constructed that are differentially sensitive to particular time patterns in their inputs. Assemblies can also be formed that emit particular temporal patterns when activated (John and Schwartz, 1978). Thus, the most significant property of such functional ensembles is the capacity for undergoing rapid and repeated global state changes (Freeman, 2000a,b). Formation of new neural assemblies is then a means by which the brain can adaptively construct what are in effect new measuring "devices" that make new distinctions on an internal milieu that is richly coupled to the external world (Cariani, 2001).

The activity of these neuronal assemblies represents the mesoscopic level of brain organization (the term has been introduced by Freeman in 1992; see also Freeman, 2000c; Freeman et al., 2001). Mesoscopic effects operating at spatial and temporal scales of 1 cm and 100 ms mediate between the two extremes of single neurons and the major lobes of the forebrain. They correspond in size to Brodmann's areas and in duration to psychophysical events that compose perceptions. Thus, mesoscopic effects provide a link between extreme local fragmentation and global uniformity (Fig. 1 B). They change continually in space and time, requiring a very close relationship between dynamic events, e.g. amplitude modulation of local field potentials, and the media through which the propagation occurs (Freeman, 1992; Skarda and Freeman, 1987).

---

[18] This is how brains do spatial ensemble averaging. There is no need to store the traces of activity.

[19] It is a set of emergent properties of abundant amounts of elements in assembly that is important. In this sense, the representation of information by neuronal assemblies is ergodic; the same as the generation of pressure by water molecules in an enclosed volume (John, 2001). Because of this, the representation of information by neuronal assemblies is also robust, meaning that damage to a single cell (or cell mortality) will not have a catastrophic effect on the representation of information. Additionally, neuronal assemblies have other key important properties, such as mechanism for noise removal, short-term memory and the instantiation of complex, nonlinear functions (Pouget et al., 2000).

There is intensive research of inherent relation between local field potentials produced by neuronal assemblies[20] and cognitive operations. Thus, it has been demonstrated that local field potentials change in motor (Vaadia et al., 1995; Donoghue et al., 1998; Lee, 2003) and sensory (de Oliveira et al., 1997; Super et al., 2003) cortices during periods in which the animal is anticipating behaviorally relevant events. Similarly, group of neurons in motor cortical areas display coherent oscillations during demanding tasks, or task epochs presumably requiring cognitive effort (Murthy and Fetz, 1996). Other studies have shown that synchrony (Steinmetz et al., 2000) and oscillations in the local field potentials (Fries et al., 2001) can be modulated by attention to a particular location in the visual field or to a particular sensory modality. These experiments suggest that coherent oscillations might be involved in the realization of cognitive operations, because they appear when the subject is preparing to process specific sensory stimuli, or is selectively processing a subset of the available sensory stimuli. Some of the more compelling data in support of this idea come from analyses of error trials. Three studies have shown that, when subjects do not execute correct responses, coherent oscillations are reduced (Woelbern et al. 2002; Lee, 2003; Super et al., 2003), suggesting that the absence of coherent oscillations reflects a failure in the flow of information. Generally speaking, "the transitions between walking and running, speaking and swallowing, sleeping and waking, fast changes of objects and scenes in the visual field and at last the staccato flow of thoughts and mental images are all realized by transient functional neuronal assemblies" (Freeman et al., 2001).

In conclusion, we should stress that functional neural cell assemblies, though powerful by themselves, are also ideal building blocks for larger cognitive structures or complex cognitive operations (see Fingelkurts and Fingelkurts, 2001; 2003; see also Kaplan et al. 1990; Holland 1998).

Operational Synchrony and Operational Modules

The recombination of subsets of activity of neuronal assemblies (elemental operations as functional building blocks) into larger spatial-temporal structures yields a vast number of potential combinations (Fig. 1 C; see also Fingelkurts and Fingelkurts, 2004), thus providing the base for a practically infinite number of mental states and thoughts of different complexity (Fingelkurts and Fingelkurts, 2003). Just as functional connectivity (or *Operational Synchrony*, Fingelkurts and Fingelkurts, 2001) forms transient neuronal assemblies, the same principal of functional connectivity can be used to create an associative links between two or more of such assemblies[21] (Fingelkurts et al., 2005a).

[20] Oscillations in the local field potentials are normally taken as evidence of coherent oscillations among the group of neurons contributing to the field potential (Averbeck and Lee, 2004).

[21] This is possible just because the mesoscopic patterns of brain activity produced by different neural assemblies all have the same "format" (Freeman, 2000c). This indicates that the several such patterns (which represent elemental cognitive operations) can be as easily integrated with each other, leading to the formation of a more complex spatial-temporal pattern – the operational module (OM) that represents complex cognitive operation (Fingelkurts and Fingelkurts, 2001). Thus, functionally, the outcome of coincident operations is an OM rather than larger ensemble of particular neurons firing in synchrony (Cariani, 1997). Here the time dimension is very important – time structure is the organizing currency of the brain-mind system. Time structure is

Neurophysiologically, each local pattern that appears as a result of neuronal assembly activity depends on its interactions with the others to which it is functionally connected (Mumford, 1994). Because the interactions between cell assemblies are inevitably mutual, the situation is not that of one assembly imposing its pattern on another, but rather of multiple assemblies acting to constrain the pattern in each other (Bressler, 1999). Pattern constraint is a potentially powerful mechanism for the formation of novel complex dynamic coordination patterns in large-scale networks. Indeed, different brain operations executed by spatially distant neuronal assembles tend to be synchronized if they happens to be at the same time, thus related to the same perceptual/cognitive act (Cleeremans, 2002). Hence, the resultant spatial-temporal pattern or *Operational Module* (OM) is the emergent product of the synchronized simple operations of a set of strongly associated neuronal assemblies (Fig. 1 C); and these OMs represent the realization of cognitive complex macrooperations[22]. Here the notion of *operational space-time* should be introduced. It is not easy to grasp exactly what we need to explain, however, such notion is important for our conceptualization. Intuitively, the operational space-time (OST) is the virtual space and time which is "constructed" by the brain each time when the particular metastable OM emerges. Formally, the OST means that for a particular complex operation, the spatial distribution of the neuronal assemblies' locations with synchronous activity at repetitive instants of time (beginnings and ends of simple operations) builds the OM. These distributed locations of neuronal assemblies are discrete and their proximity or the activity in the in-between area, delimited by the known locations, is not considered in the definition (only the exact locations are relevant). Also, between the moments in time that particular locations of the neuronal assemblies synchronize, there can be smaller subset(s) of these locations synchronized between themselves or with other neural locations, though these do not relate to the same space-time of the same OM. The sketch of this general idea is presented in figure 2.

The communication of activity from microscopic single neurons to feature-specific neural assemblies and yet to the large-scale distributed networks, been a pressing neurocognitive problem, may be elucidated through the present framework. This framework is in agreement with the Breakspear and Stam (2005) conceptualization of the brain as a constrained multiscale system in which emergent dynamics at any scale have a critical influence on the activity in larger and smaller scale structures. Thus, the "transition" of the same neural assembly into the new OM, in accordance with participation in the realization of another complex cognitive operation, must depend on the ability of this neural assembly to adapt to the main variables of the new OM. Thus, discrete parts of the neural networks (or

---

preserved within OM in a sparse and distributed form. Information processing in such OM would be statistically-mechanical in nature, implementing temporal binding of simpler operations on the all-order interval statistics of a larger operation and consequently a larger OM (Fingelkurts and Fingelkurts, 2003).

[22] Similar view may be found in Bressler (1999; 2002): Local neuronal assemblies are considered to serve as associative memories for specific elementary types of information. But each local associative memory is coupled with a number of others according to the topological ordering of functional connectivity. Thus, cognitive structure depends not only on local stores of information, but also on heightened probabilities of conjunction among domains of knowledge stored in separate cortical areas. Context for processing in each neuronal assembly, hence, is provided by constraints imposed by the states of the other assemblies with which it interacts. Of course, not every OM constitutes a mental state or thought. Moreover, even in those, which do, the large amount of purely physical brain processes contribute to the construction of OM. However, from the level of OM there is no access to the original raw data anymore (Fingelkurts and Fingelkurts, 2003).

assemblies) may gain another functional meaning when they are recruited by other OM and, therefore take part in realization of another perceptual or cognitive act (Fingelkurts, 1998; Fingelkurts and Fingelkurts, 2001; Fingelkurts et al., 2003a,b). In this process, some local networks (assemblies) in the large-scale network become temporarily coordinated (formation of OM), while others are temporarily excluded from participation in the coordination state. Furthermore, the spatial activity pattern within each coordinated local neural assembly, representing its contribution to the large-scale pattern (indexed as OM), becomes temporarily stabilized, thus implementing the metastability principle (Kelso, 1995; Kaplan, 1998; for the recent review, see Fingelkurts and Fingelkurts, 2004).

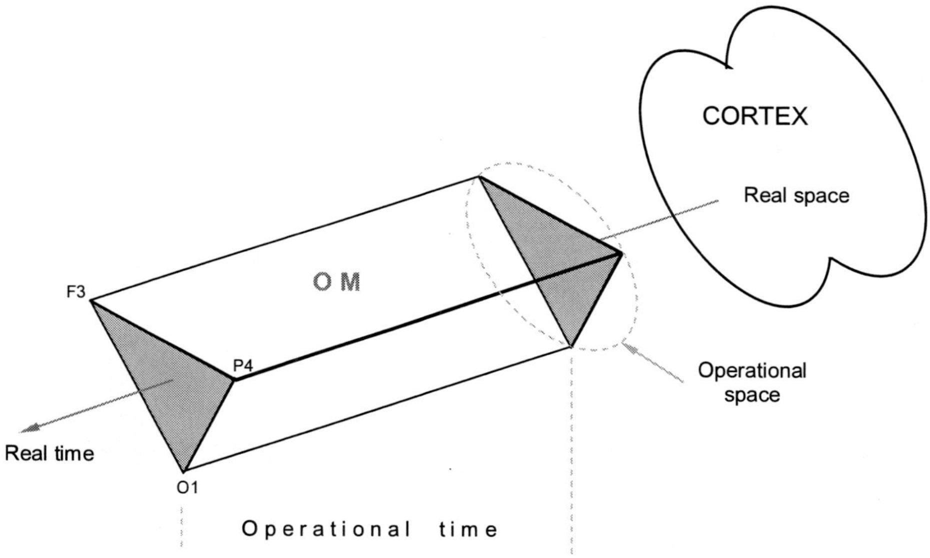

Figure 2. Operational module (OM) and operational space-time (OST). Each OM exists in the OST, which is "blind" to other possible time and space scales present simultaneously in the brain system. In the other words, all neural assemblies that do not contribute to a particular OM are temporarily and spatially excluded from the OST. F_3, is the left frontal area; P_4, is the right parietal area; and O_1, is the left occipital area. As an example, only neural assemblies in these areas (operational space) synchronize their operations on a particular (operational) time-scale.

The importance of such large-scale operational synchrony for the cognition and mind was shown experimentally. For example, it has been demonstrated that functionally distinct cortical regions might be preferentially operationally synchronized and involved in different stages of memory processing such as encoding, retrieval, and retention (for details, see Kaplan and Shishkin 2000; Fingelkurts et al., 2003a). This was expressed through a gradual increase in operational synchrony process together with a growth of cognitive loading[23] (Kaplan et al., 1997; Fingelkurts et al., 2003a). Thus, the principle finding was the existence of systematic specific functional combinations among cortical areas (OMs), which changed significantly along with the memory stages shift (Fingelkurts et al., 2003a). These findings

[23] In contrast, subjects who failed to memorize the task, showed the negative process of operational synchrony, meaning that the particular brain areas actively unsynchronized their operations (Fingelkurts, 1998).

are also in agreement with the works of McIntosh (1999), Fuster (1997), and Basar et al. (2001). In another study, using a robust illusion known as the McGurk effect (McGurk and MacDonald, 1976), it was demonstrated that the apparent synthesis of information from different modalities might be achieved through the process of operational synchrony between modality-specific and non-specific cortical areas (for a detail discussion, see Fingelkurts et al., 2003b). The temporal synchronization of cortical operations processing unimodal stimuli at different cortical sites reveals the importance of temporal features of auditory and visual stimuli for audio-visual speech integration. The main principle lies in the systematic moment-by-moment synchronization of the operations produced by different neural assemblies (Fig. 1) within the large-scale networks (Kaplan and Shishkin 2000; Bressler and Kelso, 2001). Thus, the well-timed spatiotemporal synchronization patterns (indexed by OMs) related to audio-visual integration were obtained. The subjects, who did not display the McGurk illusion (meaning that they lacked conscious multi-sensory integration), in contrast, demonstrated significant uncoupling[24] (negative values of operational synchrony) of particular brain areas (Fingelkurts et al., 2003b). These findings are in keeping with recent studies (for review, see Calvert, 2001), suggesting that multisensory integration is a process that not only facilitates detection of the multisensory stimuli by amplification of the unimodal sensory signals, but also combines these signals to form new and emergent multimodal representational percepts (O'Hare, 1991). Currently, it has been demonstrated that psychotropic drugs (in particular benzodiazepines) may significantly modify OMs and alter metastability of brain activity in healthy subjects. (Fingelkurts et al., 2004a,b).

Generally, OM has a more complex structure than operations which constitute it. OM is a gross abstraction of the brain state (Fig. 1 and Fig. 2), where much of brain state information is not transparent for the level of subjective phenomenology[25] (for detail conceptualization see Fingelkurts and Fingelkurts, 2003; see also Arbib, 2001). Such interpretation was already established by early philosopher Thomas Aquinas (reprint, 1952) who concluded that single events in the material world are not knowable, and that knowledge comes only through abstraction and generalization from the "phantasmata" of raw sensory impacts.

Properties of Operational Modules

OMs have several unique properties important for cognitive and mental activity of the brain. First is the property of *associativity*, by which the activation of a particular pattern in one local assembly co-activates linked patterns in other local assemblies (Rauschecker, 1995). This capacity is essential for joining together related information from different knowledge (or sensory) domains, such as in the association of names and visual images or auditory and visual information. However, this association is not merely a conditioning of one pattern by another, since it occurs within the overall framework of cognitive structures (Deese, 1970). The co-activation of patterns in different cortical areas is constrained by the

---

[24] Note, that the suppression of interactions between cortical areas was achieved not by inhibition responses, but rather by a sufficient degree of temporal dis-coordination of operations (see Fingelkurts et al., 2004a,b).

[25] Our OMs resembles Damasio's (2000) second-order neural patterns in several respects: It is an representation of perceived (or imagined) object (or scene) which is formed through an unfolding succession of signals related to this object/scene; it arises transiently out of interactions among a selected several neuronal assemblies; several such patterns can form composite and integrated pattern which would give rise to a new experience (we may call them the third-order neural patterns).

patterns of connectivity formed between those areas. In short, association always occurs within the context of cognitive structure (Bressler, 2002).

Second important property of OMs is *dispositionality*, a characteristic of cortical function that has been extensively discussed by Damasio (1994). What this means in the present context is that the activity patterns of some local assemblies serve a dispositional role in directing the coordination of other local assemblies. Local dispositional networks interact in the same way as local sensory or motor networks (Bressler, 2002), but the information they provide serves to specify the composition of the large-scale coordination pattern – OM in our interpretation. The recruitment of a dispositional neural assembly into an OM can thus serve to recruit additional sets of specific local assemblies. Each recruited set may contain other dispositional networks with the potential for recruiting even further sets. In this way the cortex may evolve through a series of large-scale coordination states. Thus, dispositional networks may significantly contribute to the ability of the cortex to manifest a temporal progression of logically connected mental/cognitive states (Bressler, 2002). Dispositional networks in the cortex may exist at different hierarchical levels above the primary sensory and motor areas, and different areas may potentially contribute to the orderly evolution of the cognitive states.

Another advantageous property of OM is the *intermittency*. It is the degree of coordination of the component parts over time, when this degree can abruptly increase (Bressler, 2002). Indeed, distributed sets of cortical areas may remain uncoordinated for some time, and then, with a change in cognitive state, suddenly become coordinated through a rapid increase in operational synchrony (Fingelkurts et al., 2003a,b).

The last and the most important property of OMs is their *metastability* (Kelso, 1991, 1995; Kaplan, 1998; for the resent review see Fingelkurts and Fingelkurts, 2004). Metastability may allow the cortex to enter into many different states of coordination of its constituent areas without becoming trapped in any one state (Bressler, 2002). More precisely, in a metastable regime of brain dynamics, the interdependence of separate areas is balanced between integrating and segregating activities (Kelso, 1991, 1995; Friston, 1997; Kaplan, 1998). This property provides the cortical system with the flexibility necessary to rapidly adapt at both large-scale and local levels to changing contingencies required for a cognitive function. This flexibility may be advantageous for cognition if it allows the cortex to carry out a variety of tasks simply by changing the coordination states of its networks (Bressler and Kelso, 2001). Thus, different kinds of spatial-temporal patterns (OMs) can be present/sent over the same transmission lines at different times or even interleaved together without being functionally confused (Fingelkurts and Fingelkurts, 2003).

This raises the possibility that the structure of functional organization of informational process in the brain is *isomorphic* to the operational structure of the cognition, and on a more abstract level, to the phenomenological structure of awareness and consciousness (Fingelkurts and Fingelkurts, 2001). Indeed, one can see that the structure of electrical brain field, structure of cognition and the phenomenal structure of consciousness have the same construction: the succession of discrete and relatively stable periods (OMs, cognitive acts or thoughts) separated by rapid transitive processes (abrupt changes of OMs, cognitive acts or thoughts)[26]. In this interpretation, ordered sequences of OMs generated from within the brain system would have the character of successions of mental symbols, and reformulating Bressler (2002) these would be experienced as thoughts. This phenomenon is usually referred as a "stream of thoughts"[27] (James, 1890; for resent developments see Mangan, 1993a,b; Chafe, 1994; Galin, 1994, 2000). Further, the OM's patterns that are related to goal-states would then have the character of system imperatives to adjust behavior, and thus would be experienced as desires and pains; and actions would be experienced through their effects on perceptions, sensory, and hedonic states (Bressler, 2002).

In the framework of operational architectonics (OA) framework, OMs (being by themselves the result of synchronized operations going on in different brain structures) could be also operationally synchronized[28] between each other (on the new time scale), thus forming more abstract and more complex OM that constitutes new integrated subjective experience (Fingelkurts and Fingelkurts, 2003; this idea coheres with O'Brien and Opie, 1999b). When two or more active OMs are cross-correlated and synchronized through continuous operational synchrony, a further complex OM[29] arises that maps these two (or more) independent simple OMs to each other within the operational time, which in its own turn is mapped onto real time. Different properties of the perceived scene thus can be integrated in order to form an operational whole, which now has higher level of abstractness[30]. The opposite process is also possible when complex OM could be decomposed to simpler OMs, whereas each of which would give rise to a distant subjective experience. However, the price for this decomposition is narrowly *focused attention* and consequently the *focused mental (conscious) state* (von der Malsburg, 1997). Thus, attention could be the possible mechanism that guides decomposition or construction of OMs of different complexity[31] (for detail conceptualization, see Fingelkurts and Fingelkurts, 2003).

Practical Implementation

In the light of our discussion, what is the appropriate method for functional brain imaging, considering that this method should have the capability of revealing the mesoscopic level of brain organization, which is directly involved (as it has been discussed earlier) in the realization of cognition and, eventually, consciousness? As it was already mentioned above, the time-scale of mesoscopic level (the level of neuronal assemblies) is of milliseconds, while the spatial resolution is about a centimeter. Electroencephalography (EEG) and

---

[26] For similar ideas see also O'Brien and Opie, 1999a,b.

[27] According to this metaphor, consciousness is always changing, but it presents us with a series of substantive thoughts that are themselves momentarily stable and unified (James, 1890).

[28] This is the self-organizing dynamic process (for the review see Fingelkurts and Fingelkurts, 2001).

[29] It is important to stress here, that complex OM does not have instructive power upon simpler OMs, it is just a new cognitive state in its own right.

[30] The property of abstractness gives particular advantages for adaptive behavior of the organism: If only a few signals from the relevant objects are available, categorical (abstracted) knowledge can allow for an adequate response to a wide range of stimuli and thus permit adaptive behavior (Edelman, 1987).

[31] See also Taylor (2002) for the view that consciousness can be regarded as created by suitably specific processes arising from the movement of attention.

magnetoencephalography (MEG) are the only methods that satisfy simalteneously to both these time and space scales (Freeman et al., 2001). EEG/MEG detect fast changes in the gross synchronous activity of thousands of cells in selected areas on the cortical surface, thus collecting information from the relevant level of brain organization (Revonsuo, 2001). However, classical approaches to EEG/MEG analysis reveal only limited knowledge of what is going at the level of neural assemblies (Fingelkurts et al., 2005a). The main reason for that is that the studies are designed in a way that they avoid the temporal structure of the phenomenon under investigation. Recordings of brain activity are generally averaged over hundreds of repeated trials or more, in order to eliminate fluctuations in ongoing activity (the "noise") that are not correlated with stimulus presentation (for a critical discussion see Fingelkurts et al., 2002; Fingelkurts et al, 2003c). Thus, an additional question arises: Which of known EEG/MEG analysis approaches can derive the information about operations (discrete events) of neural assemblies and estimate the inherent temporal/dynamical correlations (functional connectivity) among them?

Estimation of Neuronal Assemblies

Neurons that constitute neural assemblies, sum their electrical fields in passing across the extracellular resistance, giving rise to extraneuronal potential differences manifested in the EEG, which correspond to the local field potentials (Freeman et al., 2001). The fact that neurons are able to synchronize their subthreshold oscillations (excitatory postsynaptic potential, EPSP and inhibitory postsynaptic potential, IPSP), leading to fixed states of an overall neuronal assembly and to rapid transitions between such states, was shown experimentally and in computational models (Makarenko and Llinas, 1998). Generally, the overall pattern of correlated activity is very sensitive to fluctuations and it may be swiftly rearranged during rapid shift (Kirillov and Makarenko, 1991; for review, see Singer et al., 1997). As it was demonstrated *in vitro*, the intervals of local fixed potentials are manifested in the oscillatory waves, which are the result of neuronal clustering (Leznik et al., 2002). At the EEG level these intervals are reflected in defined periods (segments) of *quasi-stationary activity*[32] (Fig. 3) operating in different frequency ranges (for review, see Kaplan and Shishkin, 2000; Kaplan et al., 2005). In this case, it is possible to consider one segment as the single event in EEG-phenomenology (Fingelkurts and Fingelkurts, 2001). Within the duration of one segment, the neuronal assembly that generates the oscillations is in the steady stationary state (Brodsky et al., 1999). The transition from one segment to another reflects the changes of the generator system microstate or changes in the activity of the two or more systems (Jansen et al., 1988; Kaplan and Shishkin, 2000). Thus, in order to detect such rapid transitions the task is to divide the EEG signal into stationary segments by estimating the

[32] Yet in 1972 year, it was experimentally shown in detail by Elul, that EEG is a product of (de)synchronized neurons within a cellular assembly (Elul, 1972a,b). EEG waves recorded from the scalp are integrated excitatory postsynaptic potentials (EPSP's) and inhibitory postsynaptic potentials (IPSP's) of neuronal membranes. Since they reflect extracellular currents caused by synchronized neural activity within the local brain volume (John, 2002), the EEG signal within quasi-stationary segments is the envelope of the probability of non-random coherence (so called a "common mode") in the neuronal ensembles near to the recording electrodes.

points of transition. These instants within short-time window, when the EEG amplitude is changed abruptly, are identified as *rapid transition processes* (RTP) (Kaplan et al., 2005). RTP is supposed to be of minor length, and therefore can be treated as a point or near-point[33] (Fig. 3; see also Fingelkurts and Fingelkurts, 2001). The issue of segmental description of brain activity has been addressed by several researchers (for review see Barlow, 1985). However, virtually all such segmentation approaches have a number of inherent limitations (for a detailed review and discussion see Kaplan and Shishkin, 2000 and Kaplan et al., 2001).

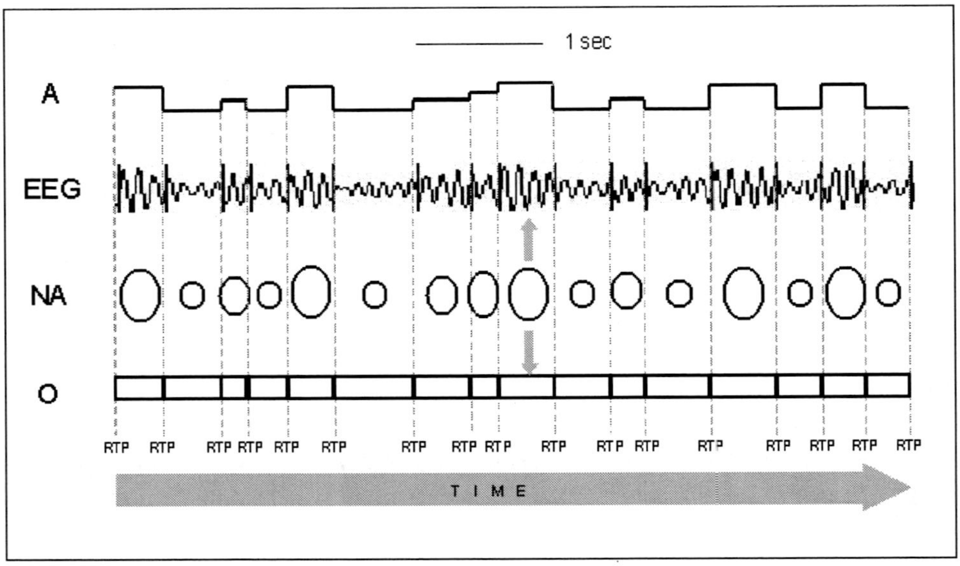

Figure 3. Correspondence between neuronal assemblies and EEG segments. A, amplitude of EEG segments; EEG, electroencephalogram; NA, neuronal assemblies of different size; O – operations of different duration; RTP, rapid transition periods (boundaries between quasi-stationary EEG segments).

To overcome the disadvantages of classical methods of segmentation, the novel technology of the adaptive *non*parametric EEG/MEG segmentation was developed (Kaplan et al., 1997). This method (SECTION 01®, suggested by A. Kaplan, Moscow State University) is performed in two stages (Fig. 4 A). The *first stage* is performed in two steps. During the first step, the native EEG/MEG values were converted into the module. Second step corresponds to the basic procedure of segmentation: The main idea is in comparison of the ongoing EEG/MEG amplitude absolute values averaged in the sliding *test*-window and EEG/MEG amplitude absolute values averaged in the sliding *level*-window (test window << level window). The duration of windows is short (6-800 ms) and dependent on the analyzed frequency range and sampling rate of the signal; the shift of both windows is equal to one data-point. The use of short time windows is motivated by the need for tracking non-

[33] Note, that mathematically it is not important in which time-window the amplitude transition is estimated. What is important, – it is the speed of such transition. Experimentally it was found, that amplitude transition in the RTP area is always very rapid – not less than twofold, if comparison is made between amplitude values in the close area before RTP and immediately after it (Fingelkurts, 1998).

stationary transient cortical processes on a sub-second time scale. As a result of averaging in sliding test- and level-windows, two new sequences (test – t and level – l) are constructed from the initial one, and are placed on the same time-scale (Fig. 4 A). The time-instants corresponding to the crossing of t- and l-time-series become a preliminary estimate of RTP.

The aim of the *second stage* is to estimate the statistically significant RTPs. For that the two conditions should meet (Fig. 4 B). First condition estimates the steepness of a change (Fig. 4 B, a): the EEG/MEG amplitude values are averaged at the t-time-series within n data-points before (M_{-n}) and after (M_{+n}) preliminary RTP. If the result of subtraction ($M_{+n} - M_{-n}$) is statistically significant (the Student criteria, $p < 0.05$ with coefficient 0.3), then this first condition is accepted and second condition should be tested. Second condition (Fig. 4 B, b) must be fulfilled in order to eliminate possible "false alerts" associated with anomalous peaks in the EEG/MEG amplitude. The five points of the digitized EEG/MEG following this preliminary RTP must have a statistically significant difference between averaged amplitude values in the t- and l- time-series (the Student criteria, $p < 0.05$ with coefficient 0.1). Only if these two criteria are met, the preliminary RTP is assumed as actual.

Using this technique, the sequence of RTPs with statistically proven ($p < 0.05$, Student t-test) time coordinates can be determined for each EEG/MEG location individually for each analyzed EEG/MEG epoch. RTPs or jumps in EEG/MEG amplitude in such a way are, in fact, the markers of boundaries between concatenated quasi-stationary segments. By varying the parameters of this technique it is possible to obtain the segments corresponding to a more or less detailed structure of the EEG/MEG. Therefore, there are prospects for the description of the structural EEG/MEG organization as a hierarchy of segmental descriptions on different time scales (Kaplan and Shishkin, 2000). The modeling experiments and theoretical concepts behind this analysis are described elsewhere (Kaplan, 1998; Kaplan and Shishkin, 2000; Fingelkurts et al., 2005; Kaplan et al., 2005).

After quasi-stationary segments (indexed by RTP) are obtained, several characteristics (attributes) of segments (Kaplan and Borisov, 2003) can be calculated separately for each channel (Fig. 3):

1. Average amplitude (A) within each segment (μV^2) – as generally agreed, indicates mainly the volume or *size of neuronal population.*
2. Average length (L) of segments (ms) – illustrates the functional life span of neuronal population or the *duration of operations* produced by this population.
3. Coefficient of amplitude variability (V) within segments (%) – shows the *stability of local neuronal synchronization* within neuronal population or assembly.
4. Average amplitude relation (AR) among adjacent segments (%) – indicates the neuronal assembly behavior – growth (*recruiting of new neurons*) or distraction (*functional elimination of neurons*).
5. Average steepness (S) among adjacent segments (estimated in the close area of RTP) (%) – reflects the *speed* of neuronal population growth or distraction.

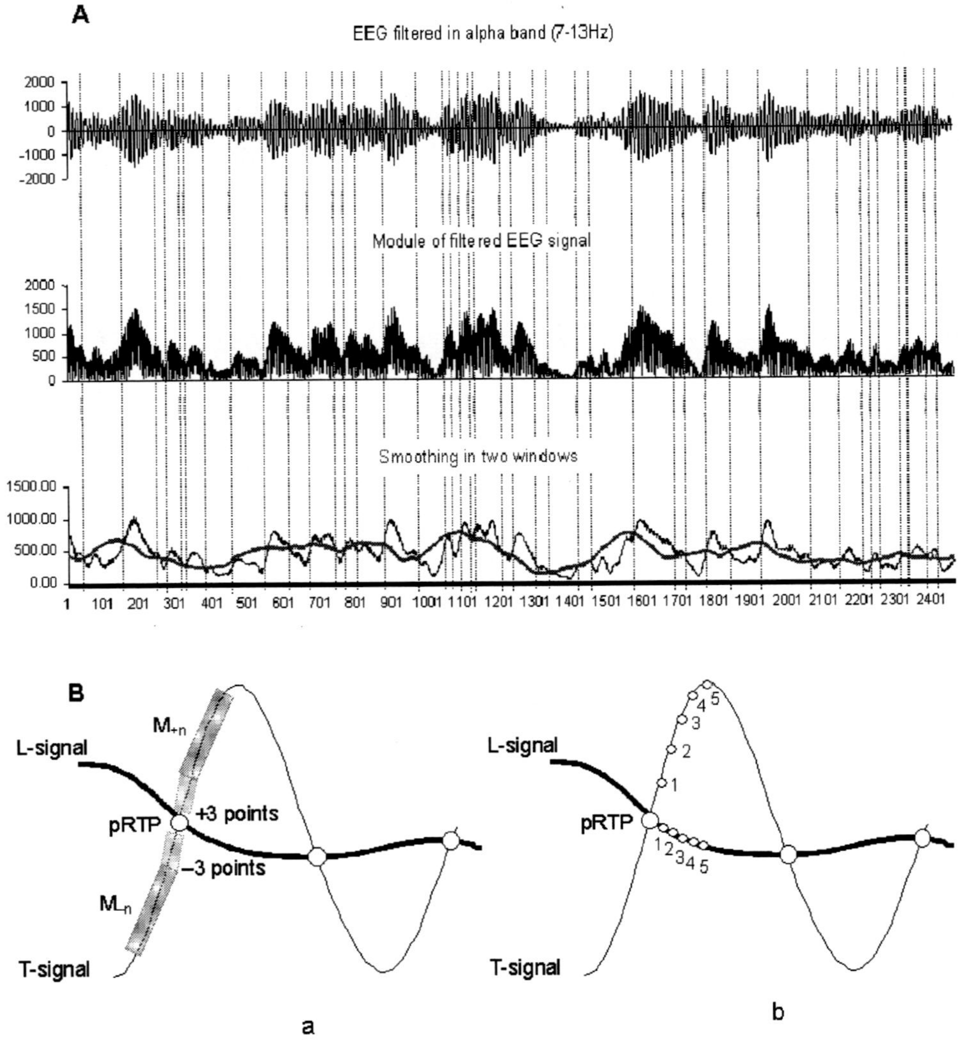

Figure 4. Nonparametric adaptive level segmentation of EEG/MEG (schematic presentation). *A*, First stage of segmentation (two steps). On the horizontal axis the data-points of digitized signal is shown. On the vertical axis the amplitude of the signal is shown in μV^2. Vertical dotted lines indicate the time coordinates of preliminary RTPs. *B*, Second stage of segmentation: two conditions for estimation the statistical significance of preliminary RTP (pRTP). Explanation in the text.

The comparison of the same segment attributes between different experimental conditions or functional states is performed using Wilcoxon matched pairs *t*-test. These attributes reflect different aspects of local processes in the cortex and thus permit assessing the mesolevel description of cortex interactions (interactions within transient neuronal assemblies) through large-scale EEG/MEG estimates (for experimental support and detailed discussion see Fingelkurts et al., 2004b; Kaplan et al., 2005).

Estimation of Functional Connectivity and/or OM

Considering that complex cognitive operations arise from combined synchronous operations of many neural assemblies, the measure of functional connectivity should be capable to estimate such synchrony. Traditionally, coherence and correlation have been the main methods to assess the degree of functional connectivity between brain areas (Thatcher et al., 1986). Recently, several new methods for detecting functional connectivity between cortical areas have been introduced: Partial directed coherence (Baccala and Sameshima, 2001), dynamic imaging of coherent sources (Gross et al., 2001), structural equation models for fMRI (Friston and Buchel, 2000), and phase synchrony (Tass, 1999). However, all these methods have several limitations (for a discussion, see Fingelkurts et al., 2005a).

The novel approach (JUMPSYN 01®, suggested by A. Kaplan, Moscow State University) overcomes the disadvantages of conventional methods, and can reveal inherent functional interrelationships between cortical areas different from those measured by correlation, coherence and phase analysis (for a discussion and modeling experiments see Kaplan et al., 2005; Fingelkurts et al., 2005a).

The technology for estimation of functional brain connectivity through the index of EEG/MEG structural synchrony (ISS) is as follows. Each rapid transitional process (RTP) in the *reference* EEG/MEG channel (the channel with the minimal number of RTP from any pair of EEG/MEG channels) is surrounded by a short "window" (ms). It is taken that any RTP from another (*test*) channel coincided if it fell within this window. The ISS for pairs of EEG/MEG channels can be estimated using this procedure. The ISS is computed as follows:

$$\mathbf{ISS} = \boldsymbol{m}_{windows} - \boldsymbol{m}_{residual},$$

$$\text{where } m_{windows} = 100 * \frac{sn_w}{sl_w}; \; m_{residual} = 100 * \frac{sn_r}{sl_r};$$

sn_w – total number of RTPs in all windows (window for synchronization) in the test channel;

sl_w – total length of EEG/MEG recording (in data points) inside all windows in the test channel;

sn_r – total number of RTPs outside the windows (window for synchronization) in the test channel;

sl_r – total length of EEG/MEG recording (in data points) outside the windows in the test channel.

It is obvious, however, that even in the absence of any functional interrelations between EEG/MEG locations there should be a certain stochastic level of RTPs coupling, which would reflect merely occasional synchrony. The values of such stochastic inter-location relations should be uniform and substantially lower than in the actual presence of functional interrelation between different of EEG/MEG channels. Because of unknown statistical properties of the RTPs coincidence, the construction of thresholds is necessary. The time-variant thresholds were established by the use of surrogate data. Thus, to arrive at a direct estimation of a 5% level of statistical significance of the ISS ($p < 0.05$), computer simulation of RTP's synchronization is undertaken based on random shuffling of time segments marked by RTPs (500 independent trials). These share the properties of the experimental data (number of RTPs in each EEG/MEG channel of analyzed pair, number of segments, and number of windows of synchronization), but the time coordinates of RTPs were altered randomly in each trial so as to destroy the natural temporal structure of the data. Justification for this approach can be found in Fingelkurts et al. (2004a). However, other approaches are also possible (see for example Bullmore et al., 2001).

As a result of 500 times repeated random reshuffling of the time segments marked by RTPs the stochastic level of RTPs coupling (ISS_{stoh}), and the upper and lower thresholds of ISS_{stoh} significance (5%) are calculated. These values represent an estimation of the maximum (by module) possible stochastic rate of RTPs coupling (confidence levels). Only those values of ISS which exceeded the upper (*active coupling*) and lower (*active decoupling*) thresholds of ISS_{stoh} have been assumed to be statistically valid ($p < 0.05$). Thus, the ISS tends towards zero where there is no synchronization between the EEG/MEG segments and has positive or negative values where such synchronization exists (Fig. 5). Positive values indicate 'active' *coupling* of EEG/MEG segments (synchronization of EEG/MEG segments is observed significantly more often than expected by chance), whereas negative values mark 'active' *decoupling* of segments (synchronization of EEG/MEG segments is observed significantly less than expected by chance). From a qualitative perspective, the coupling of EEG/MEG segments corresponds to the phenomenon of synchronization of brain operations or *Operational Synchrony* – OS (for review, see Fingelkurts and Fingelkurts, 2001, 2003).

It is obvious also that there should be the synchronization of segments in a more than two EEG (or MEG) locations, assuming that same set of neuronal assemblies may co-operate in different combinations along the execution of a cognitive and mental acts (Fingelkurts and Fingelkurts, 2003, 2004). Thus, transient synchronization of brain operations (indexed by structural synchrony in EEG/MEG) going on in several cortical areas would construct a so-called *operational module* (OM) (Kaplan, 1995; see also Fingelkurts and Fingelkurts, 2001; for experimental support see Fingelkurts et al., 2003a; 2004b), which constitutes the unified and metastable neural state (for a detail see Fig. 2 and the previous section of this Chapter). OM means that the set of the neuronal assemblies synchronously participated in the same cognitive act during the analyzed period. The criterion for defining an OM is a sequence of the same *synchrocomplexes* (SC). Whereby, SC is a set of EEG/MEG channels in which each channel forms a paired combination (high values of ISS) with all other EEG/MEG channels in the same set (Fig. 6); meaning that all pairs of channels in an SC have to have significant index of structural synchrony (Fingelkurts et al., 2003a; 2004b; see also Fingelkurts and Fingelkurts 2003).

The result of structural synchrony measure is automatically drowned upon computer OS maps (Fig. 7). The changes in operational synchrony maps should only considered relevant if these changes appeared consistently in a majority of the trials and subjects (not less than 85% of occurrence) under the experimental conditions being analyzed. This permits to overcome the common problem of multiple comparisons between maps that exists due to the large number of electrode pairs in the maps (Rappelsberger and Petsche, 1988).

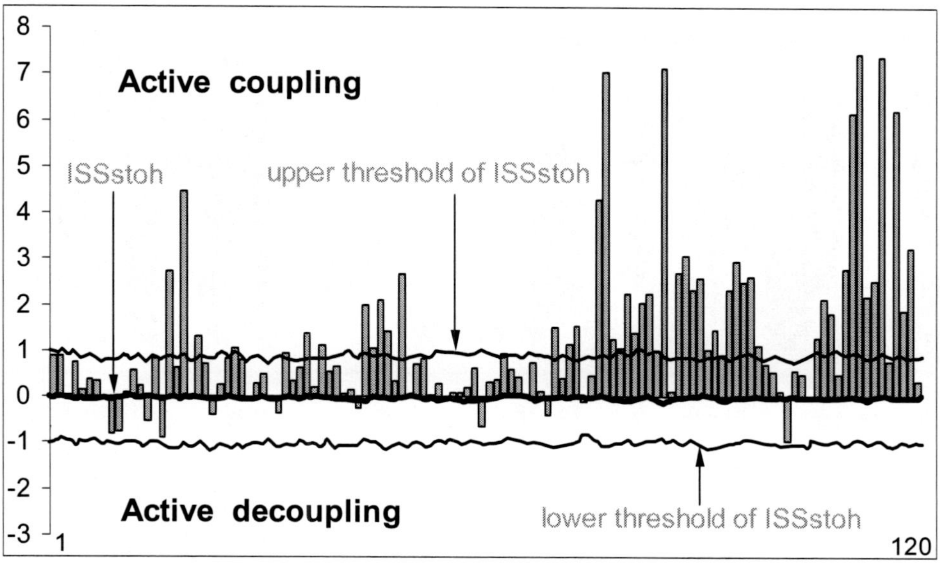

Figure 5. Schematic illustration of the index of structural synchrony (ISS) and its stochastic levels. As an example, the calculations of ISS are shown for 16 EEG channels. The *Y*-axis displays the ISS values found in the experiment (illustrated as gray bars). The *X*-axis displays the 120 possible pair combinations of 16 EEG channels (1 = O1-O2, 2 = O1-P3, 3 = O1-P4, 4 = O1-T5, ... 115 = F4-Fz, 116 = F4-F7, 117 = F4-F8, 118 = Fz-F7, 119 = Fz-F8, 120 = F7-F8). Figure is reproduced from the Fingelkurts et al. 2004, Human Brain Mapping ©.

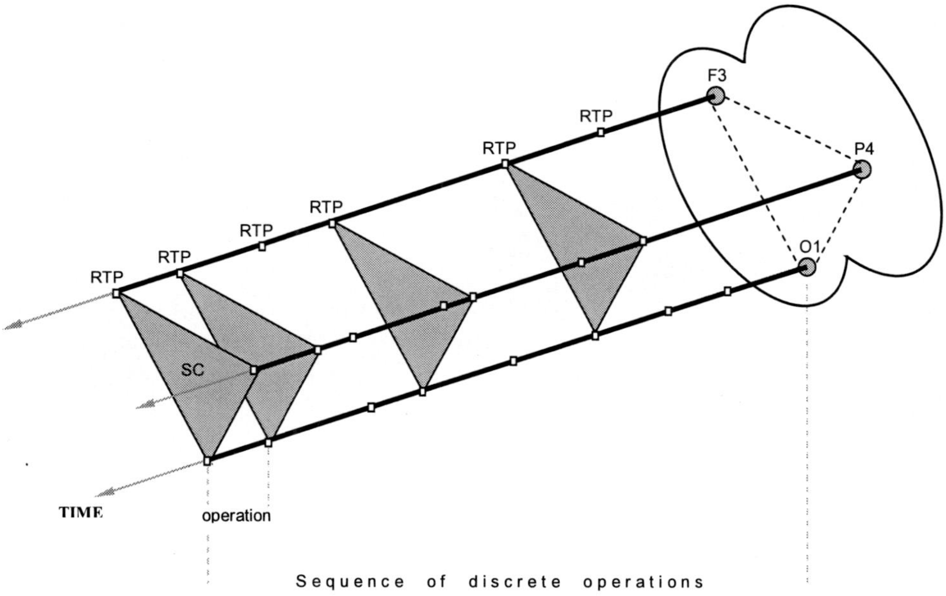

Figure 6. Estimation of OM. *RTP*, rapid transition periods, – are the boundaries between EEG/MEG quasi-stationary segments (at electromagnetic level) and the boundaries between neural operations (at the phenomenological level). F_3, is the left frontal area; P_4, is the right parietal area; and O_1, is the left occipital area. Only neural assemblies in these areas synchronize their operations on a particular time-scale. *SC*, momentary synchrocomplex, – the synchronization of RTPs between different local EEG/MEG at a particular moment.

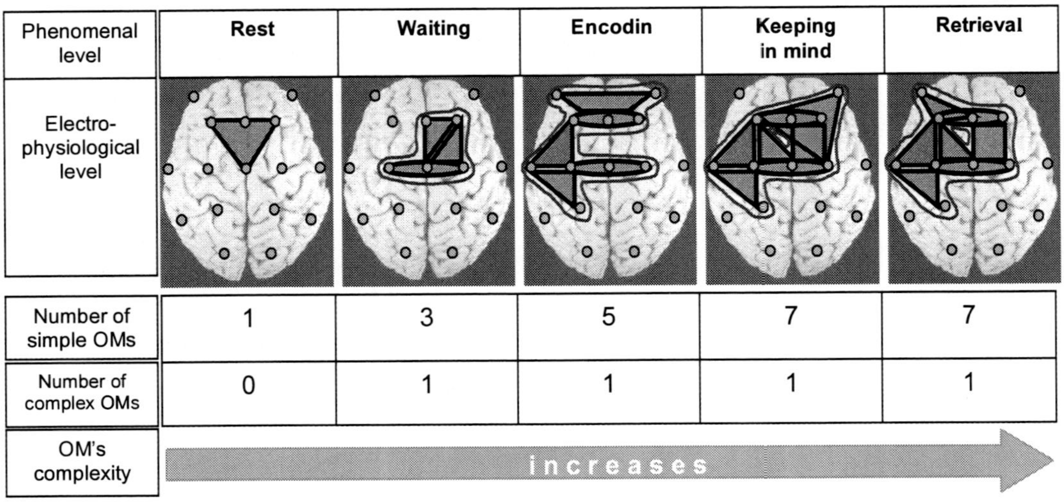

Figure 7. Isomorphism between functional structures of phenomenological experience and electromagnetic brain field. Phenomenological level illustrates the ever-changing stream of cognitive acts (in limit, thoughts or images) where each momentarily stable pattern is a particular cognitive operation. Thus, stream of phenomenal experience has a composite structure: It contains stable nuclei (or cognitive operations/thoughts/images) and transitive fringes (or periods). At the EEG/MEG level these processes are reflected in the chain of periods of short-term metastable states (or operational modules – OM) of the whole brain and its individual subsystems (grey shapes), when the numbers of degrees of freedom of the neuronal networks are maximally decreased. Red shapes illustrate complex OMs. Changes from one cognitive act to another are achieved through rapid transitional periods. Experimental data are presented from the experimental study by Fingelkurts et al., 2003a.

It was demonstrated, that the metastable topological combinations in the EEG/MEG field do exist (Fig. 7) and appeared to be correlated with and dependent on the subjects' individual level of anxiety (Shishkin et al., 1998), cognitive tasks (Fingelkurts et al., 2003b), multisensory perception (Fingelkurts et al., 2003a), and on the pharmacological influence (Fingelkurts et al., 2004a,b), large ontogeny shifts (differences between children and adults) (Borisov, 2002), and on the changes in the functional state of the brain during schizoid diseases (Kaplan and Borisov, 2002). These data not only increase our knowledge about fundamental brain mechanisms, but also provide sensitive indexes which can serve as additional diagnostic markers of some psychiatric and brain disorders (Fingelkurts et al., 2005b).

Conclusion

This Chapter outlines the Operational Architectonics (OA) framework of brain and mind functioning (Fingelkurts and Fingelkurts, 2001) with emphasis on neuronal assemblies and their operations (mesoscopic level). This framework captures a strong intuition about the brain mechanisms that constitute perception, cognition and consciousness. Practical methods of imaging the mesoscopic level of brain organization were described. These methods allow analyzing with an incredible detail the operational behavior of local neuronal assemblies and their joint activity in the form of unified and metastable operational modules. We argue that the level of brain organization revealed by these methods corresponds to the phenomenal level of cognition and consciousness.

Acknowledgements

We have owed a large intellectual debt to Prof. Alexander Kaplan, who supported our interest in the fundamental questions in neuroscience during our student years. We wish also to thank Prof. Walter Freeman, Prof. Antti Revonsuo, Prof. Erol Basar, Prof. Hermann Haken, Prof. Steve Bressler, and Prof. Yurii Alexandrov for their very useful contribution in the discussion of related subjects. Special thanks to Viktor Ermolaev, Boris Darkhovsky, and Carlos Neves for software development and/or technical and mathematical support.

References

Alexandrov, Yu. I. (1999). Psychophysiological regularities of the dynamics of individual experience and the "stream of consciousness." In C. Taddei-Feretti, & C. Musio (Eds.), *Series on biophysics and biocybernetics. Neural basis and psychological aspects of consciousness* (vol. 8 – Biocybernetic, pp. 201-219). Singapore-New Jersey-London-Hongkong: World Scientific.

Andrews, T. J., White, L. E., Binder, D., & Purves, D. (1996). Temporal events in cyclopean vision. *Proceedings of the National Academy of Sciences of the United States of America, 93,* 3689-3692.

Anokhin, P. K. (1973). *Biology and neurophysiology of conditioned reflex and its role in adaptive behavior.* Oxford: Pergamon Press.

Anokhin, P. K. (1978). *Philosophical aspects of the theory of functional systems.* Moscow: Nauka (in Russian).

Aquinas St. Thomas. (1952:1272). Treatise on Man. In: D. J. Sullivan (Rev.), *Summa Theologica, Translated by Fathers of the English Dominican Province* (vol. 19, pp. 378-487). Chicago, IL: Great Books Series, Encyclopedia Britannica.

Arbib, M. A. (1981). Perceptual structures and distributed motor control. In V. Brooks (Ed.), *Handbook of physiology: Motor control* (vol. 3, pp. 1449-1480). Bethesda, MD: American Physiological Society.

Arbib, M. A. (1989). *The metaphorical brain 2: Neural nets and beyond.* New York: John Wiley.

Arbib, M. A. (2001). Co-evolution of human consciousness and language. In E. P. Marijuan (Ed.), *Cajal and consciousness: Scientific approaches to consciousness on the centential of ramon y Cajal's textura* (vol. 929, pp. 195-220). New York, NY: Annals of the NYAS.

Averbeck, B. B., & Lee, D. (2004). Coding and transmission of information by neural ensembles. *Trends in Neurosciences, 27,* 225-230.

Baars, B. J. (1988). *A cognitive theory of consciousness*. New York: Cambridge University Press.

Baars, B. J. (1997). In the theatre of consciousness: Global workspace theory, a rigorous scientific theory of consciousness. *Journal of Consciousness Studies, 4,* 292-309.

Baccala, L. A., & Sameshima, K. (2001). Partial directed coherence: a new concept in neural structure determination. *Biological cybernetics, 84,* 463-474.

Bauer, R., & Dicke, P. (1997). Fast cortical selection: A principle of neuronal self-organization for perception? *Biological cybernetics*, 77, 207-215.

Bak, P., & Chialvo, D. R. (2001). Adaptive learning by extremal dynamics and negative feedback. *Physical Review E, 63,* 031912.

Barlow, J. S., (1985). Methods of analysis of nonstationary EEGs, with empahasis on segmentation techniques: A comparative review. *Journal of Clinical Neurophysiology, 2,* 267-304.

Basar, E., Basar-Eroglu, C., Karakas, S., & Schurmann, M. (2001). Gamma, alpha, delta, and theta oscillations govern cognitive processes. *International Journal of Psychophysiology, 39,* 241-248.

Basar, E. (2004). Macrodynamics of electrical activity in the whole brain. *International Journal of Bifurcation and Chaos, 14,* 363-381.

Beer, R. D. (2000). Dynamical approaches to cognitive science. *Trends in Cognitive Sciences, 4,* 91-99.

Bechtel, W. (2002). Decomposing the mind-brain: A long-term pursuit. *Brain and Mind, 3,* 229–242.

Bi G., & Poo, M. (2001). Synaptic modification by correlated activity: Hebb's postulate revisited. *Annual Review of Neuroscience, 24,* 139-166.

Bickle, J., Worley, C., & Bernstein, M. (2000). Vector subtraction implemented neurally: A neurocomputational model of some sequential cognitive and conscious processes. *Consciousness and Cognition, 9,* 117-144.

Borisov, S. V. (2002). *Studying of a phasic structure of the alpha activity of human EEG.* Ph.D. Dissertation. Moscow: Moscow State Univ., pp. 213. (in Russian).

Braitenberg, V. (1978). Cell assemblies in the cerebral cortex. In R. Heim, & G. Palm (Eds.), *Theoretical approaches to complex systems: Lecture notes in mathematics* (vol. 21). Springer.

Breakspear, M., & Stam, C. J. (2005). Dynamics of a neural system with a multiscale architecture. *Philosophical Transactions of the Royal Society B, 360,* 1051-1074.

Bressler, S. L. (1999). The dynamic manifestation of cognitive structures in the cerebral cortex. In A. Riegler, M. Peschl, & A. von Stein (Eds.), *Understanding Representation in the Cognitive Sciences* (pp. 121-126). New York: Kluwer Academic/Plenum Publishers.

Bressler, S. L. (2002). Understanding cognition through large-scale cortical networks. *Current Directions in Psychological Science, 11,* 58-61.

Bressler, S. L., & Kelso, J. A. S. (2001). Cortical coordination dynamics and cognition. *Trends in Cognitive Sciences, 5,* 26-36.

Broca, P. (1861). Remarques sur la siège de la faculté de la parole articulée, suivies d'une observation d'aphémie (perte de parole). *Bulletin de la Société d'Anatomie, 36,* 330–57.

Brodsky, B. E., Darkhovsky, B. S., Kaplan, A. Ya., & Shishkin, S. L. (1999). A nonparametric method for the segmentation of the EEG. *Computer Methods and Programs in Biomedicine, 60,* 93-106.

Brown, T. H., Kairiss, E. W., & Keenan, C. L. (1990). Hebbian synapses: Biophysical mechanisms and algorithms. *Annual Review of Neuroscience, 13,* 475-511.

Bullmore, E., Long, C., Suckling, J., Fadili, J., Calvert, G., Zelaya, F., Carpenter, T. A., & Brammer, M. (2001). Colored noise and computational inference in neurophysiological (fMRI) time series analysis: Resampling methods in time and wavelet domains. *Human Brain Mapping, 12,* 61-78.

Buzsaki, G. (2004). Large-scale recording of neuronal ansembles. *Nature Neuroscience, 7,* 446-451.

Buzsaki, G., Horvath, Z., Urioste, R., Hetke, J., & Wise, K. (1992). High-frequency network oscillation in the hippocampus. *Science, 256,* 1025-1027.

Calvert, G. A. (2001). Crossmodal processing in the human brain: Insights from functional neuroimaging studies. *Cerebral Cortex, 11,* 1110-1123.

Carello, C., Turvey, M. T., Kugler, P. N. & Shaw, R. E. (1984). Inadequacies of the computer metaphor. In M. S. Gazzaniga (ed.), *Handbook of cognitive neuroscience* (pp. 229-248). New York: Plenum Press.

Cariani, P. (1994). As if time really mattered: temporal strategies for neural coding of sensory information. In K. Pribram (Ed.), *Origins: Brain and self-organization* (pp. 208-252). Hillsdale, NJ: Lawrence Erlbaum.

Cariani, P. (1997). Emergence of new signal-primitives in neural systems. *Intellectica, 2,* 95-143.

Cariani, P. (2001). Symbols and dynamics in the brain. *Biosystems, 60,* 59-83.

Chafe, W. L. (1994). *Discourse, consciousness, and time: The flow and displacement of conscious experience in speaking and writing*. Chicago: Univ. of Chicago Press.

Chalmers, D. J. (1995). Facing up to the problems of consciousness. *Journal of Consciousness Studies, 2,* 200-219.

Chalmers, D. J. (2002). Consciousness and its place in nature. In D. Chalmers (Ed.), *Philosophy of mind: Classical and contemporary readings*. Oxford. URL = http://jamaica.u.arizona.edu/~chalmers/papers/nature.html

Choe, Y. (2002). Second order isomorphism: A reinterpretation and its implications in brain and cognitive sciences. In W. D. Gray, & C. D. Schunn (Eds.), *Proceedings of the 24th annual conference of the cognitive science society* (pp. 190-195). Erlbaum.

Churchland, P. S. & Sejnowski, T. J. (1992). *The computational brain*. Cambridge: MIT Press.

Cleeremans, A. (2002). *The unity of consciousness: Binding, integration, dissociation.* Oxford: Oxford Univ. Press.

Crick, F., & Koch, C. (2003). A framework for consciousness. *Nature Neuroscience, 6,* 119-126.

Damasio, A. R. (1994). *Descartes' error*. New York: G. P. Putnam's Sons.

Damasio, A. R. (2000). *The feeling of what happens. Body, emotion and the making of consciousness*. London: Vintage.

Damasio, A. R., & Damasio, H. (1999). Brain and language. In *The Scientific American Book of the Brain* (pp. 29-41). Guilford, Connecticut: The Lyons Press.

Deacon, T. W. (1989). Holism and associationism in neuropsychology: An anatomical synthesis. In E. Perecman (Ed.), *Integrating theory and practice in clinical neuropsychology*. Erlbaum.

Deese, J. (1970). *Psycholinguistics*. Boston: Allyn and Bacon.

deCharms, R. C. (1998). Information coding in the cortex by independent or coordinated populations. *Proceedings of the National Academy of Sciences of the United States of America, 95,* 15166-15168.

deCharms, R. C., & Merzenich, M. M. (1996). Primary cortical representation of sounds by the coordination of action-potential timing. *Nature, 381,* 610–613.

deCharms, R. C., & Zador, A. (2000). Neural representations and the cortical code. *Annual Review of Neuroscience, 23,* 613–647.

de Oliveira, S. C., Thiele, A., & Hoffmann, K. P. (1997), Synchronization of neuronal activity during stimulus expectation in a direction discrimination task. *The Journal of Neuroscience, 17,* 9248–9260.

Donoghue, J. P., Sanes, J. N., Hatsopoulos, N. G., & Gaal, G. (1998). Neural discharge and local field potential oscillations in primate motor cortex during voluntary movements. *Journal of Neurophysiology, 79,* 159–173.

Dreyfus, H. L. (1992). *What computers still can't do: A critique of artificial reason.* Cambridge, Massachusetts: MIT Press.

Edelman, G. M. (1987). *Neural Darwinism: The theory of neuronal group selection.* New York: Basic Books.

Edelman, G. M., & Tononi G. (2000). *A Universe of consciousness: How matter becomes imagination.* New York: Basic Books.

Efron, E. (1970). The minimum duration of a perception. *Neuropsychologia, 8,* 57-63.

Eichenbaum, H. (1993). Thinking about brain cell assemblies. *Science, 261,* 993-994.

Eliasmith, C. (1996) The third contender: A critical examination of the dynamicist theory of cognition. *Philosophical Psychology, 9,* 441-463.

Elul, R. (1972a). The genesis of the EEG. In C. C. Pfeiffer, & J. R. Smythes (Eds.), *International review of neurobiology* (vol. 15, pp.227-272). New York: Academic Press.

Elul, R. (1972b). Randomness and synchrony in the generation of electroencephalogram. In H. Petsche, & M. A. B. Brazier (Eds.), *Synchronization of EEG activity in epilepsies* (pp. 59-77). Vienna: Springer Verlag.

Epstein, H. T. (1999). Other brain effects of words. *The Behavioral and Brain Sciences, 22,* 287-288.

Erdi, P. (2000). On the 'dynamic brain' metaphor. *Brain and Mind, 1,* 119-145.

Erdi, P., & Barna, G. (1984). Self-organizing mechanism for the formation of ordered neural mappings. *Biological Cybernetics, 51,* 93-101.

Fingelkurts, An. A. (1998). *Time-spatial organization of human EEG segment's structure.* Ph.D. Dissertation, Moscow: Moscow State Univ., p. 415 (in Russian).

Fingelkurts, An. A., & Fingelkurts, Al. A. (2001). Operational architectonics of the human brain biopotential field: Towards solving the mind-brain problem. *Brain and Mind, 2,* 261-296.

Fingelkurts, An. A., & Fingelkurts, Al. A. (2003). Operational architectonics of perception and cognition: A principle of self-organized metastable brain states. *VI Parmenides workshop – Perception and thinking*, Institute of Medical Psychology. April 5-10, Elba/Italy (invited full-text contribution). URL = http://www.bm-science.com/team/art24.pdf

Fingelkurts, An. A., & Fingelkurts, Al. A. (2004). Making complexity simpler: Multivariability and metastability in the Brain. *The International Journal of Neuroscience, 114,* 843-862.

Fingelkurts, An. A., Fingelkurts, Al. A., & Kähkönen, S. (2005a). Functional connectivity in the brain – is it an elusive concept? *Neuroscience and Biobehavioral Reviews, 28,* 827-836.

Fingelkurts, An. A., Fingelkurts, Al. A., & Kähkönen, S. (2005b). New perspectives in pharmaco-electroencephalography. *Progress in Neuropsychopharmacology & Biological Psychiatry, 29,* 193-199.

Fingelkurts, Al. A., Fingelkurts, An. A., Krause, C. M., & Sams, M. (2002). Probability interrelations between pre-/post-stimulus intervals and ERD/ERS during a memory task. *Clinical Neurophysiology, 113,* 826-843.

Fingelkurts, An. A., Fingelkurts, Al. A., Krause, C. M., Kaplan, A. Ya., Borisov, S. V., & Sams, M. (2003a). Structural (operational) synchrony of EEG alpha activity during an auditory memory task. *NeuroImage, 20,* 529-542.

Fingelkurts, An. A., Fingelkurts, Al. A., Krause, C. M., Möttönen, R., & Sams, M. (2003b). Cortical operational synchrony during audio-visual speech integration. Brain and Language, 85, 297-312.

Fingelkurts, Al. A., Fingelkurts, An. A., Krause, C. M., & Kaplan, A. Ya. (2003c). Systematic rules underlying spectral pattern variability: Experimental results and a review of the evidence. *The International Journal of Neuroscience, 113,* 1447-1473.

Fingelkurts, An. A., Fingelkurts, Al. A., Kivisaari, R., Pekkonen, E., Ilmoniemi, R. J., & Kähkönen, S. (2004a). Enhancement of GABA-related signalling is associated with increase of functional connectivity in human cortex. *Human Brain Mapping, 22,* 27-39.

Fingelkurts, An. A., Fingelkurts, Al. A., Kivisaari, R., Pekkonen, E., Ilmoniemi, R. J., & Kähkönen, S. (2004b). Local and remote functional connectivity of neocortex under the inhibition influence. *Neuroimage, 22,* 1390-1406.

Fodor, J. (1987). *Psychosemantics*. Cambridge, MA: MIT Press.

Fodor, J., & Pylyshyn, Z. (1988). Connectionism and cognitive architecture: A critique. *Cognition, 28,* 3-71.

Freeman, W. J. (1992). Tutorial on neurobiology – from single neurons to brain chaos. *International Journal of Bifurcation and Chaos, 2,* 451–482.

Freeman, W. J. (2000a). Brains Create Macroscopic Order from Microscopic Disorder By Neurodynamics in Perception. In P. Århem, C. Blomberg, & H. Liljenström (Eds.). *Disorder versus Order in Brain Function: Essays in Theoretical Neurobiology* (chapter 7, pp. 205-219). Singapore: World Scientific Publishing Co.

Freeman, W. J. (2000b). A proposed name for aperiodic brain activity: Stochastic chaos. *Neural Networks, 13,* 11–13.

Freeman, W. J. (2000c). Mesoscopic neurodynamics: From neuron to brain. *Journal of Physiology Paris, 94,* 303-322.

Freeman, W. J., & Barrie, J. M. (1993). Chaotic oscillations and the genesis of meaning in cerebral cortex. *The IPSEN foundation symposium on Temporal Coding in the Brain,* Paris, 11 October.

Freeman, W. J., Kozma, R., & Werbos, P. J. (2001). Biocomplexity: Adaptive behavior in complex stochastic dynamical systems. *Biosystems, 59,* 109-123.

Freeman, W. J., Chang, H. J., Burke, B. C., Rose, P. A., & Badler, J. (1997). Taming chaos: stabilization of aperiodic attractors by noise. *IEEE transactions on Circular Systems-I. Fundamental Theory Applications, 44,* 989–996.

Fries, P., Reynolds, J. H., Rorie, A. E., & Desimone, R. (2001). Modulation of oscillatory neuronal synchronization by selective visual attention. *Science, 291,* 1560–1563.

Friston, K. J. (1997). Transients, metastability and neural dynamics. *Neuroimage, 5,* 164-171.

Friston, K. J. (2000). The labile brain. I. Neuronal transients and nonlinear coupling. *Philosophical Transactions of the Royal Society of London. Series B. Biological Sciences, 355,* 215–236.

Friston, K. J., & Buchel, C. (2000). Attentional modulation of effective connectivity from V2 to V5/MT in humans. *Proceedings of the National Academy of Sciences of the United States of America, 97,* 7591-7596.

Fuchs, A., Jirsa, V. K., & Kelso, J. A. S. (2000). Theory of the relation between human brain activity (MEG) and hand movements. *Neuroimage, 11,* 359–369.

Fuchs, A., Kelso, J. A. S., & Haken, H. (1992). Phase transitions in the human brain: Spatial mode dynamics. *International Journal of Bifurcation and Chaos, 2,* 917–939.

Fujii, H., Ito, H., Aihara, K., Ichinose, N., & Tsukada, M. (1996). Dynamical cell assembly hypothesis–theoretical possibility of spatiotemporal coding in the cortex. *Neural Networks, 9,* 1303-1350.

Fuster, J. M. (1997). Network memory. *Trends in Neurosciences, 20,* 451-459.

Galin, D. (1994). The structure of awareness: Contemporary applications of William James' forgotten concept of "the fringe". *Journal of Mind and Behavior, 15,* 375-402.

Galin, D. (2000). Comments on Epstein's neurocognitive interpretation of William James's model of consciousness. *Consciousness and Cognition, 9,* 576-583.

Geissler, H.-G. (1987). The temporal architecture of central information processing: evidence for a tentative time-quantum model. *Psychological Research, 49,* 99-106.

Geissler, H.-G. (1997). Is there a way from behavior to non-linear brain dynamics? On quantal periods in cognition and the place of alpha in brain resonances. *International Journal of Psychophysiology, 26,* 381-393.

Georgopoulos, A. P. (1990). Neural coding of the direction of reaching and a comparison with saccadic eye movements. *Cold Spring Harbor Symposia on Quantitative Biology, 55,* 849–59.

Gho, M., & Varela, F. J. (1988). A quantitative assessment of the dependency of the visual temporal frame upon the cortical rhythm. *Journal of Physiology, 83,* 95-101.

Glicksohn, J. (2001). Temporal cognition and the phenomenology of time: A multiplicative function for apparent duration. *Consciousness and Cognition, 10,* 1-25.

Gross, J., Kujala, M., Hämäläinen, M., Timmermann, L., Schnitzler, A., & Salmelin, R. (2001). Dynamic imaging of coherent sources: Studying neural interactions in the human brain. *Proceedings of the National Academy of Sciences of the United States of America, 98,* 694-699.

Haken, H. (1991). *Synergetic Computers and Cognition.* Berlin: Springer.

Haken, H. (1999). What can synergetics contribute to the understanding of brain functioning? In C. Uhl (Ed.), *Analysis of neurophysiological brain functioning* (pp. 7-40). Berlin: Springer-Verlag.

Hatsopoulos, N. G., Ojakangas, C. L., Paninski, L. & Donoghue, J. P. (1998). Information about movement direction obtained from synchronous activity of motor cortical neurons. *Proceedings of the National Academy of Sciences of the United States of America, 95,* 15706-15711.

Hebb, D. (1949). *The organization of behavior*. New York: Wiley.

Hirsh, I. J., & Sherrick, C. E. J. (1961). Perceived order in different sense modalities. *Journal of Experimantal Psychology, 62,* 423-432.

Holland, J. H. (1998). *Emergence: From chaos to order*. Addison-Wesley.

Honavar, V. (1994). Symbolic artificial intelligence and numeric artificial neural networks: Toward a resolution of the dichotomy. In R. Sun, & L. Bookman (Eds.), *Computational architectures integrating symbolic and neural processes* (pp. 351-388). New York: Kluwer.

Ivanitsky, A. M., & Nikolaev, A. R. (1999). Homogeneous neural networks cannot. *The Behavioral and Brain Sciences, 22,* 293.

James, W. (1890). *The principles of psychology: Vol. I.* New York: Dover.

Jansen, B. H., & Cheng, W. K. (1988). Structural EEG analysis: an explorative study. *International Journal of Bio-Medical Computing, 23,* 221-237.

Jirsa, V. K., Fuchs, A., & Kelso, J. A. S. (1998). Connecting cortical and behavioral dynamics: bimanual coordination. *Neural Computation, 10,* 2019–2045.

John, E. R. (1990). *Machinery of the mind.* Boston, MA: Birkhauser.

John, E. R. (2001). A field theory of consciousness. *Consciousness and Cognition, 9,* 10, 184-213.

John, E. R. (2002). The neurophysics of consciousness. *Brain Research. Brain Research Reviews, 39,* 1-28.

John, E. R., & Schwartz, E. L. (1978). The neurophysiology of information processing and cognition. *Annual Review of Psychology, 29,* 1-29.

Kaplan, A. Ya. (1995). On the frame architecture of central information processing: EEG analysis. *The Fourth IBRO World Congress of Neuroscience* (p. 438).

Kaplan, A. Ya. (1998). Nonstationary EEG: Methodological and experimental analysis. *Uspehi Physiologicheskih Nayk (Success in Physiological Sciences), 29,* 35-55 (in Russian).

Kaplan, A. Ya., & Shishkin, S. L. (2000). Application of the change-point analysis to the investigation of the brain's electrical activity. In B. E. Brodsky, & B. S. Darkhovsky (Eds.), *Nonparametric statistical diagnosis: Problems and methods* (chapter 7, pp. 333-388). Dordrecht (the Netherlands): Kluwer Academic Publishers.

Kaplan, A. Ya., & Borisov, S. V. (2002). The differences in structural synchrony of the brain electrical field in alpha range between normal control and schizophrenic adolescents. *(Human Brain Mapping 2002 Meeting). Neuroimage,* Poster No. 10472.

Kaplan, A. Ya., & Borisov, S. V. (2003). Dynamic properties of segmental characteristics of EEG alpha activity in rest conditions and during cognitive load. *Zhurnal Vysshei' Nervnoi' Deiatel'nosty im I. P. Pavlova (I. P. Pavlov Jouranl of Higher Nervous Activity), 53,* 22-32 (in Russian).

Kaplan, A. Ya., Fingelkurts, Al. A., Fingelkurts, An. A., & Darkhovsky, B. S. (1997). Topological mapping of sharp reorganization synchrony in multichannel EEG. *American Journal of Electroneurodiagnostic Technologies, 37,* 265-275.

Kaplan, A., Röschke, J., Darkhovsky, B., & Fell, J. (2001). Macrosructural EEG characterization based on nonparametric change point segmentation: Application to sleep analysis. *Journal of Neuroscience Methods, 106,* 81-90.

Kaplan, A. Ya., Fingelkurts, An. A., Fingelkurts, Al. A., Borisov, S. V., & Darkhovsky, B. S. (2005). Nonstationary nature of the brain activity as revealed by EEG/MEG: Methodological, practical and conceptual challenges. *Signal Processing,* (in press).

Kaplan, S., Weaver, M., & French, R. (1990) Active symbols and internal models: Towards a cognitive connectionism. *AI and Survey, 4,* 51–71.

Katchalsky, A., Rowland, V., & Blumenthal, R. (1974). Dynamic patterns of brain cell assemblies. *Neurosciences Research Program Bulletin, 12,* 3-87.

Kelso, J. A. S. (1991). Behavioral and neural pattern generation: The concept of Neurobehavioral Dynamical System (NBDS). In H. P. Koepchen (Ed.), *Cardiorespiratory and motor coordination.* Berlin: Springer-Verlag.

Kelso, J. A. S. (1995). *Review of dynamic patterns: The self-organization of brain and behavior*. Cambridge, MA: MIT Press.

Kelso, J. A. S., Bressler, S. L., Buchanan, S., De Guzman, G. C., Ding, M., Fuchs, A., & Holroyd, T. (1992). A phase transition in human brain and behavior. *Physics Letters A, 169,* 134–144.

Kirillov, A. B., & Makarenko, V. I. (1991). Metastability and phase transition in neural networks: statistical approach. In A. V. Holden, & V. I. Kryukov (Eds.), *Neurocomputers and attention* (vol. 2, pp. 825-922). Manchester: Manchester University Press.

Koenig, T., & Lehmann, D. (1996). Microstates in language-related brain potentials show noun-verb differences. *Brain and Language, 53,* 169-182.

Kogan, A. B., & Choraian, O. G. (1977). Elementary neuronal ensembles as the basis for the functional organization of the brain. *Zhurnal Vysshei' Nervnoi' Deiatel'nosty im I. P. Pavlova (I. P. Pavlov Jouranl of Higher Nervous Activity), 27,* 922-930 (in Russian).

Kristofferson, A. B. (1967). Successiveness discrimination as a two-state, quantal process. *Science, 158,* 1337-1339.

Lee, D. (2003) Coherent oscillations in neuronal activity of the supplementary motor area during a visuomotor task. *The Journal of neuroscience, 23,* 6798–6809.

Lehmann, D. (1971). Multichannel topography of human alpha EEG fields. *Electroencephalography and Clinical Neurophysiology, 31,* 439-449.

Lehmann, D., Ozaki, H., & Pal, I. (1987). EEG alpha map series: Brain micro-states by space oriented adaptive segmentation. *Electroencephalography and Clinical Neurophysiology, 67,* 271-288.

Lehmann, D., Strik, W. K., Henggeler, B., Koenig, T., & Koukkou, M. (1998). Brain electrical micro-states and momentary conscious mind states as building blocks of spontaneous thinking. I. Visual imagery and abstract thoughts. *International Journal of Psychophysiology, 29,* 1-11.

Leznik, E., Makarenko, V., & Llinas, R. (2002). Electrotonically mediated oscillatory patterns in neuronal ensembles: An in vitro voltage-dependent dye-imaging study in the inferior olive. *Journal of Neuroscience, 22,* 2804-2815.

Lichtheim, L. (1885) On aphasia. *Brain, 7,* 433–484.

Maass, W., & Bishop, C. M. (1999). *Pulsed neural network.* Cambridge: MIT Press.

Makarenko, V., & Llinas, R. (1998). Experimentally determined chaotic phase synchronization in a neuronal system. *Proceedings of national Academy of Sciences of the United States of America, 95,* 15747-15752.

Mangan, B. B. (1993a). Taking phenomenology seriously: The "fringe" and its implications for cognitive research. *Consciousness and Cognition, 2,* 89-108.

Mangan, B. B. (1993b). Some philosophical and empirical implications of the fringe. *Consciousness and Cognition, 2,* 142-154.

Marr, D. (1991). *From the retina to the neocortex: Selected papers of David Marr.* Boston: Birkhäuser.

McCulloch, W. S. (1965). *Embodiments of mind.* Cambridge: MIT Press.

McGurk, H., & MacDonald, J. W. (1976). Hearing lips and seeing voices. *Nature, 264,* 746-748.

McIntosh, A. R. (1999). Mapping cognition to the brain through neural interactions. *Memory, 7,* 523-548.

McIntosh, A. R. (2000). Towards a network theory of cognition. *Neural Networks, 13,* 861-870.

Merzenich, M. M., & deCharms, C. (1996). Neural representations, experience, and change. In R. Llinas, & P. S. Curchland (Eds.), *The mind brain continuum* (pp. 61-81). Cambridge: MIT Press.

Milner, P. M. (1957). The cell assembly: Mk. II. *Psychological Review, 64,* 242–252.

Mountcastle, V. (1967). The problem of sensing and the neural coding of sensory events. In G. C. Quarton, T. Melnechuk, & F. O. Schmitt (Eds.), *The neurosciences: A study program.* New York: Rockefeller University Press.

Mountcastle, V. B. (1998). *Perceptual neuroscience: The cerebral cortex.* Harvard University Press.

Mumford, D. (1994). Neuronal architectures for pattern-theoretic problems. In C. Koch, & J. L. Davis (Eds.), *Large-scale neuronal theories of the brain.* Cambridge, Ma: MIT Press.

Murthy, V. N., & Fetz, E. E. (1996). Oscillatory activity in sensorimotor cortex of awake monkeys: Synchronization of local field potentials and relation to behavior. *Journal of Neurophysiology, 76,* 3949–3967.

Newell, A., & Simon, H. A. (1976). Computer science as empirical enquiry: Symbols and search. *Communications of the Association for Computing Machinery, 19,* 113-126.

Nunez, P. L. (2000). Toward a quantitative description of large-scale neocortical dynamic function and EEG. *The Behavioral and Brain Sciences, 23,* 371-437.

O'Brien, G., & Opie, J. (1999a). A Connectionist theory of phenomenal experience. *The Behavioral and Brain Sciences, 22,* 127-148.

O'Brien, G., & Opie, J. (1999b). Putting content into a vehicle theory of consciousness. *The Behavioral and Brain Sciences, 22,* 175-196.

O'Hare, J. J. (1991). Perceptual integration. *Journal of Washington Academy of Sciences, 81,* 44-59.

Owen, B. M., & Lee, D. N. (1986). Establishing a frame of reference for action. In M. G. Wade, & H. T. A. Whiting (Eds.), *Motor developments: Aspects of coordination and control.* Dordrecht: Martinus Nijhoff.

Paillard, J. (1971). Les déterminants moteurs de l'organisation spatiale. *Cahiers de Psychologie, 14,* 261-316.

Paillard, J. (1990). Basic neurophysiological structures of eye-hand coordination. In C. Bard, M. Fleury, & L. Hay (Eds.), *Development of eye-hand coordination across the life span* (pp. 26-74). Columbia, Sc: South Carolina University Press.

Paillard, J. (1991). Knowing where and knowing how to get there. In J. Paillard (Ed.), *Brain and space* (chapter 24, pp: 461-481). Oxford: Oxford University Press.

Palm, G. (1982) *Neural assemblies.* Springer.

Palm, G. (1990). Cell assemblies as a guideline for brain research. *Concepts in Neuroscience, 1,* 133-147.

Palm, G. (1993) On the internal structure of cell assemblies. In A. Aertsen (Ed.), *Brain theory: Spatiotemporal aspects of brain function.* Elsevier.

Pascual-Marqui, R., Michel, C., & Lehmann, D. (1995). Segmentation of brain electrical activity into microstates. *IEEE Transaction on Biomedical Engineering, 42,* 658-665.

Perkell, D. H., & Bullock, T. H. (1968). Neural coding. *Neurosciences Research Program Bulletin, 6,* 221-348.

Petersen, S. E., & Fiez, J. A. (1993). The processing of single words studied with positron emission tomography. *Annual Review of Neuroscience, 16,* 509–530.

Phillips, C. G., Zeki, S., & Barlow, H. B. (1984). Localization of function in the cerebral cortex: Past, present, future. *Brain, 107,* 328-61.

Phillips, W. A., & Singer, W. (1997). In search of common foundations for cortical computation. *The Behavioral and Brain Sciences, 20,* 657-722.

Piatelli-Palmarini, M. (1980). *Language and learning: The debate between Jean Piaget and Noam Chomsky.* Cambridge, MA: Harvard University Press.

Pöppel, E. (1988). *Mindworks: time and conscious experience.* Boston: Harcourt Brace Jovanovich.

Pouget, A., Dayan, P., & Zemel, R. (2000). Information processing with population codes. *Nature Reviews Neuroscience, 1,* 125-132.

Prigogine, I. (1980). *From being to becoming: Time and complexity in the physical sciences.* San Francisco: Freeman.

Pulvermueller, F. (1999). Words in the brain's language. *The Behavioral and Brain Sciences,* 22, 253–336.

Pulvermueller, F., Preissl, H., Eulitz, C., Pantev, C., Lutzenberger, W., Elbert, T., & Birbaumer, N. (1994). Brain rhythms, cell assemblies and cognition: Evidence from the processing of words and pseudowords. *PSYCOLOQUY, 5,* brain-rhythms.1.pulvermueller.

Raichle, M. E. (1999). Visualizing the mind. In *The Scientific American Book of the Brain* (pp. 43-53). Guilford, Connecticut: The Lyons Press.

Rapp, P. (1993). Chaos in the neurosciences: Cautionary tales from the frontier. *Biologist, 40,* 89–94.

Rappelsberger, P., & Petsche, H. (1988). Probability mapping: Power and coherence analysis of cognitive processes. *Brain Topography, 1,* 46-54.

Rauschecker, J. P. (1995). Reverberations of Hebbian thinking. *Behavioral and Brain Sciences, 18,* 642-643.

Revonsuo, A. (2000). Prospects for a scientific research program on consciousness. In T. Metzinger (Ed.), *Neural correlates of consciousness* (pp. 57-75). Cambridge, MA: MIT Press.

Revonsuo, A. (2001). Can functional brain imaging discover consciousness in the brain? *Journal of Consciousness Studies, 8,* 3-23.

Rieke, F., Warland, D., de Ruyter van Steveninck, R., & Bialek, W. (1997). *Spikes: Exploring the neural code*. MIT Press, Cambridge.

Ryder, D., & Favorov, V. (2001). The new associationism: A neural explanation for the predictive powers of cerebral cortex. *Brain and Mind, 2,* 161-194.

Schyns, P. G., Goldstone, R. L., & Thibaut, J.-P. (1998). The development of features in object concepts. *Behavioral and Brain Sciences, 21,* 1-54.

Schwartz, A. B. (1994a). Direct cortical representation of drawing. *Science, 265,* 540–542.

Schwartz, A. B. (1994b). Distributed motor processing in cerebral cortex. *Current Opinion in Neurobiology, 4,* 840–846.

Searle, J. R. (1992). *The rediscovery of mind.* Cambridge, Massachusetts: MIT Press.

Sejnowski, T. J., & Tesauro, G. (1989). The Hebb rule for synaptic plasticity: Algorithms and implementations. In J. H. Byrne (Ed.), *Neural models of plasticity: Experimental and theoretical approaches* (pp. 94-103). San Diego, CA: Academic.

Shishkin, S. L., Darkhovsky, B. S., Fingelkurts, Al. A., Fingelkurts, An. A., & Kaplan, A.Ya. (1998). Interhemisphere synchrony of short-term variations in human EEG alpha power correlates with self-estimates of functional state. In *Proc. 9-th World Congress of Psychophysiology* (pp. 133). Italy, Tvaormin, Sicily.

Shvyrkov, V. B. (1990). *Neurophysiological study of systemic mechanisms of behavior*. New Delhi: Oxonian press PVT.LTD.

Singer, W. (1994). Time as coding space in neocortical processing: A hypothesis. In M. S. Gazzaniga (Ed.), *The cognitive neurosciences*. Cambridge, MA: MIT Press.

Singer, W. (1995). Development and plasticity of cortical processing architectures. *Science, 270,* 758–764.

Singer, W. (2001). Consciousness and the binding problem. *Annals of the NY Academy Science, 929,* 123-146.

Singer, W., & Gray, C. M. (1995). Visual feature integration and the temporal correlation hypothesis. *Annual Review in Neuroscience, 18,* 555–586.

Singer, W., Engel, A. K., Kreiter, A. K., Munk, M. H. J., Neuenschwander, S., & Roelfsema, P. R. (1997). Neural assemblies: necessity, signature and detectability. *Trends in Cognitive Sciences, 1,* 252-261.

Skarda, C. A., Freeman, W. J. (1987). How brains make chaos in order to make sense of the world. *The Behavioral and Brain Sciences, 10,* 161–195.

Steinmetz, P. N., Roy, A., Fitzgerald, P. J., Hsiao, S. S., Johnson, K. O., & Niebur, E. (2000). Attention modulates synchronized neuronal firing in primate somatosensory cortex. *Nature, 404,* 187–190.

Strik, W. K., & Lehmann, D. (1993). Data-determined window size and space-oriented segmentation of spontaneous EEG map series. *Electroencephalography and Clinical Neurophysiology, 87,* 169-174.

Stroud, J. M. (1955). The fine structure of psychological time. In H. Quastler (Ed.), *Information theory in psychology: Problems and methods* (pp. 174-205). Glencoe, Ill.: The Free Press.

Super, H., van der Togt, C., Spekreijse, H., Lamme, V. A. (2003). Internal state of monkey primary visual cortex (V1) predicts figure-ground perception. *The Journal of Neuroscience, 23,* 3407–3414.

Tallon, C., Bertrand, O., Bouchet, P., & Pernier, J. (1995). Gamma-range activity evoked by coherent visual stimuli in humans. *European Journal of Neuroscience, 7,* 1285–1291.

Tallon-Baudry, C., Bertrand, O., Delpuech, C., & Pernier, J. (1996). Stimulus specificity of phase-locked and non-phase-locked 49 Hz visual responses in humans. *Journal of Neuroscience, 16,* 4240–1249.

Tass, P. A. (1999). Phase resetting in medicine and biology (pp.247-248). Berlin: Springer.

Taylor, J. G. (2002). Paying attention to consciousness. *Trends in cognitive sciences, 6,* 206-210.

Thatcher, R. W., Krause, P. J., Hrybyk, M. (1986). Cortico-cortical associations and EEG coherence: A two-compartmental model. *Electroencephalography and Clinical Neurophysiology, 64,* 123-143.

Thomas, G. J. (1984). Memory: Time binding in organisms. In L. R. Squire, & N. Butters (Eds.), *Neuropsychology of Memory* (pp. 374-84). London: Guilford Press.

Thompson, E., & Varela, F. J. (2001). Radical embodiment: Neural dynamics and consciousness. *Trends in Cognitive Science, 5,* 418-425.

Triesch, J., & von der Malsburg, C. (2001). Democratic integration: Self-organized integration of adaptive cues. *Neural Computation, 13,* 2049-2074.

Tsuda, I. (2001). Toward an interpretation of dynamic neural activity in terms of chaotic dynamical systems. *The Behavioral and Brain Sciences, 24,* 793-810.

Turing, A. M. (1952). The chemical basis of morphogenesis. *Philosophical Transactions of the Royal Society of London B, 237,* 37–72.

Ukhtomsky, A. A. (1935). *Lability as a condition of urgency and coordination of neural acts: Collected works* (vol. 2). Leningrad University Press.

Uttal, W. R. (1973). *The psychobiology of sensory coding*. New York: Harper and Row.

Vaadia, E., Haalman, I., Abeles, M., Bergman, H., Prut, Y., Slovin, H., & Aertsen, A. (1995). Dynamics of neuronal interactions in monkey cortex in relation to behavioural events. *Nature, 373,* 515–518.

van Gelder, T. (1995). What might cognition be, if not computation? *The Journal of Philosophy, 91,* 345-381.

Van Gelder, T., & Port, R. (1995). It's about time: An overview of the dynamical approach to cognition. In R. F. Port, & T. van Gelder (Eds.), *Mind as motion: Explorations in the dynamics of cognition* (pp. 1-41). Cambridge, MA: MIT Press.

Varela, F. J., Toro, A., John, E. R., & Schwartz, E. L. (1981). Perceptual framing and cortical alpha rhythm. *Neuropsychologia, 19,* 675-686.

Varela, F., Lachaux, J-P., Rodriguez, E., & Martinerie, J. (2001). The brainweb: Phase synchronization and large-scale integration. *Nature Reviews Neuroscience, 2,* 229-239.

von Baer, K. E. (1864). Welche Auttasung der lebendigen Natur ist die richtige? Und wie ist diese Auttasung auf die Entomologie auzuwenden? In. H. Schmitzdorff (Ed.), *Reden gehalten in wiss: Versammlungen und kleine Aufsätze vermischten Inhalts* (pp. 237-287). S:t Petersburg: Verlag der kaiserl, Hofbuchhandlung.

von der Malsburg, C. (1981). The correlation theory of brain function. *MPI Biophysical Chemistry, Internal Report 81-2*. Reprinted in E. Domany, J. L. van Hemmen, & K. Schulten (Eds.), *Models of neural networks II* (1994), Berlin: Springer.

von der Malsburg, C. (1999). The what and why of binding: The modeler's perspective. *Neuron, 24,* 95-104.

Vvedensky, N. E. (1906). *Excitation and inhibition in the reflex apparatus during strychnine poisoning*. (Reprinted in Russian as Completed collected works, vol. 4., 1953). Leningrad University Publishing House.

Watanabe, M., Nakanishi, K., Aihara, K. (2001). Solving the binding problem of the brain with bi-directional functional connectivity. *Neural Networks, 14,* 395-406.

Wernicke, C. (1874). *Der aphasische symtomencomplex: Eine psychologische studie auf anatomischer basis*. Kohn und Weigert.

Woelbern, T. Eckhorn, R., Frien, A., Bauer, R. (2002). Perceptual grouping correlates with short synchronization in monkey prestriate cortex. *NeuroReport, 13,* 1881–1886

Woodworth, R. S. (1938). *Experimental psychology*. Holt.

Zak, M. (1993). Terminal model of Newtonian dynamics. *International Journal of Theoretical Physics, 32,* 159–190.

In: Brain Mapping Research Progress
Editors: Ines C. Girard and Jade S. Andre

ISBN: 978-1-60456-784-7

Chapter IX

Neural Mechanisms in Anxiety and Panic

Marcus Lira Brandão* and Julia Maria dos Santos
Laboratório de Psicobiologia, FFCLRP, campus USP, Ribeirão Preto, SP, Brasil
Instituto de Neurociências & Comportamento - INeC, Ribeirão Preto, SP, Brasil

Abstract

Depending on the nature of the aversive stimuli or threatening conditions different types of fear responses are elaborated in the brain. Conditioning procedures using light, tones and contexts used as conditioned stimuli associated to unconditioned stimuli of moderate intensity causes orientated and active forms of defense reaction. Organized and oriented defense reactions seem to be linked to anxiety. On the other hand, intense fear conditioning or past experience with stressful situations originate active but disorganized forms of defensive responses that ensures emotional states of different nature. The faulty performance of these animals in the fear-potentiated startle and contextual fear procedure show similarities with panic attacks in man. A sequential pattern of defense reaction made up of arousal, immobility, escape and an incapacitating immobility is also seen when the prey are exposed to potential, distal and proximal signals emitted by the approaching predator. Efforts have been made to characterize the neural circuits recruited in the organization of the defensive reactions during these conditions. The prefrontal cortex, hippocampus and ventral periaqueductal gray are mainly involved in the integration of anxiety-like responses whereas the dorsal periaqueductal gray constitutes the main neural substrates for the integration of aversive states related to panic. In this chapter we summarize the evidence linking the brain's defense systems to the concept of anxiety-panic. The neural substrates of aversion in the hypothalamus seem to be in the middle of these processes. As a working hypothesis, it is advanced that past experience with stressors may lead to an emotional shift from the neural circuits responsible for the production of the usual defensive responses to environmental stressful events in higher

* Correspondence concerning this article should be addressed to M.L. Brandão Laboratory of Neuropsychopharmacology, FFCLRP, campus USP, av Bandeirantes 3900, 14049-901, Ribeirão Preto, SP, Brazil. FAX: 55 16 36024830; e-mail: mbrandao@usp.br.

brain structures towards disturbed or maladaptive defense responses related to panic attacks in brainstem structures. Therefore, prior experience with stressor events may shift orientated, active and organized motor patterns of appropriate defensive behaviors in response to contextual aversive stimuli towards non-oriented, fragmentary and uncoordinated motor acts. With great probabilities the switch mechanisms for these processes are part of the neural substrates of defense located at the level of the amygdala and the hypothalamus.

Keywords: fear, GAD, panic, periaqueductal gray matter, hypothalamus, amygdala

Introduction

Anxiety has been defined as a subjective state induced by an aversive condition of unknown origin. The word anxious derives from the Greek root angst, meaning to "press tight" or strangle. A common anxiety situation refers to the reaction to a frighten loud noise accompanied by an increased heart rate, tensed muscles, and an acute sense of orientation and intense arousal in order to determine the source of the noise. Normally, these aversive stimuli triggers normal defense processes, called "the fight-flight reaction" that prepare the individual to either protect itself or fight or even to flee a dangerous situation. This reaction is considered pathological when it becomes exaggerated and compromises the work and/or social performance of the individual.

Anxiety Disorders are categorized by the Diagnostic and Statistical Manual of Mental Disorders, 4th edition (DSM-IV), published by the American Psychiatric Association in a large number of disorders where the primary feature is abnormal or inappropriate anxiety. Among them the generalized anxiety disorder (GAD), panic and post-traumatic stress disorder (PTSD) will be focused in this chapter. Often anxiety gets generalized to other situations, not related to any specific event and can then become overwhelming, in which case is called generalized anxiety disorder. Typically GAD develops over a period of time and as its name implies GAD is evidenced by general feelings of anxiety such as excessive worry accompanied by mild heart palpitations and dizziness. GAD may not be noticed until it is significant enough to cause problems with the normal life of the person. PTSD always follows a traumatic event which causes intense fear and/or helplessness. Typically the symptoms develop shortly after the event, but may take years. The PTSD symptoms include re-experiencing the trauma through nightmares, obsessive thoughts, and flashbacks (feeling as if the person is actually in the traumatic situation again). There is an important avoidance component, where the individual avoids situations, people, and/or objects which remind the traumatic event (e.g., a person might avoid driving or being a passenger in a car after a serious car accident). Finally, there is increased anxiety in general, possibly with a heightened startle response (e.g., individuals startle easily by noises).

Panic disorder is characterized by sudden attacks of intense fear or anxiety, usually associated with numerous physical symptoms such as heart palpitations, rapid breathing or shortness of breath, blurred vision, dizziness and racing thoughts. Often, the symptoms of this disorder come on rapidly and without an identifiable stressor accompanied by the feeling of imminent death. Generally, the term anxiety has been used as a synonymous of generalized anxiety disorder. To ease the communication with the reader we will keep the use of the term anxiety in the sense of GAD.

In this chapter we will focus on the neurobiology of fear and anxiety giving special emphasis on recent laboratory findings that have contributed to our understanding of the neural mechanisms underlying these conditions. It is expected that data obtained with the use of animal models of anxiety could also be relevant for the disclosure of the alterations of the neural processes underlying GAD, panic and PTSD.

Anxiety Versus Fear

While anxiety is an aversive and subjective state of unknown origin, fear has identifiable origin and causes. The dichotomy between anxiety and fear has become clearer when the first has been related to cognition while fear has been considered a more primitive reaction. It has been suggested that anxiety serves primarily to signal the brain to activate a physical response that will eliminate its source. The experience of anxiety is, in general, consequent to previous exposure of the individual to the same aversive situation, which leads to a conditioned, learned response to the aversive condition and is the expression of activation of higher brain structures. For example, when a person approaches a cliff and feels he is not in complete control of the situation gets aroused and anxious and retreats to control the situation again. On the other hand, fear is a basic, unconditioned, innate response to dangerous situations and is the expression of the activation of mechanisms of defense in the brainstem. Thus, anxiety in this context has been related to higher brain structures while fear seems to be elaborated in brainstem structures.

In the beginning of the last century William James and Carl Lange drew our attention to the fact that the perception of the physiological reaction initiated by the emotional stimulus automatically provides the feedback that defines the emotional feelings. On this view, to feel afraid is to feel one's heart pound, one's palms sweat, one's breathing become faster, and so on. All these physiological changes – like the sweating or piloerection responses – are due to the activity of the autonomic nervous system. Emotions feel different from other states of mind because they have these bodily responses that give rise to internal sensations, and different emotions feel different from one another because they are accompanied by different bodily responses and sensations. According to this theory, each emotion has a particular signature. If we extend the scope of this theory to the physiological events controlled by the other great branch of the nervous system – the skeletal nervous system responsible for movements of the trunk and limbs – the paradoxical nature of this theory discloses in a statement like this: we do not run because we are afraid, we feel afraid because we run. Together, both assessment and physiological activation, act in concert to produce our emotions. The physiological arousal triggered by the stimulus causes unique bodily sensations and the corresponding emotion with its unique quality. The individual should be able to recognize differences between the patterns of physiological change observed in the different emotions. One good and healthy consequence of the physiological arousal is to feel ready for action. The rather limited degree of correlation between particular emotions and events in the autonomic nervous system and endocrine system somehow reduced the importance of the James-Lange theory. However, it has been recognized by many authors that bodily responses and sensations in the experience of anxiety have important role to play in the neurobiology of anxiety. In this context, the James-Lange theory may still be useful in the study of the pathophysiology of the emotions. As such, disturbances in the processing of internal physiological stimuli may determine a faulty strategy to face imminent danger. For instance, one of them could be the paralysis that results from the tightness of the neck, shoulders, arms, and legs; and still other the predominant emotion would be the feeling of being strangulated in the throat, the heart leaping out of the chest or have a knot in the gut. Also of particular importance for this chapter is the concept of "emergency reaction" proposed by Walter Cannon and Philip Bard in the 1920s. According to these authors, emotional stimuli have two separate effects; they excite the feeling of emotion in the cortex and the expression of emotion through the activation of the sympathetic division of the autonomic nervous system. Thus, the feeling of emotion is the result of the activity in neural mechanisms within the brain, without the need of the "brain reading" of the bodily response. The Cannon-Bard theory views emotional experience and emotional expression as parallel processes that have no direct causal relation. Therefore, the physiological responses accompanying different emotions should be the same regardless of the particular emotional state that is experienced.

Today, it has become clearer that cognition fills the gap between the specificity of feedback (James – Lange) and the non-specificity of felt experiences (Cannon-Bard) in the genesis of an emotional experience. There has been good agreement that to understand anxiety and fear, the appraisal of a situation is of fundamental importance. The meaning of the stimulus plays an important role in the cognitive assessment we make of dangerous situations. The majority of the animal models of anxiety focus on its somatic-emotional component, because the cognitive processing is not easily approached. However, a crucial issue for modeling each condition in laboratory animals is not the defensive reaction *per se* but may be related to the earlier stages of the processing of information. As such, to interpret a given input as signifying potential, distal or proximal danger/threat is of utmost importance for the organization of the appropriate response. Thus, animal models focusing on adaptive responses of animals to distal or potential *versus* actual or proximal threat may be modeling different types of anxiety.

In the study of the neurobiology of anxiety we should bear in mind that not necessarily all forms of threat trigger the same body signal, which is relayed to higher brain structures, where the activation of their neural substrates would implement an appropriate course of action. The action dependent on cognitive analysis goes against the basic biological requirements for an immediate, precise, and unequivocal response to threat. Indeed, as it will be seen later a great deal of evidence even points to antagonistic effects of planned, organized and cognitive acts against immediate, disorganized bodily responses of the defensive reaction to threatening situations.

Another point of interest on this issue is related to the context in which we feel threatened and anxious. If we assess that we can escape or fight back; we will feel one set of physical sensations. If, on the other hand, we feel threatened and perceive that we cannot escape or fight back; then we feel something quite different. Both the assessment of danger and the perception of our capacity to respond are not primarily conscious. Blanchard et al.

(1969, 1972) showed that whereas the wild rats preferentially flee away to an approaching experimenter when an escape route is available, freezing is the preferential response in an experimental setting when an escape route is not available. Thus, contrary to the prevalent idea that freezing is a response to distal threats, it can also be a defensive behavior against proximal aversive stimuli too.

A specific combination of autonomic and motor patterns may be used for conditioned responses, a different combination for unconditioned freezing, and a still different pattern for escape. In the following paragraphs of this chapter we will report that when an animal has experienced prior stress events in the same context where it faces dangerous situations high levels of fear ensues with a fall in the motor capacity to deal with it. What is the real biological meaning of these defensive responses? Is it stress, fear, anxiety or panic? We present in this chapter recent evidence collected in this and other laboratories that bring some contribution to the answers to these questions.

The Dichotomy between Anxiety and Panic

Anxiety and panic show similar dichotomy as anxiety and fear. They have also been regarded as different entities based on clinical and laboratory evidence. Anxiety is a subjective state of discomfort with behavioral and autonomic manifestations with a slow onset while panic is characterized by a sudden sensation of imminent death with more pronounced neurovegetative changes. During panic attack, along with the usual autonomic reactions, patients report sudden apprehension and intense fear of going crazy or dying, but although they often report the intention of escape and phobic avoidance of places and situations in which the panic attack occurred, the usual behavior evoked by them is characterized by defensive immobility (Brandão et al., 2003).

Other clinical evidence presented in favor of the dissociation between panic and anxiety is the poor therapeutic response of panic to benzodiazepines in contrast with the good therapeutic response of anxiety generalized disorders to chlordiazepoxide, diazepam, midazolam and other anxiolytic benzodiazepine compounds. On the other hand, in contrast with anxiety, panic attacks have been shown to be sensitive to chronic treatments with the selective serotonin reuptake inhibitors such as fluoxetine, tianeptine and others.

Also from the neurobiological viewpoint a dichotomy similar to that pointed out above for anxiety/fear comes out for anxiety and panic. Anxiety in this context has been related to higher brain structures, such as the frontal cortex, hippocampus and amygdala while panic has been considered as a more primitive reaction and elaborated in brainstem structures, such as the superior colliculus, dorsal periaqueductal gray and cuneiform nucleus. It has been suggested that anxiety serves primarily to signal the brain to activate a physical response that will eliminate the source of potential or distal threatening stimuli. As we will see afterwards panic is a feeling of imminent death with neurovegetative alterations along with an involuntary, somatic and often paralyzing brainstem response which results from a disturbance in the processing of internal physiological signals and, hence, could not serve to the purpose of activating brain mechanisms to deal with the proximal threatening stimuli. Therefore, while panic seems to be a general disturbance in the processing of internal stimuli and, as such, be a maladaptive response to face imminent danger, anxiety has an adaptive role insofar as it is a response to stimuli from the external world or an arrangement in the processing of internal physiological stimuli as a strategy to face threatening situations. While there seems to be no considerable dispute on that anxiety has, indeed, an adaptive value many neurobiologists do not agree on the notion of maladaptive function of panic. Table I summarizes the main differences between these two conditions.

One aspect that neurobiologists that investigate the neural substrates of fear agree is that although the neural mechanisms underlying anxiety and panic disorder are dissociated they overlap at some extent. The search for the mechanisms, structures or circuits that serve as commutator or switch for these processes has pointed out the hypothalamus as a strong candidate to this role. It has been established long ago that the hypothalamus plays a key role in the expression of defense reaction. In fact, innumerable studies have been performed showing that the defensive hypothalamic zone is composed of the anterior hypothalamic nucleus (AHN), the dorsomedial portion of the ventromedial nucleus (VMHDM), the dorsomedial hypothalamus (DMH) and the dorsal premammillary nucleus (PMD), which are highly interconnected and are involved in integrating innate defensive responses to environmental threats (Canteras, 2002; Di Micco et al., 2002). Recent study from this laboratory has suggested that gabaergic mechanisms of the DMH and PMD have selective involvement in unconditioned fear. On the other hand, the AHN and VMHDM appear to be mainly involved in conditioned fear (Santos et al., 2008). Thus, whereas the DMH and PMD are known to be part of the caudal-most parts of the medial hypothalamic defensive system which integrates unconditioned fear, systems mediating conditioned fear select the VMHDM and AHN nuclei, which belong to the rostral-most medial hypothalamic defensive area.

Table I. Levels of defense, predominant behavior and neural substrates associated to anxiety and panic

	Type of Danger	Behavior		Critical Structures			*Treatment*
		Predominant	Freezing				
Anxiety	Potential	Immobility	Conditioned	Pre-frontal cortex	Amygdala	Hippocampus	*Benzodiaze-pines*
				Hypothalamus			
Panic	*Proximal*	*Escape*	*Unconditioned*	*Dorsal periaqueductal gray*			*Selective serotonin reuptake inhibitors*

How to approach these issues in the laboratory when we do not have a communication channel with the animals? To do this we start from the Darwinian principle that the defense reaction displayed by animals is a good model of anxiety because its roots in man may be found in the defensive behaviors of the animals when they face dangerous situations. This behavioral expression of panic in man is very similar to the freezing responses displayed by experimental animals facing severe threat situations. In this case, however, this immobility is tense accompanied by autonomic alterations different from the passive immobility of the anxiety-like conditions.

Different Kinds of Fear

To introduce this topic let's summarize the hierarchical model for defensive strategies the animal displays when facing the predator. The defensive strategies adopted by an animal will depend of the distance of the predator. A characteristic organization of the conditioned defensive behavior may be observed when an animal unexpectedly gets in an unknown territory, the first thing that happen is an arousal reaction to the potential threat that interrupts any motor patterns that were already in execution and then prepares the animal for the defensive behaviors. Little defensive behavior from the prey is usually observed when the predator is very far away. The animal crouches reflexively; the eyes narrow somewhat as to increase the perception of what is going on through the activation of the parasympathetic autonomic nervous system. The initial arrest-crouch response minimizes detection by the predators. At a closer distance, the rat might engage in antidetection behavior such as freezing or hiding. If the initial signal in the open field had been from the predator itself, like a sound or its sight, a very different reaction would have been evoked: its head turns automatically in the direction of the signal in an attempt to localize and identify it. The neck, back, legs, and feet muscles coordinate so that the whole body turns. This initial action pattern, first to the potential and then to the distal threat, is an instinctive orientation preparing the animal to respond adequately to many possible contingencies. When the predator is in contact with the rat escape might predominate, or it fights back, possibly followed by tonic immobility (Klemm, 1990). When the predator approaches the prey has to change the strategy. By the time a rat is next to a predator, it might be too late to perform successful behaviors in order to avoid to be detected. If this is the case, in the presence of intense danger signals, the rat should implement another defensive strategy such as moving to a safe place if an escape route is available or fight back if it is not. In any event, the outcomes will depend on the particular set of neural regulatory mechanisms that trigger the corresponding set of muscles, viscera, and autonomic nervous system that cooperate in the preparation of the defense. This pattern of defense reaction is also based on genetic predispositions so that arousal, immobility, freezing or escape may be the appropriate choice depending on the particular danger stimulus the animal faces. In this sense, it is important to take note that the rat's defense system may have been phylogenetically ineffective as a proximal defense reaction for predators and, as such it is uncoordinated, disorganized and incomplete. Figure 1 presents a general model with sequential defensive responses as the predator approaches the prey.

Nowadays, a procedure called contextual fear conditioning (CFC) has been widely used as an animal model of anxiety. In this test, the time animals spend freezing when they are placed in a context (background stimuli, CS) in which they had previously received footshocks is considered a good index of anxiety. Biologically, immobility is a potent adaptive strategy used by animals when they are re-exposed to dangerous situations or are presented with neutral signals that had been previously paired with an unconditioned stimulus

(UCS), such as footshocks (Fanselow, 1994). Animals are immobilized in a sustained pattern of neuromuscular activity and high autonomic and brain wave activity. Sympathetic and parasympathetic responses are also concurrently activated, like brake and accelerator, working against each other. Ethologists have found wide adaptive value in these immobility responses. Indeed, freezing makes prey less visible avoiding attacks from predators.

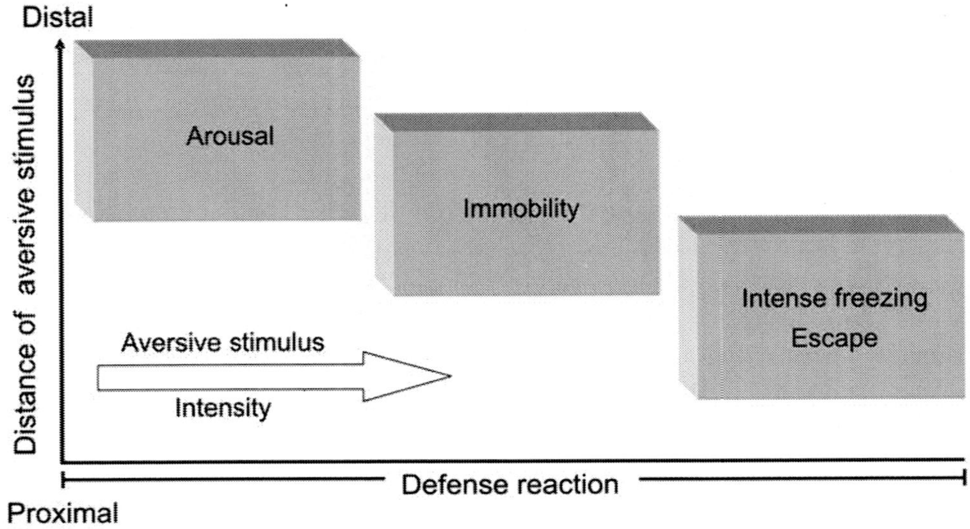

Figure 1. Hierarchical organization of defensive behaviors displayed by preys to increasing proximity of the predators. Similar pattern of defense reaction is observed to increasing intensity of electrical current applied to the dorsal periaqueductal gray (dPAG).

It has been suggested that the immobility induced by contextual fear, which is integrated in the ventral periaqueductal gray (vPAG), courses with little muscle tone, and the animal does not appear ready to jump or run (LeDoux, 1995; Carrive, 1995). Indeed, electrical or chemical stimulation of the vPAG causes immobility along with cessation of ongoing movement. This vPAG-evoked immobility is a hyporeactive type of immobility, which has been described as "quiescent immobility" and is considered to be phasic (Walker and Carrive, 2003). Consistent with this, we have shown that electrolytic and excitotoxic lesions of the vPAG reduced freezing evoked by re-exposure of rats to the same box in which it has previously received electric footshocks (Vianna et al., 2001). Immunohistochemical studies confirmed that contextual fear is associated with marked increase in Fos expression in the vPAG (Carrive et al., 1997). On the contrary, an active and tense freezing is induced by electrical or chemical stimulation of the dorsal periaqueductal gray (dPAG). Several studies using c-fos have shown that the dorsal parts of the PAG are activated by immediate threatening stimuli (Sandner et al., 1993; Canteras and Goto, 1999; Lamprea et al., 2002). As can be seen in Figure 2 lesions of the vPAG significantly reduce the conditioned contextual immobility but does not change the freezing and escape responses induced by electrical or chemical stimulation of the dPAG (Vianna et al., 2001). Thus, it is unlikely that the increase in muscle tone responsible for the tense freezing posture is mediated by vPAG.

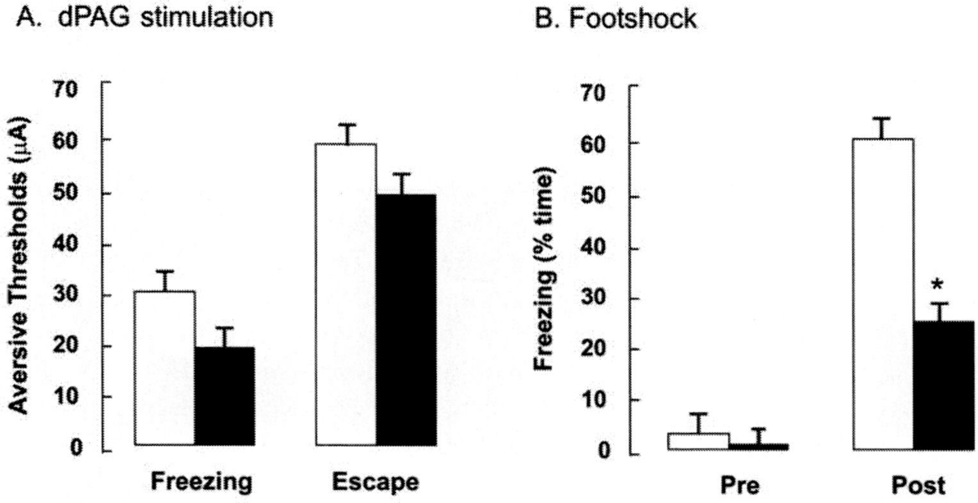

Figure 2. Aversive thresholds and percentage of time spent freezing by rats with sham (open columns) or ventral periaqueductal gray (vPAG - closed columns) lesions and submitted to electrical stimulation of the dPAG at freezing or escape thresholds (left) or placed in a contextual conditioning procedure using footshocks as unconditioned stimuli (right). Pre and Post represent measures taken before and 24 h after the conditioning procedure.

Exposure to the context where rats received footshocks 24-h earlier is also an aversive manipulation that causes freezing behavior concomitant with fear-potentiated startle (McNish et al., 1987; Walker and Carrive, 2003; Silva et al., 2003). This can be easily observed by the increase in the amplitude of the startle reflex observed in rats submitted to contextual fear conditioning alone (Phillips and Le Doux, 1992; Frankland and Yeomans, 1995; McNish et al., 1997). As discussed in the precedent paragraphs, while freezing behavior varies directly with shock intensity, startle to loud noise responds in a non-monotonic way to increasing contextual freezing generated by weak and strong conditioning with footshocks. This situation is not easily understood for those that only see a positive correlation between the strength of the conditioning stimulus and the conditioned response.

In our laboratory, using this simple conditioning procedures we observed that conditioned freezing in response to background conditioned stimuli (context - CS) is stronger than that obtained in classical conditioning paradigms with the use of tone or light (foreground stimuli). Also, rats that have being submitted to the association of moderate footshocks plus contextual cues show potentiated startle to a loud noise when the contextual signals are presented alone. On the contrary, a depression of the startle response to loud noises may ensue when these animals are submitted to an associative conditioning using higher intensity of footshocks. The amount of freezing measured in both situations, however, correlates positively with the intensity of the shocks applied in the conditioning sessions. In other words, conditioned freezing varies directly with shock intensity. The moderate conditioning might exert more powerful control than the intense conditioning over either a conditioned or an unconditioned preparatory response to danger. In the latter case, the contextual cues condition very well in the sense of becoming a reliable signal for shock but condition poorly as to its ability to elicit overt conditioned defensive behavior. The intense fear would turn on the motor systems for the preparatory response to a level higher than that supported by the system to increase the magnitude of conditioned startle so that instead of the enhanced fear potentiated startle a depression of the startle reflex may ensues in high fear conditions.

It is thought that context is a good CS that elicits some form of conditioned responses other than freezing or some form of unconditioned response that interferes with the startle response on re-exposure to the context. Specifically, when paired with unconditioned stimuli (USs) of higher intensity, context CSs often evoke more freezing (defensive immobility) than do moderate conditioning (Santos et al 2005). An interesting explanation for this difference is that moderate and intense conditionings have similar conditioned values but they support different forms of defensive behavior. Although there is no direct evidence to support this idea, probably, both types of conditioning might control conditioned responses that differ in form or control different forms of behavior (Figure 3).

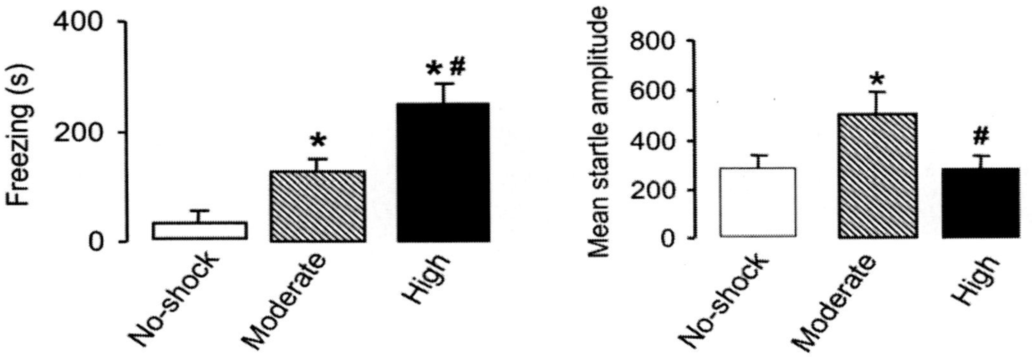

Figure 3. Different fear responses in rats submitted to moderate (five footshocks of 0.3 mA, 1s) and high (five footshocks 0.6 mA, 1s) levels of contextual fear conditioning. A: Time (s) of freezing. B. Mean startle amplitude to 30 loud sounds (100 dB, 1s) in the same chamber where rats were previously submitted to moderate and high fear conditioning. Mean ± S.E.M. * $p<0.05$ different from No-shock group. # $p<0.05$ different from moderate fear conditioning group.

The mechanisms underlying this dissociation could be related to those that influence response topography. Taking into account the considerations advanced above that the high and moderate CSs could differ in their ability to interfere with the fear potentiated startle we could envisage a parallel with what happens with the prey's defense response when the predator approaches. This makes sense if we consider that freezing increases at the same extent as the predator evolves from distances considered distal to proximal ones. However, the strategies a rat implements in this latter condition when it is in an open field as described in the beginning of this section would be difficult to recognize when testing the rat in a conditioning chamber that has no escape routes or places of safety.

Developing still further the above mentioned hypothesis that low levels of aversion trigger behavioral mechanisms different from those triggered by higher levels the present findings can be considered in the theory stated elsewhere that defensive behaviors are hierarchically organized and different behaviors within this class are provoked by aversive stimuli of different intensities (Blanchard et al., 1969, 1972). For example, arousal/immobility is the result of mild or distant threatening stimuli whereas freezing behavior is the outcome of stronger or nearer stimuli. Likewise, in the present experiment, conditioned contextual fear alone triggered mechanisms similar to those that mediate arousal/moderate immobility while conditioning with high level of stress may trigger an intense freezing that precede more vigorous behaviors. Consequently, the first case would make the animals more able to receive all kinds of sensorial information and more prone to a motor activity whereas in the second case the animal could have already made great physical struggle what would make the animals less able to exert further physical activity in response to the loud noise. Consistent with this hypothesis, a recent study from this laboratory demonstrated that rats exposed to a standard elevated plus-maze with conventional wooden walls showed higher levels of freezing than when exposed to a modified plus-maze with transparent walls in which they display more exploratory activity and lower levels of fear (Anseloni et al., 1995). Also, we have recently reported that prior electrical stimulation of the midbrain tectum, at aversive thresholds, caused an increase in fear-like behaviors with a concomitant reduction in the exploratory activity of rats in the elevated plus-maze (Pandossio et al., 2001).

In summary, the aversive circumstance to which an animal is exposed is determinant for the type of defense reaction. In the case of the contextual fear conditioning, a sensorial mapping of the context is first made through a pattern of neural firing that is registered in phylogenetically primitive brain regions. For instance, neurons of deeper layers of the superior colliculus are in good position for processing the sensory synthesis that plays a prominent role in attentive behavior and orienting reflexes which are basic components of defensive behaviors; neurons in the central nucleus of the inferior colliculus process acoustic information of aversive nature before they are sent to the medial geniculate nucleus of the thalamus and then to the temporal lobe; and neural substrate in the dorsal columns of the periaqueductal gray receive tactile or nociceptive information related to the aversive stimulus. A recognition pattern is then formed in subcortical structures and triggers the preparation for defensive responding before it is registered in consciousness. Access to memory information of previous experiences with similar situations influences these responses activating preset patterns of defensive behaviors. These outcomes will depend on the particular set of neural regulatory mechanisms that trigger the corresponding set of muscles, viscera, and autonomic nervous system that cooperate in the preparation of the defense. This pattern of defense reaction is also based on genetic predispositions so that arousal, immobility, freezing or escape may be the appropriate choice depending on the particular danger stimulus the animal faces. Therefore, according to these considerations the response selection of defensive behaviors from a phylogenetic perspective varies with the proximity of the predator.

Past Stressful Experiences Change the Nature of the Fear Responses

As discussed in the previous section of this chapter, it is established that animals that have been conditioned with light or tone respond with an enhanced potentiated startle when they are exposed to loud sounds in the presence of the light or tone-CS alone. The same happens when the context of the experimental chamber is used as the CS after conditioning that used shocks of moderate intensity. Rats given the same shock treatment but in a context different to that used for test, did not respond more than non-shocked groups. Therefore, exposure to discrete stimulus such as light or tone or contextual stimuli used as CS after conditioning procedures of moderate intensity leads to enhancement of the startle reflex to loud sounds. This successful response, i.e. active and enhanced defense reaction, clearly suggests that shock sensitization of startle is due to these CS (light, tone and context). Indeed, animals possess a variety of orientation, arousal and defensive responses that allows them to respond automatically to potentially dangerous situations rapidly and fluidly. It has been suggested that the aversive state generated in the animals submitted to this procedure is an anxiety-like state and this procedure has been considered an animal model of anxiety. However, a complete different pattern of response emerges when rats are submitted to conditioning procedure in which context is associated to past experience with high stress levels in that context; no enhancement or even a depression of the startle reflex is obtained (Nobre et al 2003; Santos et al 2005). It has been suggested that the aversive state generated in the animals submitted to this procedure is a fear-like state and this procedure has been considered an animal model of panic.

The observed lack of enhancement of startle reflex in rats with previous experience of high levels of stress more likely reflects a performance deficit. If this response reflected a lack of fear, one would expect this to be equally evident across other fear measures. However this is not the case here since when freezing was recorded as an additional measure of conditioned fear, animals trained after exposure to high stress events also presented significant freezing behavior, despite lower levels of startle in the same animals. These results suggest that fear itself is maintained, indeed elevated, in this group of animals and that the loss of enhancement of startle reflex with this kind of conditioning reflects a performance rather than learning deficit. This performance hypothesis had already been advanced by Davis and Astrachan (1987) with the use of light CS instead of background stimuli as in the present work. Based on this and other findings Davis and his group have proposed that fear may be linearly related to the intensity of shock used during training, but that the magnitude of potentiated startle may be non-monotonically related to fear (Walker et al 1997). For example, moderate fear levels may produce maximal fear-potentiated startle, whereas higher levels might switch animals to a different mode of defensive responding that do not include fear-potentiated startle as a component behavior. In conformity with this possibility the present results clearly show that a previous history of stress sensitizes defensive mechanisms with weakening of physical strength in reaction to subsequent submission to other aversive stimuli. Animals previously exposed to stress-inducing procedures have been reported to display subsequent behavioral passivity, even when these animals are submitted to only a mild stressor (Van Dijken et al., 1992). This is not to say that the stressor exposure procedure causes a general debilitating effect on motor activity since animals submitted to the forced swim test after stressful experience displayed higher immobility but the struggle phase of the test was even enhanced (Molina et al., 1994). As further confirmation of these findings, sensitization to subsequent aversive stimuli in animals with a past history of stress has been largely documented by hormonal, neurochemical and immunological studies (Weiss et al., 1981; Irwin et al., 1986; Caggiula et al., 1989; Antelman et al., 1990).

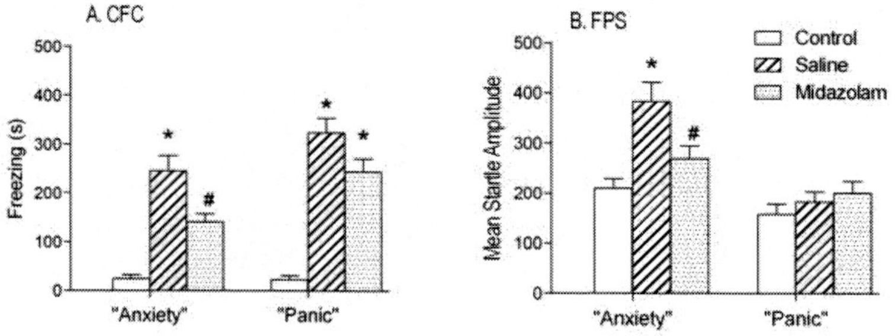

Figure 4. Different sensitivity to the anxiolytic effects of midazolam (0.5 mg/kg, IP) on anxiety-like (moderate fear conditioning) and fear-like states (high fear conditioning) assessed by time of freezing measured in a context fear conditioning (CFC-left) and fear-potentiated startle (FPS-right) procedures with rats submitted to loud sounds in the same chamber where they previously had been conditioned. In both conditions, control groups did not receive footshocks. The effects of saline and midazolam were evaluated in test sessions. Mean time of freezing or startle amplitude ± S.E.M. * $p<0.05$ different from control group (No-shock). CFC: context fear conditioning. FPS: fear potentiated startle. # $p<0.05$ different from saline group (moderate fear group). The benzodiazepine midazolam shows anxiolytic effects only in rats submitted to moderate levels of fear.

Another hypothesis is a parallel between the non-monotonic function and the generation of two distinct states of anxiety generated by stress associated to contextual fear conditioning. These behavioral effects may be related to fear states different from the anxiety state induced by contextual conditioned stimuli alone acquired by the previous pairing to footshocks. Indeed, midazolam caused an anxiolytic-like effect on the contextual fear-potentiated startle at a dose that did not produce any effect al all on the depression of the startle in rats previously conditioned with high level of fear (Figure 4). The resistance of this group of rats to the anxiolytic effects of midazolam is a good evidence for the distinction between anxiety and this form of fear. This may represent an emotional shift from low to high fear levels, which leads to change in the responsivity of the animals to benzodiazepines. As a working hypothesis we will name these two forms of emotional reactivity as “anxiety-like” and “panic-like” responses. Past experience with intense stressful stimuli seems to paradoxically bring the alterations lower than the baseline level. Importantly, baseline responses (i.e. startle to noise alone) were unaffected. Thus, the relative ineffectiveness of contextual stimuli paired with footshock in rats pre-exposed to intense fear stimuli cannot be attributed either to ceiling effects produced by a baseline elevation or to a general suppression of startle responses. As we can seen in Figure 4, the level of freezing was even higher in the fear-depressed startle (“panic-like”) group than the fear-potentiated (“anxiety-like”) startle group. From a neurological point of view, it is recognized that there could be two different types of anxiety: anxiolytic-sensitive and anxiolytic-insensitive. Where the flight-or-fight response is appropriate, freezing will be relatively maladaptive; where freezing is appropriate, attempts to flee or fight are likely to be maladaptive. Biologically, immobility is a potent adaptive strategy where active escape is prevented. When, however, it becomes a preferred response pattern in situations of activation in general, it is profoundly debilitating. Although, much work still need to be done we cannot help comparing the present results with the phenomenon of one-trial tolerance to midazolam in the elevated plus-maze test. In this condition re-exposure of rats to the height and open spaces of the apparatus causes the development of anxiolytic-insensitive fear states (Cruz-Morales et al., 2002).

The findings from these works have suggested that post-traumatic stress occurs when the animal shows an inability to deal with previously experienced aversive events, that is, when a given situation becomes both dangerous and inescapable.

Neural Substrates

Evidence from many sources has been obtained in support of the notion that the medial hypothalamus, dPAG, superior and inferior colliculi constitute the main neural substrates for the integration of unconditioned aversive behaviors in the brain (Graeff 1990, 1994, Brandão et al., 1994, 1999). Indeed, gradual increases in the intensity of electrical stimulation of these structures causes in progressive manner alertness, arousal, turnings, freezing and escape in the same way as the predator approaches the prey from a distant to a nearer or proximal position (Figure 2). As this set of structures shares this functional role in the organization of defensive behaviors and have two-way projections it has been called "brain aversion system" or "brain defense system" or still "fight-flight system" (Graeff 1990, 1994; Gray and MacNaughton, 2000; Brandão et al., 2003). This circuit acts to generate the basic changes necessary for the expression of any emergency response, from arousal to full-blown fight or flight (Brandão et al. 1994, 1999; Graeff, 1990, 1994). Orientation and turning toward the source of dangerous signal and other defensive postures are turned on just prior to the onset of freezing. This freezing behavior, however, unlike that related to vPAG previously described, is tonic and accompanied of hypertension, tachycardia, piloerection, micturition and defecation. This tonic freezing is prevalent and also thought to be linked to the activation of neural circuits of panic. The tonic freezing, fight or escape are sequentially the usual defense response consequent of the activation of this system. It has been shown that four interesting features make the arousal system unique (Schmitt et al., 1985; Brandão et al., 1986): 1) turning and freezing are not common responses induced by activation of the amygdala, which, by its turn, cause an oriented, flexible and well-coordinated escape response; 2) stimulation of the dPAG causes uncoordinated and explosive escape response; 3) sensory changes, such as sensorial neglect to tactile stimulation and serotonergic analgesia, are fragrant responses specific for the neural substrates of aversion in dPAG; 4) as already described, a tonic freezing that outlasts the dPAG stimulation has characteristics distinct from the conditioned freezing. In this latter case, it could well be that where fight and escape have been unlikely, the nervous system reorganizes to tonic immobility.

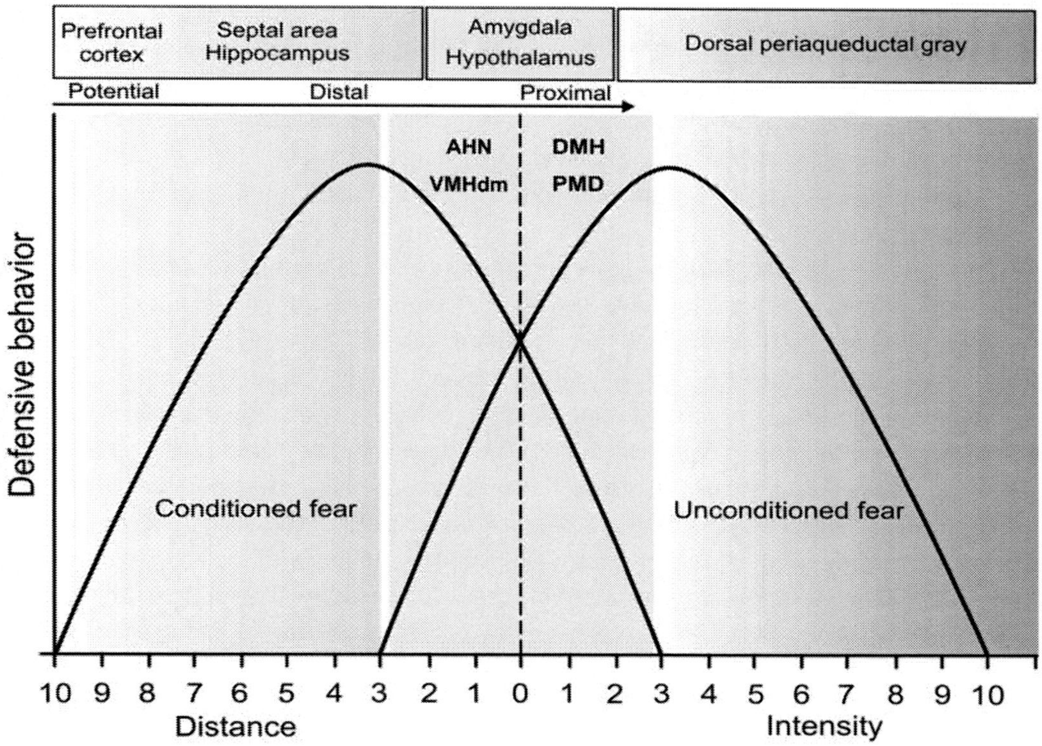

Figure 5. Defensive behaviors displayed by rats in function of the distance and intensity of the threatening stimuli and structures involved in the organization of the associated emotional behavior. Potential or distal danger stimuli elicit conditioned freezing when avoidance or escape is not available. The proximal aversive stimuli cause unconditioned freezing, which can evolve to freezing or escape depending on the experimental settings. The anterior hypothalamic nucleus (AHN) and the ventromedial, dorsomedial part of the hypothalamic nucleus (VMHDM) may act together with rostral brain structures to produce conditioned fear, whereas dorsomedial nuclei (DMH) and dorsal premammilary nuclei (PMD) would be more related to the organization of unconditioned fear. The neural substrates for conditioned and unconditioned fear may overlap. See text for more details.

It has been proposed that when orienting and defensive behaviors are carried out smoothly and effectively, anxiety-related neural substrates of the amygdala and hippocampus are activated. This generates a normal pattern of reaction to aversive situations that incorporates the curiosity, approach or avoidance. Otherwise, high levels of fear or past experience with traumatic events de-structure this defensive strategy and lead to the defensive pattern characteristic of the dPAG activation, generating a panic-related, thwarted and disorganized anxiety response. Therefore, the ability in becoming anxious is proportional to the ability in displaying active, adequate, defensive responses and to deal effectively with danger. Biologically, orientation, preparation and defense reaction are natural steps of an adaptive response to stimuli that puts at risk the organism survival. On the other hand, uncoordinated, explosive responses accompanied by sensation of imminent death are not adaptive strategies to cope with danger. As pointed out earlier, it seems likely now that distinct subsets of hypothalamic neurons could mediate different aspects of the defensive responses and serve as a kind of switch or commutator between neural processes associated with conditioned fear (anxiety-related) and unconditioned fear (panic-related). Whereas the anterior hypothalamus and ventromedial nucleus of the hypothalamus are called into play during anxiety-related processes the dorsomedial and dorsal premammilary nuclei of the hypothalamus are activated by unconditioned stimuli. Current studies are under way to determine how these systems are interrelated. A hypothetical scheme for the involvement of these hypothalamic nuclei in conjunction with other structures in the organization of fear is presented in Figure 5.

Recently, Walker and Carrive (2003) proposed that the freezing induced by contextual fear conditioning procedures is made up of two components: a phasic initial stage of a hyporeactive-hypotensive immobility pattern and a delayed stage of a rapid hyperreactive immobility pattern when the animal is tense and ready for action but temporarily immobilized. The phasic component seems to be related to "anxiety-like states" and the second component seems to be linked to "fear-like states". From what has been discussed so far, the "anxiety-like" response may also be considered phasic and anxiolytic-sensitive and the "panic-like" one may be tonic and anxiolytic-insensitive. Thus, two pathways should subserve each component of this process. One pathway dealing with the arousing properties of the stimulus would turn on motor systems and induce activity. The other pathway would deal with some of the aversive properties of the context including its inescapability and it would turn off motor systems, that is, it would impose freezing by acting as a brake on the other pathway. According to this model, the two pathways would be activated at the same time and competing against each other to set up the appropriate motor response. The neural substrates of the brain aversion system responsible for this switch in the nature of the defense reaction could be the medial hypothalamus. When by any reason the escape is not possible and the defensive preparedness for flight, concomitant with the feeling of danger, is disturbed the emotional state of the animal change abruptly. This emotional change also reflects a shift in the neural mechanisms that will command this new defense reaction. Response may go to a non-directed flight, fight or tonic freezing. In other words, when the normal orientation and defensive escape resources have failed to resolve the situation, the defense mechanisms switch to non-directed flight, fight or freezing, which has been linked to the dorsal aspects of PAG. A schematic of the diverse emotional stimuli, the associated defensive behaviors and neural substrates for this multifaceted process is presented in Figure 5.

It is tempting to speculate that past experience with stressors also leads to an emotional shift switching the neural circuits responsible for the production of the defensive response to an aversive context. Panic is the secondary emotional anxiety state that is evoked when the orientated and organized processes for dealing with the danger are not successful. Disturbances in the normal organization of defense responses or the ability to integrate the whole pattern of a defense reaction may result in intense freezing or disorganized defensive responses, which are the corollary of the panic attacks.

Conclusion

The defense reaction displayed by animals is a good model of anxiety. In fact, the roots of anxiety in man may be found in the defensive behaviors of the animals when they face dangerous situations. Anxiety has often been linked to the physiology and experience of these defensive reactions. In general, when an animal is attacked by a predator it will first attempt to escape through directed-oriented running. However, if the escaping animal is cornered so that escape is diminished, it may run in an uncoordinated and disorganized manner, without a directed orientation, or it may attempt to fight. There are many forms of anxiety. In animal models of generalized anxiety discrete signals, such as light, tones or the context paired previously with unconditioned aversive stimulus (US) trigger appropriate mechanisms that enhance the defense reactivity of the animals. Therefore, where escape or avoidance is possible, the organism responds with an active pattern of coping. On the other hand, in animal models of anxiety in its panic form fear stimuli that originate active but disorganized patterns of defensive response ensure emotional states of different nature. Depending on the intensity and/or the proximity of the danger the response may be running, escape, often uncoordinated and explosive or even incapacity of expressing appropriate reactions to emotional challenges. What structure or neural circuits are called into play in these situations? Whereas anxiety-related responses have been associated to rostral regions of the brain, the neural substrates of panic-related responses appear to be mainly linked to structures located at more caudal areas of the brain The integration of these two neural systems appears to rely on the defensive neural substrates of the hypothalamus. Thus, whereas DMH and PMD are known to be part of the caudal-most region of the medial hypothalamic defensive system, which integrates unconditioned fear, systems mediating conditioned fear select the AHN and VMHDM nuclei that belong to the rostral-most portion of the hypothalamic defense area. Thus, distinct subsets of neurons in the hypothalamus could mediate different aspects of the defensive responses. A shift in the emotional states passing through the hypothalamus may occur depending on the intensity of the threatening situation or danger stimuli. As a working hypothesis, it is advanced that past experience with stressors may lead to this emotional shift. In this case, active forms of defensive response are not entirely organized and an emotional state of different nature ensues. Therefore, intense fear or past experience with trauma plays a significant role in the organization of the defensive behavior in that it may shift oriented and organized motor patterns for preparing adequate defensive behaviors into faulty defense reaction.

References

American Psychiatric Association. *Diagnostic and Statistical Manual of Mental Disorders*, 4th edition. American Psychiatric Association, Washiton, DC, 1994.

Antelman, SM; Cunnick, JE; Lysle, DT; Caggiula, AR; Knopf ,S; Kocan, DJ; Rabin, BS; Edwards, DJ. (1990).Immobilization 12 days (but not one hour) earlier enhanced 2-deoxy-D-glucose induced immunosuppression; evidence for stressor –induced time dependent sensitization of the immune system. *Progress in Neuropsychopharmacology Biological Psychiatry, 14*, 579-590, 1990.

Anseloni, VZ; Messias, G; Brandão, ML. (1995). Behavioral and pharmacological validation of the elevated plus maze constructed with transparent walls. *Brazilian Journal of medical and Biological Research, 28*, 597-601.

Blanchard, DC; Blanchard, R J. (1969). Crouching as an index of fear. *Journal of Comparative Physiology Psychology, 67*, 370–375.

Blanchard, D C; Blanchard, R J. (1972). Innate and conditioned reactions to threat in rats with amygdaloid lesions. *Journal of Comparative Physiology Psychology, 81*, 281–290.

Brandão, ML; DiScala, G; Bouchet, MJ; Schmitt, P. (1986). Escape behavior produced by the blockade of glutamic acid decarboxilase (GAD) in mesencephalic central gray or medial hypothalamus. *Pharmacology Biochemistry & Behavior, 24*, 497-502.

Brandão, ML; Anseloni, VZ; Pandóssio, JE; De Araújo, JE; Castilho, VM. (1999). Neurochemical mechanisms of the defensive behavior in the dorsal midbrain. *Neuroscience and Biobehavioral Reviews, 23*, 863-875.

Brandão, ML. (1994). Neural substrate of defensive behavior in the midbrain tectum. *Neuroscience and Biobehavioral Reviews, 18*, 339-346.

Brandão, ML; Troncoso, AC; Silva, MAS; Huston, JP. (2003). The relevance of neuronal substrates in the midbrain tectum to anxiety and stress: empirical and conceptual considerations. *European Journal of Pharmacology, 463*, 225-233.

Caggiula, AR; Antelman, SM; Aul, E; Knopf, S; Edwards, DJ. (1989). Prior stress attenuates the analgesic response but sensitizes the corticosterone and cortical dopamine response to stress 10 days later. *Psychopharmacology, 99*, 223-237.

Canteras, NS; Goto, M. (1999). Fos-like immunoreactivity in the periaqueductal gray of rats exposed to a natural predator. *Neuroreport, 10*, 413-418.

Canteras, N.S. (2002). The medial hypothalamic defensive system: hodological organization and functional implications. *Phamacology Biochemistry and Behavior, 71,* 481-491.

Carrive, P; Leung P; Harris, J; Paxinos, G. (1997). Conditioned fear to context is associated with increased fos expression in the caudal ventrolateral region of the midbrain periaqueductal gray. *Neuroscience, 78*, 165-177.

Cruz-Morales, SE; Santos, NR; Brandão, ML. (2002). One-trial tolerance to midazolam is due to enhancement of fear and reduction of anxiolytic-sensitive behaviors in the elevated plus-maze retest in the rat. *Pharmacology Biochemistry & Behavior, 72*, 973-978.

Davis, M; Astrachan, DI. (1978). Conditioned fear and startle magnitude: Effects of different footshock and backshock intensities used in training. *Journal of Experimental Psychology: Animal Behavioral Processes, 4*, 95-103.

DiMicco, J.A.; Samuels, B.C.; Zaretskaia, M.V.; Zaretsky, D.V. (2002). The dorsomedial hypothalamus and the response to stress: part renaissance, part revolution. *Pharmacology Biochemistry and Behavior, 71,* 469–480.

Fanselow, M.S. (1994). Neural organization of the defensive behavior system responsible for fear. *Psychonom Bull Rev 1*, 429-438.

Fendt, M; Koch, M; Schnitzler H-U. (1994). Lesions of the central gray block the sensitization of the acoustic startle response in rats. *Brain Research, 661*,163–173.

Frankland, PW; Yeomans, JS. (1995). Fear-potentiated startle and electrically evoked startle mediated by synapses in rostrolateral midbrain. *Behavioral Neuroscience, 109*, 669–680.

Graeff, FG. (1994). Neuroanatomy and neurotransmitter regulation of defensive behaviors and related emotions in mammals. *Brazilian Journal of Medical and Biological Research, 27*, 811-829.

Graeff, FG. (1990). Brain defense systems and anxiety. In: Burrows, GD; Roth, M; Noyers, Jr (eds), *Handbook of Anxiety*. Amsterdam: Elsevier Science Publishers, pp. 307-354.

Gray, A; McNaughton, N. Fundamentals of the septo-hippocampal system. In: Gray, JA; McNaughton, N. (editors). *The Neuropsychology of Anxiety: An enquiry into the functions of septo-hippocampal system,* 2nd edition. Oxford: Oxford University Press, 2000, pp 204-232.

Irwin, J; Ahluwalia, P; Anisman, H. (1986). Sensitization of norepinephrine activity following acute and chronic footshock. *Brain Research, 379*, 98-103, 1986.

Klemm, WR. Historical and introductory perspectives on brainstem-mediated behaviors. In: Klemm, WR; Vertes, RP (editors*). Brainstem mechanisms of behavior*. New York: John Wiley & Sons, Inc., 1990, pp. 3-32.

Lamprea, MR; Cardenas, FP; Vianna, DM; Castilho, VM; Cruz-Morales, SE; Brandão, ML. (2002). The distribution of fos immunoreactivity in rat brain following freezing and escape responses elicited by electrical stimulation of the inferior colliculus. *Brain Research, 950*, 186-94.

LeDoux JE. (1995). Emotion: clues from the brain. *Annual Reviews of Psychology, 46*, 209-235.

Levine, P.A.; Frederick, A. (1997). Waking the tiger: Healing trauma: The innate capacity to transform overwhelming experiences. North Atlantic Books, 250 pp.

McNish, KA; Gewirtz, JC; Davis, M. (1997). Evidence of contextual fear after lesions of the hippocampus: A disruption of freezing but not fear-potentiated startle. *Journal of Neuroscience, 17*, 9253-9360.

Molina VA; Heyser; CS; Spear LP. (1994). Chronic variable stress or chronic morphine facilitates immobility in a forced swim test: Reversal by naloxone. *Psychopharmacology, 114*, 433-440.

Nobre, MJ; Sandner, G; Brandão, ML. (2003). Enhancement of acoustic evoked potentials and impairment of startle reflex induced by reduction of GABAergic control of the neural substrates of aversion in the inferior colliculus. *Hearing Research, 184*, 82-90.

Pandóssio JE; Molina VA; Brandão ML. (2000). Prior electrical stimulation of the inferior colliculus sensitizes rats to the stress of the elevated plus-maze test. *Behavioral Brain Research, 109*, 19-25.

Phillips, RG; LeDoux, JE. (1992). Differential contributions of amygdala and hippocampus to cued and contextual fear conditioning. *Behavioral Neuroscience, 106*, 274-285.

Sandner, G; Oberling, P; Silveira, MCL; Di Scala, G; Rocha, B; Bagri, A.; Deportere, R. (1993). What brain structures are active during emotions? Effects of brain stimulation elicited aversion on c-fos immunoreactivity and behavior. *Behavioural Brain Research, 58*, 9-18.

Schmitt, P; DiScala, G; Brandão, ML; Karli, P. (1985). Behavioral effects of microinjections of SR95103, a new GABA - A antagonist, into medial hypothalamus or the mesencephalic central gray. *European Journal of Pharmacology, 117*, 149-158.

Sigmundi RA; Bouton ME; Bolles RC. (1980). Conditioned freezing in the rat as a function of shock intensity and CS modality. *Bulletin of the Psychonomic Society, 15*, 254-256.

Sigmundi, RA; Bolles, RC. (1983). CS modality, context conditioning and conditioned freezing. *Animal Learning Behavior, 11*, 205-212.

Santos, JM; Gárgaro, AC; Oliveira, AR; Masson, S; Brandão, ML (2005). Pharmacological dissociation of moderate and high contextual fear as assessed by freezing behavior and fear-potentiated startle. *European Journal of Neuropsychopharmacology*, 15, 239-246.

Santos, JM ; Macedo, CE ; Brandão, ML. Gabaergic mechanisms of hypothalamic nuclei in the expression of conditioned fear. *Neurobiology of Learning & Memory,* 90:560-568, 2008

Silva, RCB; Gárgaro, AC; Brandão, ML. (2004). Differential regulation of the expression of contextual freezing and fear-potentiated startle by 5-HT mechanisms of the median raphe nucleus. *Behavioural Brain Research, 151*, 93-101.

Van Dijken, HH; ·Van Der Heyden, JAM; Mos, J; Tilders, FJH. (1992). Inescapable footshocks induce progressive and long-lasting behavioral changes in male rats. *Physiology Behavior, 51*, 787-794.

Vianna, DML; Landeira-Fernandez, J; Brandão, ML. (2001). Dorsolateral and ventral regions of the periaqueductal gray matter are involved in distinct types of fear. *Neuroscience and Biobehavioral Reviews, 25*, 711-719.

Walker, P; Carrive P. (2003). Role of ventrolateral periaqueductal gray neurons in the behavioral and cardiovascular responses to contextual fear and poststress recovery. *Neuroscience, 116*, 897-912.

Walker, DL; Cassella, JV; Lee, Y; De Lima, TCM; Davis, M. (1997). Opposing roles of the amygdala and dorsolateral periaqueductal gray in fear-potentiated startle. *Neuroscience and Biobehavioral Reviews, 21*, 743–753.

Weiss, JM; Goodman, PA; Losito, BG; Corrigan, S; Charry, JM; Bailey, WM. (1981). Behavioral depression produced by an uncontrollable stressor: relationship to norepinephrine, dopamine and serotonin levels in various regions of the rat brain. *Brain Research Review, 3*, 167-205.

In: Brain Mapping Research Progress
Editors: Ines C. Girard and Jade S. Andre

ISBN: 978-1-60456-784-7

Chapter X

Phase Synchronization at Different Frequency Bands Induced by the Emotional Film Stimuli of Happiness, Sadness and Fear

Tommaso Costa, Elena Rognoni,
Dario Galati and Manuella Crini
Department of Psychology, University of Turin, Italy

Abstract

The neural large-scale dynamics and the connectivity pathways among spatially separated neural groups are conceived as a fundamental brain mechanism to integrate and process information.

The new measures of nonlinear interdependencies applied to EEG recordings, such as phase synchronization, have been recently shown to be highly sensitive to detect the dynamical change underlying the brain functions.

In the present chapter, the patterns of interdependency among different brain regions were investigated extracting the Synchronization Index (SI) from EEG response to different emotional and non-emotional film stimuli. The three basic emotions of happiness, fear and sadness were induced with the goal to investigate the synchronization patterns at different frequencies bands specifically associated with the valence dimension (positive vs. negative) and with the distinct basic emotional systems.

The comparisons among the experimental conditions showed several significant SI changes. The results demonstrated an overall decrease of SI during emotional stimulation compared to neutral, indicating an increase of complexity in the cortical dynamics. Further differences were found among the specific emotions, involving a distinct couple of electrodes with topographical effects at the frequencies bands examined. During happiness, we found a large pattern of synchronization in the left frontal hemisphere, especially in delta and theta waves, while fear, compared to neutral stimuli, showed a higher right synchronization, especially in beta waves. Largely different SI patterns emerged in the comparisons between the two negative emotions of fear and sadness, suggesting that the basic emotions are mediated by specific synchronized activity. The observed emotion-related SI change supports the view that coupling-decoupling patterns among the neural networks may be a relevant neural mechanism for the emotional processing and that SI nonlinear analysis may contribute to describe how the brain generates the emotion.

Introduction

Neural Synchronization

The intricate connectivity among functionally specialized groups of neurons is an outstanding characteristic of mammalian brains, which are primarily characterized by the ability to integrate information (Tononi and Edelman, 1998). According to the functional integration approach (Frackowiak et al., 2004), the distributed networks of neurons transiently linked by reciprocal dynamic connections, defined neural assemblies (Hebb, 1949), are thought to be the basic functional mechanism mediating the wide sort of behaviors and mental processes. Integration is based on the positive and negative feedback among neural structures on different scale levels: on a small scale, the reentrant processes occurred at the level of cells and cell assemblies, while on a large scale, there were loops formed by reciprocal projections among brain structures distributed along the entire neuraxis, including limbic, cortical, and brain stem structures (Lewis, 2005).

Over the past years, a large body of empirical studies employing electro- and magneto-encephalography (EEG, MEG) or functional Magnetic Resonance Imaging (fMRI) have begun to explore the functional integration among the reentrant circuits and the neural networks on higher levels of brain functioning. In particular, the neurophysiological techniques such as EEG and MEG are highly suitable to capture these macroscopic spatial temporal dynamics, whose prevalent feature is the presence of metastable spatio-temporal pattern of neural activity distributed over many distinct brain regions.

Numerous mathematical methods have been devised to extract information on the various modes of reciprocal interaction from the EEG oscillations.

Since biological systems such as the neural networks are likely to be nonlinear, dissipative and stochastic systems (Rosenblum et al., 2004), nonlinear analysis may be particularly useful to describe the large-scale dynamics of the brain, as well as to define how much the system is deterministic or stochastic (Stam, 2005).

The phase synchronization among participating neuronal groups is one of the new nonlinear measures that has been proposed to play a key role in the integrative brain functions (Singer, 1999; Tononi and Sporns, 2003; Hebb, 1949). It specifically detects the interdependencies of instantaneous phases of two time series (Rosenblum et al., 1996). According to Boccaletti et al. (2002), a broad neurophysiological definition for neural synchronization refers to "the adjustment of time-varying properties between two or many subsystems (either equivalent or nonequivalent) to a common behavior through a coupling or an external forcing (periodical or noisy)" (see also Brown and Kocarev, 2000). Phase synchronization is characterized by a non uniform distribution of the phase difference between two signals, with the important advantage that it not only occurs between linear oscillators, but also between irregular and chaotic systems (Pecora and Carroll, 1990) and when the amplitudes of coupled chaotic oscillators remain uncorrelated (Rosenblum et al., 1996).

Much effort has recently been focused on detecting and quantifying synchronization within non-stationary noisy systems (Pikovsky et al., 2001). In such systems, the traditional cross-correlation technique may not assure appropriate detection in all cases of interdependency. Recent advances in synchronization analyses turn out to detect the direction of coupling between two systems, defining which signal becomes synchronized with another one and otherwise (Rosenblum and Pikovsky, 2001).

Direct evidence supporting phase synchrony as a basic mechanism for brain integration has recently been provided in relation to memory (Klimesh, 1999), learning (Singer, 1993), visual perception (Bressler et al. 1993; Rodriguez et al. 1999), binding processes (Tallon-Baudry and Bertrand, 1999), selective attention (Desmedt and Tomberg, 1994; Klimesch et al., 1998; Tallon-Baudry et al., 2001) and musical hearing (Bhattacharya, 2001). Although several cognitive processes have been linked to synchronization change, emotions have received relatively little attention in synchronization EEG studies. Nonetheless, synchronization may offer a highly informative tool to investigate the neural process underlying the emotion, that is overall recognized as a complex and multi-componential response produced by the different interconnecting neural systems. As the emotion involves cognitive, behavioral, expressive, sensory-motor and psychophysiological components, as it is mediated by largely distributed neural circuits extended along the cerebral neuraxis exerting effect on cortical dynamics detectable by synchronization analysis on EEG signals. In accordance with these considerations, investigations on synchronized activity performed by nonlinear analysis methods may extensively contribute to describe how emotions are generated and organized in the brain.

The Models of Emotion

How can we define emotion? Since James posed the question in 1884, the definition of emotion has been long debated and, at the same time, holds one of the most relevant issues for psychological disciplines and neuroscience. Emotion holds a salient evolutionary function regulating the adaptation to the environment; furthermore, emotion deeply interacts and influences a lot of psychological processes such as perception, memory, attention and reasoning, representing an essential function of the whole system. On this basis, it seems unrealistic to achieve a full model of the mind, behavior and brain, excluding emotion.

Several theories have attempted to provide a comprehensive definition of emotion and describe the complex emotional domain. Three main models of emotion represent the theoretical backgrounds to investigate the distinct neuroanatomical underpinnings of emotion: the dimensional models, the discrete multi-systems models and the dual systems models of approach and withdrawal.

Dimensional Emotions

In the past the cognitive approach to the studies of emotion in humans has developed the so-called dimensional theory that considers all emotions to be organized around a limited number of underlying dimensions: the valence or pleasantness dimension distinguishes positive (or pleasant) and negative (or unpleasant) emotions, and arousal dimension distinguishes emotion in terms of bodily activation (excitement) or deactivation (calm) (e.g. Russell, 1980). This account of emotion is based on results obtained by factor analysis on verbal assessments of emotional experiences. Several neuroimaging investigations supported a neural specialization associated with emotions with different subjective valence and arousal values (for a meta-analytic review, see Murphy et al., 2003). Lang and co-workers (1998a) have developed a neurobiological model of emotional dimensions, often referred to as the "bio-informational theory of emotion". Emotions are viewed as action dispositions, containing cognitive, motivational, physiological and behavioural components. These dispositions are organized as being either consummatory/appetitive tendencies or defensive/aversive tendencies. Consequently, this approach is associated with a two dimensional model of emotion: the valence dimension is related to variations on the level of the two motive systems, i.e. "appetitive" and "aversive"; the arousal dimension, adds to the two-dimensional affective space a component that modulates the emotional behaviour with respect to activation or intensity (Lang et al., 1998b). The two systems are thought to have different neural substrates, namely widespread networks involving a number of neocortical and subcortical structures. Variations in arousal are considered to reflect changes in the activation intensity of the aversive or appetitive subsystems.

Discrete Emotions

In opposition with dimensional approach, some theorists hypothesized a limited number of emotions that differ one from another, called "basic" emotions, from which the wide range of more complex emotions are derived (e.g., Ekman, 1992). According to this theorization, basic emotions are innate, universal and biologically given, selected along the evolutionary history of species for their specific adaptive function in promoting the survival and adaptation goal. Each emotion is characterized by specific physiological, behavioural and expressive patterns, that predispose the adaptive response, as well as by universal signals, antecedent events, distinctive thoughts, memories and images, different subjective experiences. According to the evolutionary approach, basic emotions share automatic appraisal, presence in other primates, quick onset, brief duration and unbidden occurrence (Ekman, 1992).

The basic emotions are though to be generated by specific and at least in part dissociable central affective programs involving widely distributed neural circuits, that mediate the several components of response and integrate all the process that, from perception to appraisal, contribute to emotion (e.g. Ekman and Davidson, 1994; Panksepp, 1998).

The definition of the types and the number of basic emotional system is of crucial interest for affective neuroscience. Neuroimaging researches have recently supported a neural specialization for distinct basic emotions such as fear, sadness, happiness, anger and disgust (Murphy et al., 2003; Barrett and Wager, 2006).

The Approach - Withdrawal Emotional System

Further models argue that the broad emotional domain may be organized around the basic and evolutionarily ancient systems of approach and withdrawal, associated to specific action tendencies (Davidson, 2003). The approach system facilitates appetitive or goal-directed behavior; it mainly generates the approach-related positive affect (like desire but not satisfaction), and also some negative affect that, like anger, predispose to approach the stimuli. The withdrawal system predisposes an organism to draw away from aversive stimuli, generating avoidance- related negative affect, such as fear and disgust (Davidson and Irwin, 1999).

Emotions and EEG Cortical Dynamics

Emotion have been stimulating the neurophysiological research on EEG cortical dynamics investigated both in the domain of amplitudes and frequencies with linear measures, and with nonlinear measures that capture the dynamical complexity of the system and the mutual synchronization across cortical areas. The power spectral analysis measures the event-related de-synchronization (ERD) and synchronization (ERS) – in other words, the decrease and the increase in power distribution (Pfurtscheller and Lopes da Silva, 1999). It was consistently found that emotion induced significant alpha, theta and beta ERD as respect to neutral processing, indicating an higher level of the overall cortical activations (Krause et al., 2000), with topographical effects dependent on the valence in prefrontal and posterior regions (Aftanas et al., 2001; Aftanas et al., 1998b; Aftanas et al., 2004). Emotional states were found to exert a significant impact on EEG coherence (Tucker and Dawson, 1984; Hinrichs and Machleidt, 1992), a linear measure based on the cross- and auto-correlations of power spectral densities (Thatcher et al., 1986) and, hence, on the Fourier transform that disregards the non linear properties of EEG signal. The recent discoveries of the properties of the new nonlinear measures have producing a renewed interest in the EEG response during emotions, in order to complete the neurobiological models formulated on the basis of high spatial resolution neuroimaging techniques. Interesting findings were gathered by non-linear measures that detect the dynamical complexity of the system. Emotional stimulations were associated with a more posterior increase in dimension when compared with perceptual tasks (Aftanas et al., 1994). The dimensional complexity was proven to increase with emotional arousal, whereas no specific changes were clearly associated with emotional valence (Aftanas et al., 1997a). The estimates of nonlinear forecasting and chaoticness were shown to be associated with higher EEG predictability in posterior regions during negative emotion; in turn, the dynamical complexity increased over posterior areas during positive emotions and decreased over frontal areas (Aftanas et al., 1997b). It was claimed that dynamical complexity decreases as the brain processes become more bound to low degrees of freedom and that this effects could be due to the subcortical activation and vertical synchronization (Aftanas et al., 1998b). On this basis the findings obtained by EEG nonlinear analyses are surprisingly consistent with those obtained by neuroimaging studies referring both to localization and functional integration approach. In particular high arousing and negative emotions were found to induce an increased activity in the posterior perceptual cortical areas, such as the extrastriate cortex (Lang et al., 1998b; Surguladze et al., 2003). In a previous work (Costa et al, 2006) we investigated the patterns of EEG synchronization in response to positive and negative emotional film stimuli and we found differences in cortical activity related not only to the emotional arousal, but also to the emotional valence.

The findings collected so far consistently sustain that the enhancement of dynamical complexity could be an important functional mechanism to process emotion. The future investigations on how the neural networks become coupled and decoupled should represent a crucial issue to understand the functional organization of emotions in the brain. Nonetheless, several questions remain to be answered, in particular with reference to which effects could be attributed to different type of emotions. The most of the studies were concerned with dimensional models, disregarding more specific differences related to basic emotions with the same valence or arousal, as well as to emotions associated to approach and withdrawal systems.

Objectives and Hypotheses

The present study addressed to investigate the neural synchronization on a large scale during emotional and non emotional processing and to evaluate the specific neural dynamics related to different basic emotions. The main goal was twofold: first, we intended to assess the nonlinear phase synchronization change generally associated with emotional processing; second, we intended to evaluate the synchronization patterns induced by specific basic emotions, in order to disambiguate whether the neural distinctions could be ascribed to the valence dimension or there were more subtle differences that could be better explained by the discrete models or by approach – whitdrawal system theory.

To accomplish these goals, phase synchronization was estimated by the synchronization index (SI) on EEG response to emotional film clips of fear, happiness and sadness. In addition, psychometrical ratings were collected after the experimental conditions, in order to acquire information about self-reported emotional experience and the subjective quality of emotion. The basic emotions investigated highly differ both for the specific biological function, as it was claimed by discrete models of emotion, for their valence and arousal values on the dimensional space, and for their association with approach and withdrawal systems. Hence they allow to compare the predictions drawn from the different models of emotion.

One of the main advantages of EEG measures is their ability to allow the estimation of the functional state different frequency bands with specific functional value: the reduction or desynchronization of alpha activity (8-12 Hz) is known to be a marker of the general brain activation occurring when subjects become engaged in mental tasks (Pfurtscheller and Lopes da Silva, 1999); theta rhythm (4-7 Hz) is particularly interesting for research on emotion, for its limbic origin and its association with the cortico-hippocampal-limbic interactions (Basar et al., 1999; Basar et al., 2001); delta rhythm (0,5-4 Hz) was generally associated to a decrease of the functional state of the brain, but recently it was reported that delta power increased as subjects processed emotional stimuli (Aftanas et al., 2004); a desynchronization of the beta rhythm(13-30 Hz) that is mainly generated in the motor cortex, was observed during the motor tasks (Basar et al., 2001), as well as during emotional processing (Aftanas et al., 1998b). For each of these frequency bands the fast Fourier-based power distribution was calculated in order to have a basic information on the cortical activation, and then the nonlinear synchronization analysis was performed in order to acquire information on the more subtle dynamics underlying the emotional response.

On the basis of the theoretical and empirical backgrounds, the main hypotheses to test were that: (a) significant changes of synchronized activity occurred during emotional processing as respect to non emotional processing; (b) the valenced emotions and the basic emotions differed in their synchronized activity within the functionally specific frequency bands and with topographical effects involving in particular frontal and occipital regions, that previous researches found to be relevant structures underlying emotion.

A neural correlate of valence dimension should be reflected in differences between happiness and the two negative emotions included in the study, sadness and fear. On the contrary, if there are more specific patterns of synchronized activity correlated with the arousal, we should find primarily differences between emotional and neutral stimuli processing, with a greater distinctions related to an highly arousing and activating emotion like fear. Otherwise, the distinctions among emotions, in particular between the two negative emotion of fear and sadness, may indicate that the discrete and dissociable systems, could reflect more subtle aspects of synchronization change, not fully reducible to more general dimensions. and of the functional basis of human emotion.

Method

Participants

Thirty-one healthy, right-handed (as measured by Edimburgh Handedness Inventory (Oldfield, 1971) volunteers participated in the experiment (16 males, 15 females), ranging in age from 20 to 30 years (mean $\pm$ S.D. age, 24.5 $\pm$ 2.4). All subjects underwent a physical evaluation to screen out chronic diseases, mental disorders, medication, head injury, drug or alcohol abuse. All had normal or corrected to normal vision.

The study was carried out in accordance with the Declaration of Helsinki principles, approved by the ethics committee of the University of Turin. All subjects gave written, informed consent and were informed of their right to discontinue participation at any time.

Film Stimuli

Stimuli consisted of 48 sequences (10 sec long) representing different emotional scenarios of happiness, sadness, fear and neutral content (12 per condition). The stimuli were extracted from commercial films and then edited in order to exclude any element that differs from the target emotional content. In a pilot study the stimuli were validated by 30 judges that rated each clip on a 9-point Likert scale for the valence and arousal level and for the intensity of the basic emotions subjectively experienced. The happiness sequences depicted lovers' encounters, amusement scenes and successful moments. The sadness sequences depicted scenes of death, loss, sickness and sorrow. The fear sequences depicted people's or animals' aggressions and dangerous situations such as falling down and drowning. The neutral sequences depicted a series of routine actions. All the stimuli were in color and were presented without sound and balanced in relation to the presence of human beings and complexity.

Self-Report of Emotional Experience

A self-report was used to assess the subjective emotional response to film stimuli. Subjects had to rate the pleasantness of their own emotional experience on a 9-point Likert scale ranging to 1 (very unpleasant) to 9 (very pleasant) and the arousal level from 1 (not at all, very calm) to 9 (fully experienced emotion, very excited). Finally, they indicated the intensity of the emotional state they experienced on a rating scale, including five primary emotions in random order: happiness, sadness, anger, fear, and disgust (from 1 indicating that the emotion was not at all present, to 9 indicating that it was felt very strongly).

Procedures

The subjects were seated on comfortable chairs in the recording room and they were told to look at the TV screen placed in front of them both during the film clips and the black screen which separated each sequence.

Stimuli were presented in a block design with a regular baseline between each block. The experiment included 16 blocks including three stimuli of the same condition. Hence, there were 8 blocks for the 4 experimental conditions of neutral, happiness, sadness and fear, presented in two subsequent runs. Each run included two blocks of the same conditions. Stimuli were randomly assigned to blocks and run in random order both among and within subjects. An optimized random sequence was obtained with the restriction that no more than one block of the same condition was repeated in succession.

The experiment began with a 30-second baseline recording of resting EEG, followed by the emotional film clips in random order. Each trial consisted of: (1) a brief time (200 msec.) when a cross appeared on the screen; (2) one experimental block including three clips of the same emotional condition; (3) a 30 sec. post-film rest period.

At the end of the experimental session after a resting period, the subjects were asked to view again the stimuli and to rate the pleasantness level, the arousal or excitement level and the intensity level of the basic emotion experienced during a vision of each stimulus.

Recordings and Data Pre-Processing

EEG was recorded from 19 sites (Fp1, Fp2, F7, F8, F3, F4, Fz, C3, C4, Cz, T3, T4, T5,T6, P3, P4, Pz, O1, O2), which refer to a ground electrode to the center of the forehead.

EEG and EOG signals were amplified by a multi-channel bio-signal amplifier (bandpass 0.3-70 Hz) and A/D converted at 256 Hz per channel with a 12-bit resolution. The impedance of recording electrodes was monitored for each subject prior to data collection and the threshold was always kept below 5 KOhms. EEG data was pre-processed using ICA (Independent Component Analysis) (Jung et al., 1998) removing artifacts from the traces. ICA is generally applicable for removal of a wide variety of EEG artifacts. It simultaneously separates the EEG and its artifacts into independent components based on the statistics of the data. ICA does this without relying on the availability of one or more reference channels for each type of artifact. This avoids the problem of the potential mutual contamination of regressing and regressed channels. We applied the ICA to remove ocular artifacts. We discarded all the distinct artifactual components through visual inspection. After the ICA-component removing process, a second stage of visual inspection of the EEG data was conducted. If any further artifact was present, the data was discarded. Then, data was band-pass filtered with a forward reverse filtering algorithm in the following five frequency-bands of interest: delta (0.5-3), theta (4-7 Hz), alpha (8-12 Hz) and beta (13-30 Hz).

Extraction of Instantaneous Phase at Different Oscillations

Two signals are said to be synchronous if their rhythms coincide. In its classical sense, the term synchrony has been applied to the signal that had a dominant oscillatory mode around a chosen frequency *f*. Such a signal *x(t)* can be written in the frequency domain as:

$$\tilde{x}(f,t) = |\tilde{x}(f,t)| \exp(i\phi(f,t))$$

in which the instantaneous amplitude *a(t)* and phase $\phi(t)$ of *x(t)* appear as separated entities. From this equation the amplitude of the signal is the absolute value of the spectro-temporal representation and the phase as the complex argument:

$$\varphi(f,t) = \arg(\tilde{x}(f,t))$$

Phase synchronization is usually defined as the locking of the phase of two oscillators:

$$\varphi_{x,y} = n\phi_x(t) - m\phi_y(t) = const$$

where *n* and *m* are integers. Rosenblum et al.(1996) replaced this condition of phase locking by the weaker condition of phase entrainment:

$$|\varphi_{x,y}| = |n\phi_x(t) - m\phi_y(t)| < const$$

To investigate whether two systems show phase synchronization, it is first necessary to know their phase variables. This is non-trivial for many non-linear model systems and even more difficult when dealing with noisy time-series of unknown origin. In this work we have used the wavelet method to determine the phase of an arbitrary signal *x(t)*. Specifically, let *x(t)* be an EEG signal, then the wavelet transform is:

$$W(f,t) = \int_{-\infty}^{+\infty} x(t)\psi^{*}_{f,t}(u)du$$

where $\psi^{*}_{f,t}(u)$ is the complex conjugate of the Morlet wavelet defined by:

$$\psi_{f,t} = \sqrt{f}\exp(i2\pi f(u-t))\exp(-\frac{(u-t)^2}{2\sigma^2})$$

A good estimator of the degree of phase synchronization is the synchronization index (SI) (Rosemblum et al., 2001a; Rosemblum et al., 2001b) defined as:

$$\gamma^2_{n,m} = \langle\cos\phi_{n,m}(t)\rangle^2 + \langle\sin\phi_{n,m}(t)\rangle^2$$

where the brackets denote the average over time; it varies from 0 to 1. The advantage of this index, with respect to other ones (Rodriguez et al., 1999), is that its computation involves no parameters. In this study the changes of SI patterns were analyzed during responses to emotional-laden external stimulation, using non-emotional and emotional film stimuli differentiated for valence.

Data Analysis and Results

Behavioral Results

Figure 1 depicts the mean values and the standard deviation of the self reported valence and arousal attributed by subjects to the emotional and neutral stimuli. The ratings of pleasantness and arousal were submitted to repeated measures analyses of variance with condition as within-subject factor (4 levels: happiness, fear, sadness and neutral). The pleasantness resulted to be significantly different among conditions ($F(3, 54)= 47.76$; $p<0.05$), as well as the arousal ($F(2.3,54)= 38.97$; $p<0.05$). Mean comparisons performed as post-hoc analysis, using Bonferroni correction for multiple comparisons, showed that pleasantness was significantly higher for happiness as respect to all the other conditions ($p<.001$). The post-hoc analysis on arousal ratings showed that the significance of the overall model was due to differences between emotional conditions and neutral conditions ($p<.001$), whereas there were no significant differences among the specific emotions.

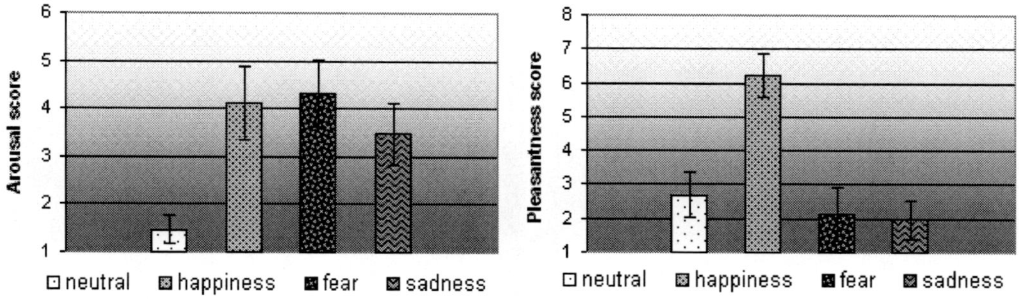

Figure 1. Mean and standard deviation of self-reported arousal (left panel) and pleasantness (right panel) of subjectively experienced emotion during the vision of the four categories of film clips.

In order to evaluate the validity of experimental conditions, a further ANOVA was performed on intensity scores given to basic emotions included in the scale, expecting that the target emotion was to be experienced more intensely than all the others. Two within-subjects factors were entered in the model: Condition (4 levels: neutral, happiness, fear, and sadness) and Emotion (5 levels: happiness, fear, anger, disgust and sadness). Results revealed a significant interaction effect of Condition X Emotion ($F(6.6; 79.4) = 65.54$, $p<.001$, $\eta^2=.84$), confirming that the emotions more intensely experienced during the vision of the stimuli were the expected ones ($p<0.001$, Bonferroni corrected).

EEG Power Distribution Results

The spectral power (μV^2) was estimated on the artefact free EEG signals segmented in overlapped epoch (1 s. each), through the Fast Fourier Transform (FFT), using a Hamming window.

Power values within each epoch were averaged, converted to power density (μV^2/Hz) and grouped into the frequency ranges of interest: delta (0,5–4), theta (4–7 Hz), alpha (8–12 Hz) and beta (13–30 Hz). A log-transformation was performed on the row data in order to normalize the distribution, then the values were averaged across the different recording sites, obtaining five clusters corresponding to regional means of interest: frontal (F), central (C), temporal (T), parietal (P) and occipital (O). In addition, two clusters were obtained to perform the analysis of frontal lateralization: right frontal ($_R$F) and left frontal ($_L$F). The averaged power distribution across the respective electrode sites were calculated for these regional means for the three frequency bands of interest and each film category. These data were then entered in the subsequent statistical analyses.

In order to test the change between conditions across the different cortical areas, a 4 X 5 repeated measure ANOVA was performed including two factors within subjects: Condition (4 levels: neutral, happiness, sadness and fear) and Localization (5 levels: frontal, central, temporal, parietal and occipital). When the sphericity assumption was not met, the Huynh-Feldt correction on degree of freedom was adopted. As expected a mean effect of Frequency was significant $F(3;72)=93.69$; $p<.001$; $\eta^2=.8$). Further, highly significant results were found for the mean effect of Condition $F(1.6;38.49)=11.65$; $p<.001$; $\eta^2=.33$), Localization

$F(2.33;72)=4.22$; $p<.05$; $\eta^2=.15$) and, more interesting, the interaction effect of Condition X Frequency $F(6.3;152.7)=5.71$; $p<.001$; $\eta^2=.2$), indicating that the specific basic emotion induced a change in cortical activation, as it is depicted in figure 2.

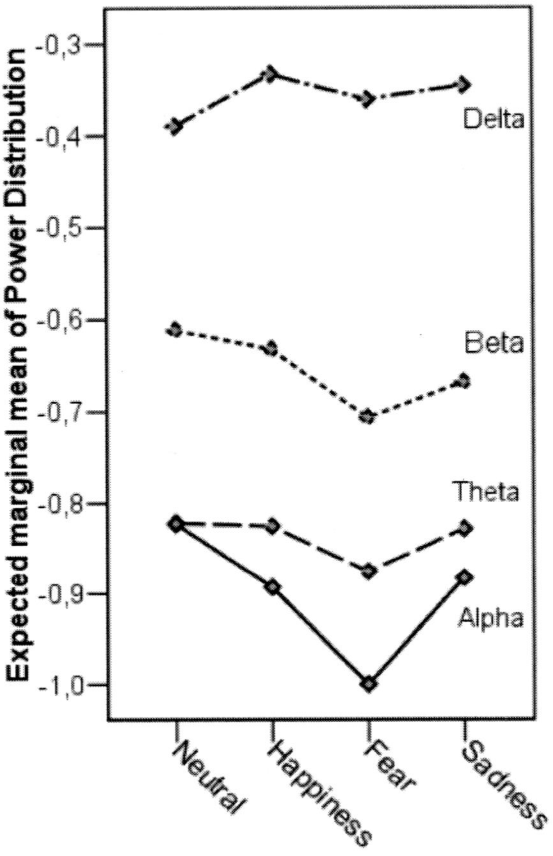

Figure 2. Expected marginal mean of the power distribution (μV^2) at the different frequency rhythms associated with processing neutral and emotional stimuli.

EEG Phase Synchronization Results

The SI was calculated at each frequency band between each electrode paired to all other electrodes, obtaining a synchronization matrix for each subject and each condition. The statistical analysis was performed independently for the different frequency bands on the synchronization matrices for all the couples of channel locations, entering the SI values into repeated-measures ANOVAs with Condition as within-subject factor (4 levels: neutral, sadness, happiness and fear). The main effect of Condition was found to be statistically significant for a number of frontal and posterior couples of electrodes. The couples of electrodes that significantly differed among conditions are depicted in figure 3.

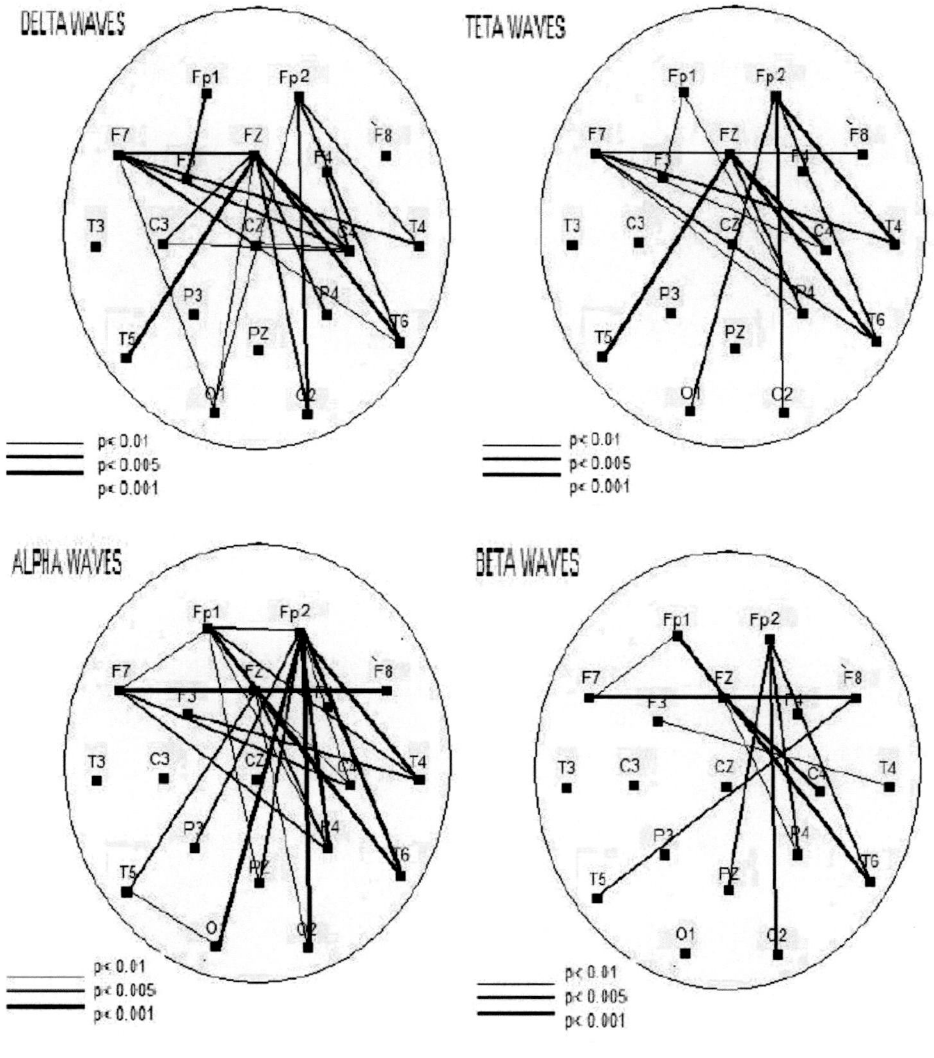

Figure 3. Images depicted the couples of electrodes whose synchronization index resulted to significantly differ among the four film clips categories at each frequency band in response. The different thickness of lines indicates the significance level of the F ratio.

Following, in order to assess the differences between conditions that contributed to the overall significance of the ANOVA models, post-hoc analyses were performed using the paired Tukey Test, that corrects for the multiple comparisons. Figure 4 depicts the synchronization patterns that resulted to be specifically associated with each emotion contrasted with neutral and figure 5 depicts the significant differences emerged from contrasts performed between the emotions.

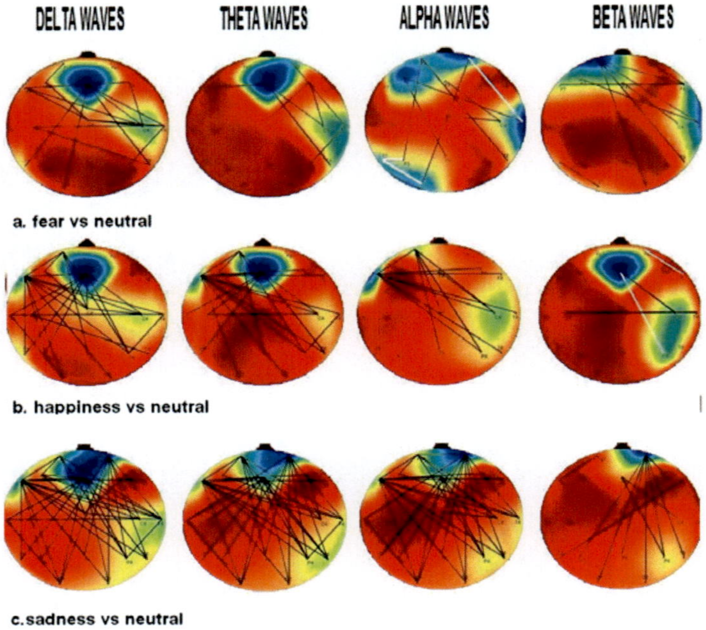

Figure 4. Map series representing significant (p<0.005) increases of SI between couples of electrodes associated with each emotion contrasted with neutral at different bands. Black lines represent a greater SI for neutral condition, while white SI represent a greater SI for emotional condition except for [a] at beta band in which SI is lower in the neutral condition respect to the fear stimuli.

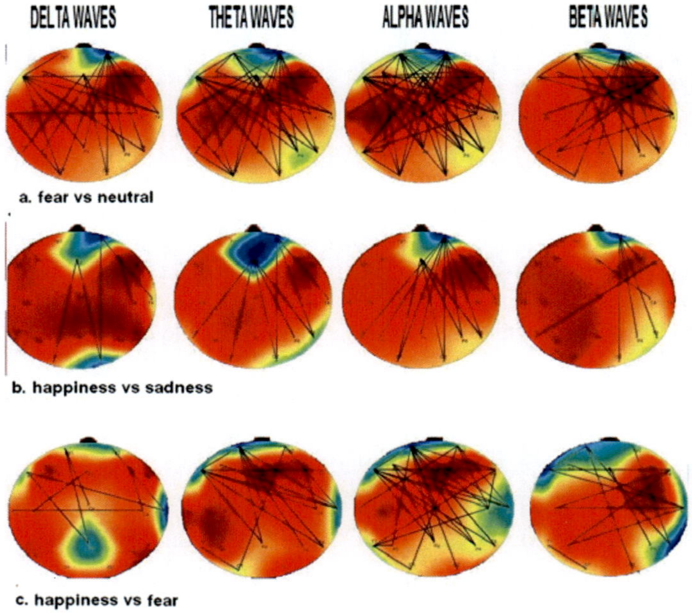

Figure 5. Map series representing significant (p<0.005) increases of SI between couples of electrodes associated with each emotion contrasted with others at different bands. The lines represent a greater SI for [a] fear contrasted with sadness; [b] happiness contrasted with sadness and [c] fear contrasted with happiness.

Discussion

The present work addressed to investigate the phase synchronization change across the local and distal EEG sites in response to film-induced basic emotions, differentiated for their valence and action tendency, in order to test which models of emotion best predicted the dynamical coupling and decoupling patterns.

The preliminary analysis on the self-reported emotional response and on the power distribution confirmed that our stimuli were able to induce the expected emotions, as well as to elicit change in the neural activity at the different frequency bands across all the cortical areas. In particular, the alpha rhythm, whose reduction is known to be a marker of the brain activation, significantly decreased during all the emotion as respect to neutral: fear resulted in the higher activation; happiness and sadness were associated with a mean level, whereas neutral response was associated to the lower level of brain activation. The observed alpha power change across conditions reflected the typical arousal level that the dimensional model ascribed to the three basic emotions here investigated (Russell, 1880). Beta and theta power also showed the expected patterns of reduction during emotion and in particular in fear. This effect was elsewhere reported (e.g., Aftanas et al., 1998b) and it was explained as a product of the cortical desynchronization induced by subcortical activity change induced by emotion (Davidson, 1990).

As respect to the power distribution analysis that informs on the quantitative brain activation change during mental engagement, the synchronization index (SI) informs on the qualitative change concerning the interconnecting patterns among different neural networks. The nonlinear analysis on synchronization deals with states in state space and not with amplitudes, power and frequencies and states may provide more information on the underlying system than amplitudes (Stam, 2005).

The present SI analysis turned out to detect at each frequency bands several significant synchronization changes during emotional and non emotional film-induction, involving local and distal couples of electrodes corresponding to different cortical regions.

In order to interpret the obtained results and compare them with previous findings, the notion of synchronization needs a clarification, as well as its relationship with the notion of dynamical complexity, that was the property more diffusely investigated in the literature on emotion. More than one meaning has been ascribed so far to complexity: nonetheless, all nonlinear analyses measures the complexity defined as degrees of freedom (or randomness) in a large system of interacting elements (Tononi et al., 1998). It refers to the lack of interactions between the elements of a dynamical system, exiting in an enhancement of the unpredictability and chaoticness of time series. As regard to a functional network, it is related to the lack of correlations between its functional sources. So, the higher the level of synchronization between functional sources in a functional network, the lower its dynamical complexity (Stam, 2005).

Like other non-linear measures of dynamical interaction, such as the Mutual Dimension (Dm), SI increases indicated an enhanced interaction between two dynamical systems or spatially separated cortical regions, corresponding to a lower dynamical complexity. Conversely, SI decrease indicates that two dynamical system become functionally separated and process more independently the information (higher dynamical complexity). A further information could be extracted from the number of synchronization changes (both increase and decrease) centred around a specific electrode, named "center of gravity" or "main processing node", whose corresponding cortical region is thought to play a specific functional role in the mental task examined (see Aftanas et al. 1998a).

Accounting for these meanings of SI, results from the present study evidenced that each emotion, compared with neutral, was accompanied by a significant decrease of synchronization across several cortical regions, indicating that the emotional processing induced an higher dynamical complexity in the EEG signals. This effect was observed at alpha, theta and delta frequency bands and it could be ascribed to the general emotional arousal. Interestingly, the significant changes mainly occurred within the frontal sites and between the frontal and occipital sites, that recent neuroimaging studies demonstrated to be associated with emotional arousal (Murphy et al., 2003; Phan et al., 2002).

According with the hypothesis stated by the authors and with the expectations drawn from the theoretical background, the observed SI changes support the view that coupling-decoupling patterns between different neural networks could be a relevant neural mechanism underlying the emotional processing and that emotion induces an increase of complexity in the cortical dynamics. This result is quietly consistent with previous evidences on the dynamical complexity of EEG response to positive and negative film-induced emotions. Aftanas and co-workers found that the Dimensional Complexity (DCx), that measures the global complexity's degree of EEG dynamics reconstructed in state space (Elbert et al.,1994), increased during both positive and negative emotional stimuli processing, as respect to neutral; furthermore, authors found that DCx positively correlated with the self-reported emotional arousal (Aftanas et al., 1998b). Similar results were obtained with different classes of nonlinear measures, such as: i) the Lyapunov exponents, that inform on the dynamical properties of the system orbiting within the attractor (Elbert et al. 1994), providing an estimate of the mean exponential divergence or convergence of nearby trajectories in phase space and expressing the sensitive dependence of the system on initial conditions (Rosenstein et al. 1993); ii) the Kolmogorov entropy metric (K2), that evaluates the degree of "chaoticness" of the system, or the average rate at which information is generated by the system, or, equivalently, the rate at which current information about system is lost (Schouten et al. 1994); iii) nonlinear forecasting, that measures the deterministic structure of the time series, through an average analysis of the temporal variations of structures in the phase space, evaluating the loss of information during the system's evolution or, in other words, quantifying the memory loss of the past states during the evolution of the system.

The Kolmogorov entropy and the principal Lyapunov exponent (L1) were found to increase after viewing positive or negative movies compared to neutral movies, indicating an enhancement of cortical dynamics during emotion, independently on valence (Aftanas et al., 1997b). The same increase of dimensional complexity with emotional arousal was also observed with different emotional induction procedures, such as the memory for personal pain (Lutzenberger et al., 1997). An enhancement of complexity was also found during the emotional imagery when compared with a cognitive task, like mental arithmetic calculus (Birbaumer et al., 1993), as a further suggestion that this effect could reflect, up to a certain level, an emotion-specific brain mechanism.

The results presented in this chapter and the previous findings converge to sustain that the neural information processing of non emotional stimuli was linked to an higher extend of degrees of freedom and, hence, to an higher predictability, while emotional processing is accompanied by an higher unpredictability and complexity of EEG signals, reflected in decreased cortical synchronization. Such a decoupling effect indicates that, at the cortical level, emotion was processed by more independent, parallel and active neural processes, involving more separated neural assemblies: it is arguable that an enlarging of the overall chaoticness, able to generate information at an higher rate, could be a functional mechanism necessary to process the salient value of emotional stimuli. Furthermore, it was underscored that decreased interconnections at the cortical level could indicate an enhancement of the functional connectivity between the given cortical area and subcortical regions (Aftanas et al. 1998b; Davidson, 1990), as well as of the vertical integration typical of emotion (Lewis, 2005). The subcortical information exchange is diffusely described during emotion by neuroimaging studies and increasing evidences have been recently collecting applying the dynamical causal model (e.g. Williams et al., 2006). In turn, processing a visual stimulus without an emotional salience could be more strongly constrained to the low degrees of freedom that characterize the information exchange among neural pathways involved at the cortical level in the perceptual object recognition.

Besides the emotional arousal effect, the present SI analysis succeeded also in detecting different synchronization patterns, at least in part specific for the basic emotions examined, as emerged from the synchronization maps associated with each single emotion contrasted with neutral, as well as from the significant contrasts between happiness, sadness and fear. The differences were both quantitative, referring to decrease or increase of SI, and qualitative, referring to the couples of electrodes involved in the SI patterns. The emotion-related effects mainly regarded (i) inter-hemispheric interactions, (ii) rostro-caudal interactions, and (iii) frontal lateralization effects.

Sadness was the emotion with the lower synchronized activity, happiness showed to be more synchronized than sadness, and fear showed the higher synchronized activity. At alpha frequency bands, and rather similarly, at delta and theta, the synchronization analyses showed that happiness and sadness, when compared with neutral, induced a wide number of significant decreases of the dynamical coupling within the left frontal region, between righ and left frontal regions and between the frontal and occipital regions. In turn, fear appeared not specifically associated with the left frontal and inter-hemispheric patterns, whereas it showed a specific change in right frontal sites.

Sadness specifically involved an overall ipsi-and controlateral decoupling across the frontal-parietal-occipital pathways, that was not observed, or there was at a lesser extend, in happiness and fear. This rostro-caudal effect was more pronounced at alpha band, with a main processing node in Fp2 and, at a lesser extend, in F7. Differently, happiness showed a specific rostro-caudal decoupling involving a more anterior left laterizated pathway (Fp1-Pz), with processing nodes in Fp1 and F7. Direct comparisons between happiness and sadness resulted in distinct patterns within the right frontal loci and between the frontal and posterior sites with right-sided processing nodes. As regard to the inter-hemispheric synchronization, sadness showed to produce a decoupling between the more anterior sites, such as the prefrontal loci Fp1-Fp2; conversely, happiness involved more posterior frontal sites and fear did not show to be associated with this network.

Fear appeared highly dissociable both from sadness and happiness, also presenting variation across the different frequency bands. At the delta and theta band, fear showed a restricted rostro-caudal desynchronization pattern and a specific right frontal pattern (F4-Cz). More interestingly, at the alpha band fear showed a specific effect of increased synchronization within the left posterior region (T5-P3 and T5-01), when compared to neutral, that did not occurred in happiness or in sadness (nor SI decrease or increase). This alpha synchronization pathway indicates lower degrees of freedom in posterior temporal and occipital areas during fear, that could be reconducted to a full visual elaboration of a stimulus with an high adaptive value.

At the beta band, fear response resulted highly different from happiness, sadness and neutral response, showing a specific increase of synchronization, involving short-distance interconnections within the right frontal regions, within posterior regions, as well as long-distance inter-hemispheric and rostro-caudal interconnections. The widely distributed EEG beta activity was found to be functionally related to increased alertness and cognitive processes (Steriade, 1999) and to emotional response, showing a desynchronization effect, in particular during highly aorusing negative emotions (Aftanas et al., 2006; Aftanas et al., 1998b). A circumscribed centrally distributed cortical beta rhythm was proven to be strongly related to motor functions and to originate from primary motor cortex (Pfurtscheller and Lopes da Silva, 1999), as well as from the supplementary motor area (Pfurtscheller et al., 2003). The emotional response of fear is strictly associated with the adaptive action tendency, that allows to face off a threath and achieve a safety condition. Considering this impelling/urgent adaptative value, the neural pathway of fear could necessarily reclutate the motor areas to prepare the movement, succeeding in cortical dynamics characterized by an higher predictability of information processing and a decreased complexity. A role of the motor component is sustained by the evidence that the significant contrasts involved the sites closed to the motor cortex (F8-F7, Fz-C4, Fp1 and F3 with T4). Furthermore, SI change during happiness, that is related to the behavioural activation as fear, showed a similar pattern of increased synchrony at beta band, although limited to the right prefrontal region (Fp2 -F8 and Fz-C4), whereas sadness, that is associated to behavioural inhibition, did not.

With regards topographical differences, previous studies reported that positive emotion induced a lower dynamical complexity over frontocortical regions, and an increase over posterior regions, whereas an opposite pattern was found for negative emotions, with a complexity increase over frontocortical regions, and a decrease over posterior regions (Aftanas et al., 1997b). Investigations on Dm reported that during positive emotion the central, parietal and posterior temporal areas became more coupled. In contrast, negative emotions produced a general dynamical decoupling over posterior regions, indicating that they were processed by more independent cortical networks (Aftanas et al., 1998a).

The present SI analysis on EEG response to happiness, sadness and fear just in part matched these findings: the increased complexity during positive emotions compared with negative was replicated considering the contrast between happiness and fear, while sadness clearly elicited a wider desynchronization. The wide posterior decoupling was instead observed during sadness, but not during fear. Hence, the present study succeeded in finding significant differences between emotions with the same valence: sadness and fear extensevely differed, but these specific patterns could not be detected in the perspective of dimensional models; rather they emerge when a more subtle distinction between basic emotions is done in the perspective of the discrete models.

The evidence that specific basic emotions with the same valence induce different EEG response could explain some of the divergences across the results collected so far. Most of the studies used video-clips with an highly arousing and aversive content (usually burn victims) inducing negative emotions linked to the withdrawal system and, in the basic emotion perspective, similar to fear and/or disgust. This type of stimuli are very different from ours, as well as the type of emotion induced. The negative emotion previously studied was similar enough, but not at all, to our film-induced fear. In fear, but not in sadness, we observed the similar synchronization increase (or dynamical complexity decrease) that previous studies found for negative emotion. Nonetheless, the present SI analysis did not find the topographical effect described elsewhere. The decreased dynamical complexity of negative emotion over frontocortical regions have been explained with the higher attentional constraints that negative emotion may put on the frontocortical activity: according to this hypothesis, the attentional resources should be allocated to process the attractive stimuli inducing pleasant emotion and retained from the aversive stimuli that subjects attempt to withdraw (Aftanas et al., 1997a; 1998a).

An alternative interpretative hypothesis refers to the different adaptive value of emotions and to their evolutionary hystory. For its basic role in the survival, fear is though to be one of the most ancient emotion: the neural substrates should be highly conserved along the evolutionary history and shared by several species as evolutionary homology (Panksepp, 1998). The adaptive value of a stimulus is evaluated by innate neural circuits underpinning the fear response, and this automatic appraisal process could be linked to more restrained processing patterns. Automatic processing pathways could imply a lesser extend of degrees of freedom of the information processing, explaining the higher synchronization and a lower dynamical complexity. Conversely, the neural substrates of happiness and sadness could be thought as more recent and more differentiated among the species, and in particular in the human beings: these two emotions could also linked to a more complex process for appraisal of the stimuli, more linked to a integration with memories and, in particular, with symbolic knowledge stored in the system (Leventhal and Scherer, 1987).

The lower frontal synchronization, and the higher complexity, of happiness and sadness, not observed in fear, suggest that these two emotions, especially sadness, could involve a larger evaluation component mediated by frontal cortex. Several findings from neuroimaging research reported that frontal regions are involved in the evaluation processes of an emotional response and in the emotional regulation through "top – down" connectivity circuits (Miller and Cohen, 2001).

Because of the urgent adaptive value of fear response, this emotion could not be necessarily linked to the evaluation process mediated by higher-level structures, such as frontal cortex, but it could be primarily elaborated by the subcortical structures such as the amygdala, as it was described by LeDoux (2000). In the present study, the film sequencies of fear depicted scenarios of danger and threath with a tipically evolutionary value, so that it could be expected that these stimuli induced an automatic elaboration in the subcortical structures with a diminished intervent of the more recent structures, like the frontal lobes. The scenarios of happiness and sadness sequences could have a more complex content that requested wider processing resources, exiting in more complex EEG dynamics.

Considering the present SI results as a whole, it has to be underscored the difference found between the two negative emotions included in the study and the higher similarity between sadness and happiness as respect to fear. In particular happiness and fear shared left-sided frontal synchronization pathways and frontal inter-hemispheric interconnections, whereas highly differed in the rostro-caudal pathways, with happiness more synchronized than sadness. The approach-withdrawal model of emotion could explain the observed dissociation between fear, on one side, and happiness and sadness, on the other side, instead of the dimensional model. Although the two models have been often overlapped reporting positive emotions to approach system and negative emotions to withdrawal system, there were some relevant differences. For example, the negative emotion of anger is associated with an approach tendency, as well as sadness is associated with a de-activation of the approach system (Davidson and Irwing, 1999; Davidson, 2003).

The present findings matched the predictions from this model of emotion: happiness and sadness were mediated by a frontal pattern that respectively showed an increase and decrease of synchronized activity. Interestingly, the lateralization pattern emerged in the present analysis is coherent with the hypothesis of a role of the left frontal region in the approach emotions, while the right frontal region would be involved in the withdrawal emotions: sadness and happiness showed several significant SI change with processing node in the left frontal hemisphere; on turn, fear showed processing nodes in the right hemisphere (mainly F4 and then Fp2).

Our results also showed that fear was associated with a larger involvement of the posterior regions in front of the larger involvement of anterior lobes in sadness and happiness, sustaining the hypothesis of a deeper involvement of the high order evaluation processes, while fear appears to be associated with a low-order sensory-motor evaluation.

Future research could advance these discoveries by including more differentiated emotions in the experimental designs, and comparing discrete emotions with the same valence. Further investigations could be concerned with disgust (negative emotion of withdrawal system) and anger (negative emotion of approach system) to disentangled the functional organization of emotion in the brain predicted by theoretical models.

Conclusion

As far as we know, the present study is the first that investigated EEG cortical responses to emotional stimulation, using the Synchronization Index as a measure of the synchronized activity within the different frequency bands. The SI index here proposed contributes to the view of nonlinear interaction process occurring in cortical activity during emotional processing: SI had been shown to be sensitive to detecting the change in cortical dynamics related to emotional processing, differentiating the neural response induced by emotional arousal, by the emotional valence and in particular by specific basic emotions.

Results of this study support the view that synchronization provides an interesting and useful tool for studying and more deeply understanding the variation in brain activity that occurs during mental processes. Moreover, it was demonstrated that synchronization change could be considered as a relevant and necessary neural mechanism to generate emotion. The application of SI analysis to the EEG has been shown to offer information beyond that provided by linear EEG measures, as well as by nonlinear measures that estimate complexity from the individual signal. A meaningful information about cortical networks functioning in relation to emotion can be obtained, and it seems to be necessary for a deep understanding of neural activity underlying emotion.

If we consider the complex nature of emotion, which involves several biological systems as well as several neural circuits at different cerebral levels, we can conclude that synchronization seems to be a relevant topic for this field of research.

The results presented in this chapter also show the importance of investigating basic emotion, with respect to the more diffusely studied emotional valence dimension. It is arguable that the valence-specific effect expected on the basis of the dimensional model of emotion do not fully explain the data. The alternative model of approach-withdrawal better fits the present data as well as the model of discrete emotions. It is possible that there are brain mechanisms underlying the valence-process and that these mechanisms are further differentiated with respect to the specific kinds of emotion. Following our results, we can conclude that the model of basic emotions is more suitable than the dimensional model.

References

Aftanas, L.I., Koshkarov, V.I., Mordvintsev, Y.N., and Pokrovskaja, V.L., (1994). Dimensional analysis of human EEG during experimental affective experience. *International Journal of Psychophysiology*, Volume: 18, pp. 67-70.

Aftanas, L.I., Lotova, N.V., Koshkarov, V.I., Pokrovskaja, V.L., Popov, S.A., and Makhnev, V.P., (1997a). Non-linear analysis of emotion EEG: calculation of Kolmogorov entropy and the principal Lyapunov exponent. *Neuroscience Letters*, Volume: 226, pp. 13-16.

Aftanas, L.I., Lotova, N.V., Koshkarov, V.I., Popov, S.A., and Makhnev, V.P., (1997b). Nonlinear forecasting measurements of the human EEG during evoked emotions. *Brain Topography*, Volume: 10, pp. 155-162.

Aftanas, L.I., Lotova, N.V., Koshkarov, V.I., and Popov, S.A., (1998a). Non-linear dynamical coupling between different brain areas during evoked emotions: an EEG investigation. *Biological Psychology*, Volume: 48, pp. 121-138.

Aftanas, L. I., Reva, N. V., Varlamov, A. A., Pavlov, S. V., and Makhnev, V. P., (2004). Analysis of Evoked EEG Synchronization and Desynchronization in Conditions of Emotional Activation in Humans: Temporal and Topographic Characteristics. *Neuroscience and Behavioural Physiology*, Vol. 34, No. 8.

Aftanas, L. I., Varlamov, A.A., Pavlov, S.V., Makhnev, V., and Reva, N., (2001). Event-related synchronization and desynchronization during affective processing: emergence of valence-related time-dependent hemispheric asymmetries in theta and upper alpha band.

International Journal of Neuroscience, 110: 197–219.

Aftanas, L.I., Lotova, N.V., Koshkarov, V.I., Makhnev, V.P., Mordvintsev Yu. N., and Popov, S.A. (1998b) Non-linear dynamic complexity of the human EEG during evoked emotions. *International Journal of Psychophysiology*, 28(1):63-76.

Aftanas, L. I., Reva, N. V., Savotina, L. N., and Makhnev, V. P.(2006). Neurophysiological Correlates of Induced Discrete Emotions in Humans: An Individually Oriented Analysis. *Journal Neuroscience and Behavioral Physiology,* Volume 36, Number 2, pp.119-130

Barrett, L.F., and Wager, T.D., (2006). The Structure of Emotion: Evidence From Neuroimaging Studies. *Current Directions in Psychological Science*, Volume 15, Number 2, pp. 79-83(5).

Basar, E., Basar-Eroglu, C., Karakas, S., and Schurmann, M., (1999). Oscillatory brain theory: a new trend in neuroscience. *IEEE England. Med. Biol. Mag.*, 18:56–66.

Basar, E., Basar-Eroglu, C., Karakas, S. and Schurmann, M., (2001). Gamma, alpha, delta, and theta oscillations govern cognitive processes. *International Journal of Psychophysiology*, 39:241-8.

Bhattacharya, J., H., Petsche, H., and Pereda, E., (2001). Long-Range Synchrony in the γ Band: Role in Music Perception. *Journal of Neuroscience*, 21(16) :6329–6337.

Birbaumer, N., Lutzenberger, W., Elbert, T., Flor, H., and Rockstroh, B., (1993). Imagery and brain processes. In: N. Birbaumer and A. Ohman (Eds.). *The Structure of Emotion*, Hogrefe and Huber, Toronto,122-138.

Boccaletti, S., Kurths, J., Osipov, G., Valladares, D.L., Zhou, C.S., (2002). The synchronization of chaotic systems, *Physics Reports,* 366 (2002), 1–101.

Bressler, S.L., Coppola, R. and Nakamura, R., (1993). Episodic multiregional cortical coherence at multiple frequencies during visual task performance. *Nature*, 366:153-156.

Brown, R., and Kocarev, L., (2000). A unifying definition of synchronization for dynamical systems. *Chaos*, Volume: 10, pp. 344-349.

Costa, T., Rognoni, E., and Galati, D. (2006). EEG phase synchronization during emotional response to positive and negative film stimuli. *Neuroscience Letters*, 406:159-164.

Crawford, H.J., Clarke, S.W. and Kitner-Triolo, M. (1996). Self-generated happy and sad emotions in low an highly hypnotizable persons during waking and hypnosis: laterality and regional EEG activity differences. *International Journal of Psychophysiol*ogy, 24: 239-266.

Davidson, R.J, Chapman, J.P., Chapman, L.J., and Henriques, J.B., (1990) Asymmetrical brain electrical activity discriminates between psychometrically-matched verbal and saptial cognitive tasks. *Psychophysiology*, 27, 528-543.

Davidson, R. J., and Irwin, W., (1999). The functional neuroanatomy of emotion and affective style. *Trends in Cognitive Sciences*, 3, 11-21.

Davidson, R.J., (2003). Affective neuroscience and psychophysiology: Toward a synthesis. *Psychophysiology*, 40 (2003), 655–665.

Desmedt, J.E., and Tomberg, C., (1994). Transient phase-locking of 40 Hz electrical oscillations in prefrontal and parietal human cortex reflects the process of conscious somatic perception, *Neuroscience Letters*, 168: 126-129.

Ekman, P, and Davidson, R.J., (1994). *The nature of emotion: fundamental questions*. Oxford University Press.

Ekman, P., (1992). An argument for basic emotions, Cognition and emotion, 3:169-200.Ekman P., (1999) Basic Emotions In T. Dalgleish and M. Power (Eds.). *Handbook of Cognition and Emotion.* Sussex, U.K.: John Wiley and Sons, Ltd.

Elbert, T., Ray, W.J, Kowalik, Z.J., Skinner, J.E., Graf, K.E., and Birbaumer, N., (1994). Chaos and physiology: deterministic chaos in excitable cell assemblies. *Physiological Reviews*, Vol 74, 1-47.

Frackowiak, R.S.J., Friston, K.J., Frith, C., Dolan, R., Friston, K.J., Price, C.J., Zeki, S., Ashburner, J., and Penny, W.D., editors, (2004). *Human Brain Function.* Academic Press, 2nd edition.

Hebb, D.O., (1949). *The Organization of Behavior.* Wiley, New York.

Hinrichs, H. M., and Machleidt, W., (1992). Basic Emotions reflected in EEG-coherences, *International Journal of Psychophysiology*, 3:225-232.

Jung, T-P., Humphries, C., Lee T-W., Makeig, S., McKeown, M.J., Iragui, V., and Sejnowski, T.J., (1998). Extended ICA Removes Artifacts from Electroencephalographic Recordings, in D. Touretzky, M. Mozer and M. Hasselmo (Eds), *Advances in Neural Information Processing Systems*, 10:894-900.

Klimesch, W., (1999). EEG alpha and theta oscillations reflect cognitive and memory performance: a review and analysis. *Brain Research Review*, 291 :169-195.

Klimesch, W., Doppelmayr, M., Russagger, H., Pachinger, T. and Schwaiger, J., (1998). Induced alpha band power changes in the human EEG and attention. *Neuroscience Letters*, 244 :73-76.

Krause, C.M., Viemerö, V., Rosenqvist, A., Sillanmäki, L., Aström, T., (2000). Relative electroencephalographic desynchronization and synchronization in humans to emotional film content: an analysis of the 4±6, 6±8, 8±10 and 10±12 Hz frequency bands. *Neuroscience Letters,* 26;286(1):9-12.

Lang, P.J., Cuthbert, B.N., and Bradley, M.M., (1998a). Measuring emotion in therapy: Imagery, activation and feeling. *Behavior Therapy*, 29, 655–674.

Lang, P.J., Bradley, M.M., Fitzsimmons, J.R., Cuthbert, B.N., Scott, J.D., Moulder, B. and Nangia, V., (1998b). Emotional arousal and activation of the visual cortex: An fMRI analysis. *Psychophysiology*, 35:199–210.

LeDoux, J., (2000). Emotion Circuits in the Brain. *Annual Review of Neuroscience,* 23, 155-184.

Leventhal, H., and Scherer, K.R., (1987). The relationship of emotion to cognition: a functional approach to a semantic controversy, *Cognition and Emotion* 1, pp. 3–28.

Lewis, M.D., (2005). Bridging emotion theory and neurobiology through dynamic systems modeling, *Behavioral and Brain Sciences*, 28: 169-194.

Lutzenberger, W., Flor, H., and Birbaumer, N., (1997). Enhanced dimensional complexity of the EEG during memory for personal pain in chronic pain patients, *Neuroscience Letters*, Volume: 266, pp. 167-170.

Miller, E.K., and Cohen, J.D., (2001). An integrative theory of prefrontal cortex function. *Annual Review of Neuroscience*, 24:167-202.

Murphy, F.C., Nimmo-Smith, I., and Lawrence, A.D., (2003). Functional neuroanatomy of emotions: A meta-analysis. *Cognitive, Affective, and Behavioral Neuroscience*, 3 (3), 207-233.

Oldfield, R.C., (1971). The assessment and analysis of handedness: the Edinburgh Inventory. *Neuropsychologia*, 6, 97-113.
Panksepp, J., (1998). Affective neuroscience: The foundations of human and animal emotions. New York: Oxford University Press.
Pecora, L.M., and Carroll, T.L., (1990). Synchronization in chaotic systems, Phys Rev Lett, Volume: 64, pp. 821-824.
Pfurtscheller, G., and Lopes da Silva, F. H., (1999). Event-related EEG/EMG synchronization and desynchronization. Basic principles. *Clinical Neurophysiology*, 110: 1842–1857.
Pfurtscheller, G., Woertz, M., Supp, G., and Lopes da Silva, F.H., (2003). Early onset of post-movement beta electroencephalogram synchronization in the supplementary motor area during self-paced finger movement in man. *Neuroscience Letters*, 20;339(2).
Phan, L.K., Wager, T., Taylor, S.F. and Liberzon, I., (2002). Functional Neuroanatomy of Emotion: A Meta-Analysis of Emotion Activation Studies in PET and fMRI. *NeuroImage*, 16:331–348.
Pikovsky, A.S., Rosemblum, M.G. and Kurths, J., (2001). *Synchronization – A universal Concept in Nonlinear Science.* Cambridge.
Rodriguez, E., George, N., Lachaux, J.P., and Martinerie, J., (1999). Perception's shadow: long-distance synchronization of human brain activity. *Nature* 397: 430-433.
Rosenblum, M., Pikovsky, A., and Kurths, J., (1996). Phase synchronization of chaotic oscillators. *Physical Review Letters*, 76:1804-1807.
Rosenblum, M., Pikovsky, A., Kurths, J., Schafer, C., and Tass, P.A., (2001a). Phase synchronization: from theory to data analysis, in F. Moss and S. Gielen (eds.), *Handbook of Biological Physics*, Elsevier Science.
Rosenblum, M.G., Pikovsky, A.S., (2001b). Detecting direction of coupling in interacting oscillators, *Physical Review*, Volume: 64, 045202.
Rosenblum, M.G., Pikovsky, A.S., Kurhts J., (2004). Synchronization approach to analysis of biological systems. *Fluctuation Noise Lett*ers, Volume: 4, pp. L53-L62.
Rosenstein, M.T., Collins, J.J. and De Luca, C.J., (1993). A practical method for calculating largest Lyapunov exponents from small data sets, *Physica D,* Volume: 65, pp. 117-134.
Russell, J.A., (1980). A Circumplex Model of Affect. *International Journal of Psychophysiology*, 39: 1161-1178.
Schouten, J., Takens, F., van den Bleek, and C.van.den, (1994). Maximum-likelihood estimation of the entropy of an attractor, *Physical Review E,* Volume: 49, pp. 126-129.
Singer, W., (1993). Synchronization of cortical activity and its putative role in information processing and learning. *Annual Review of Physiology*, 55:349-374.
Singer, W., (1999). Neurobiology: Striving for coherence. *Nature*, 397:391– 393.
Stam, C.J. (2005). Nonlinear dynamical analysis of EEG and MEG: Review of an emerging field. *Clinical Neurophysiology*, Vol: 116 Issue: 10, pp: 2266-2301
Steriade, M., (1999). Cellular substrates of brain rhythms. In: Niedermeyer E, Lopes da Silva F (eds) *Electroencephalography. Basic principles, clinical applications and related* Welds, 4th edn. Williams and Wilkins, Baltimore, pp 28–75.
Surguladz, S.A., Brammer, M.J., Young, A.W., Andrew, C., Travis, M.J., Williams, S.C.R., and Phillips, M.L., (2003). A preferential increase in the extrastriate response to signals

of danger *NeuroImage*, 19 1317–1328.

Tallon-Baudry, C., Bertrand, O., and Fischer, C., (2001). Oscillatory Synchrony between Human Extrastriate Areas during Visual Short-Term Memory Maintenance. *Journal of Neuroscience*, 21:1-5.

Tallon-Baudry, C., and Bertrand, O., (1999). Oscillatory gamma activity in humans and its role in object representation, *Trends in Cognitive Science*, 3,4:152-163.

Tononi, G. and Edelman, G.M., (1998). Consciousness and complexity. *Science*, 282:1846-51.

Tononi, G. and Sporns, O., (2003). Measuring information integration. *BMC Neuroscience*, 4-31.

Tononi, G., Edelman,G.M., Sporns, O., (1998). Complexity and coherency: integrating information in the brain, *TICS*, Volume: 2, pp. 474-484

Tucker, D.M., and Dawson, S.L., (1984). Asymmetric EEG changes as method actors generated emotions. *Biological Psychology*, 19, 63–75.

Thatcher, R.W., Krause, P.J., and Hrybyk, M., (1986). Cortico-cortical associations and EEG coherence: a two-compartmental model. *Electroencephalogr. Clin. Neurophysiol.* 64, 123–143.

Williams, L.M., Das, P., Liddell B.J., , Kemp, A.H., Rennie, C.J., and Gordon, E., (2006). Mode of Functional Connectivity in Amygdala Pathways Dissociates Level of Awareness for Signals of Fear *The Journal of Neuroscience*, 6, 26(36):9264-9271.

Index

A

Aβ, 139
aberrant, 42
abnormalities, viii, 33, 42
accelerator, 206
access, 38, 172
accumulation, 42
accuracy, 3, 6, 20, 155
acetic acid, 61, 62
achievement, 14
acid, 35, 55, 61, 62, 70, 216
acoustic, 209, 217, 218
activation, vii, viii, 1, 2, 3, 6, 9, 16, 22, 25, 30, 34, 35, 37, 39, 43, 45, 46, 47, 50, 51, 55, 58, 69, 72, 74, 97, 116, 119, 122, 123, 128, 130, 132, 133, 134, 167, 174, 201, 202, 205, 212, 213, 224, 225, 226, 232, 235, 238, 240, 243
acute, 30, 34, 58, 83, 200, 217
adaptation, 9, 10, 28, 31, 223, 224
adducts, 37, 38, 55
adjustment, 14, 142, 222
adolescents, 192
adriamycin, 53
adult, 43, 54, 56, 71, 76, 77, 82, 83, 84, 85, 86
adults, 88, 184
aerobic, viii, 33
affective experience, 241
age, 44, 66, 69, 70, 71, 124, 129, 150, 227
ageing, 41
agent(s), viii, 33, 35, 37, 40, 43, 49, 54, 161, 162
aging, 122, 128, 133
aid, 60
air, 59, 61
air-dried, 61
alcohol, 227
alcohol abuse, 227
alertness, 212, 238
algorithm, vii, x, 87, 89, 90, 97, 105, 137, 138, 139, 140, 141, 142, 145, 153, 154, 155, 229
alkali, 42
alkylating agents, 40
alkylation, 38
alpha, 52, 186, 189, 191, 192, 193, 195, 197, 225, 226, 229, 231, 235, 236, 237, 238, 242, 243
alpha activity, 186, 189, 192, 226
alternative, 25, 53, 76, 116, 139, 160, 164, 167, 239, 241
Alzheimer, viii, 33, 34, 42, 48, 50, 52, 53, 56, 120, 121, 128, 129, 130
Alzheimer disease, 52
Alzheimer's disease, viii, 33, 34, 48, 50, 53, 56
ambiguity, 6, 24
American Psychiatric Association, 200, 216
amino, 82, 84
amino acids, 82, 84
amnesia, 118, 119, 121, 128, 129, 130, 131, 132, 134, 135
amplitude, 3, 6, 9, 11, 12, 13, 14, 15, 16, 18, 19, 20, 28, 31, 93, 170, 178, 179, 180, 207, 208, 211, 229
amygdala, xi, 130, 132, 200, 203, 212, 213, 218, 219, 239
amyloid, 34, 48, 49
amyloid β (Aβ), 34
amyotrophic lateral sclerosis (ALS), 34, 48
anal, 166
analgesia, 212
analgesic, 217
analog, 30

analysis of variance, 79
anatomy, 107, 132
aneuploidy, 43
anger, 224, 225, 228, 231, 240
animal models, 56, 201, 202, 215
animal studies, 112
animals, ix, xi, 43, 59, 60, 65, 66, 69, 70, 75, 76, 78, 80, 82, 83, 117, 119, 158, 199, 202, 204, 206, 207, 209, 210, 211, 215, 228
animations, 150
anion, 34
annual, 187
anomalous, 179
ANOVA, 79, 231, 233
anoxic, 73
antagonist, 218
antagonistic, 202
antibody, 54, 62, 78, 79
antigen, 46, 80
antioxidant (s), 35, 49, 53
anxiety, vi, xi, 184, 199, 200, 201, 202, 203, 204, 206, 210, 211, 213, 214, 215, 216, 217
anxiety disorder, 200
anxiolytic, 203, 211, 214, 217
aphasia, 193
apoptosis, v, vii, viii, ix, 33, 34, 35, 36, 41, 42, 43, 45, 46, 47, 48, 49, 50, 51, 52, 53, 54, 55, 56, 57, 58, 61, 62, 63, 64, 65, 67, 69, 70, 71, 72, 73, 74, 82
apoptotic, v, vii, ix, 34, 35, 36, 42, 43, 45, 48, 52, 54, 57, 58, 61, 63, 65, 67, 68, 69, 70, 71, 72, 73, 76, 79, 82
apoptotic cells, ix, 61, 73, 76, 82
application, x, 2, 24, 29, 30, 88, 115, 118, 137, 138, 139, 141, 143, 154, 169, 241
argument, 114, 229, 243
arithmetic, 236
arousal, xi, 199, 200, 201, 205, 209, 210, 212, 224, 225, 226, 227, 228, 230, 231, 235, 236, 237, 240, 243
arousal ratings, 230
arrest, 35, 45, 46, 51, 52, 205
arterioles, 29
artery, 60
artificial, 95, 96, 108, 126, 162, 188, 191
artificial intelligence, 162, 191
ascorbic acid, 35
aspartate, 71
asphyxia, 58, 70, 71
assessment, 113, 114, 115, 119, 128, 191, 201, 202, 244
association, 37, 46, 49
associationism, 188, 195
associations, 25, 30, 126, 196, 245
assumptions, 2, 5, 8, 13, 22, 25, 118
astrocyte, 3, 17, 71, 83, 86
astrocytes, viii, 4, 9, 17, 29, 33, 80, 82, 83, 84, 85, 86
asymmetry, 25, 131, 134
asymptotic, 18
asynchronous, x, 87, 138, 141, 145, 151
ataxia, 36, 41, 42, 44, 46, 48, 49, 51, 52
ataxia telangiectasia mutated protein, 52
atherosclerosis, 52
ATM, 36, 41, 43, 45, 46, 47, 48, 49, 50, 52, 54, 55, 56
atmosphere, 59
ATP, 17, 34, 74
atrophy, 121
attacks, xi, 199, 200, 203, 206, 215
attention, x, 2, 14, 28, 87, 105, 164, 171, 176, 192, 196, 201, 223, 243
attractors, 162, 190
audio, 174, 189
autobiographical memory, x, 109, 110, 113, 114, 115, 116, 119, 120, 121, 122, 123, 124, 125, 127, 128, 129, 131, 132, 133
autocorrelation, 25
autonomic, 201, 203, 204, 205, 206, 209
autonomic nervous system (ANS), 201, 205, 209
autonomous, 162, 163
autonomy, 158
autoregressive model, 25, 29
autoregressive modeling, 29
autosomal recessive, 41
availability, 70, 76, 95, 229
averaging, 129, 166, 170, 179
aversion, xi, 199, 209, 212, 215, 218
avoidance, 200, 203, 213, 214, 215, 225
awareness, x, 109, 110, 111, 112, 117, 126, 127, 128, 158, 175, 190
axon, 159
axonal, 16, 83, 84, 86
axons, 83

B

Baars, 165, 186
background noise, 138

basic fibroblast growth factor, 85
battery, 23
Bax, ix, 49, 57, 58, 62, 63, 64, 66, 67, 68, 69, 73
Bayesian, 16, 24, 29
Bayesian estimation, 24, 29
Bcl-2, ix, 57, 58, 62, 63, 64, 66, 67, 68, 69, 71, 73
Bcl-2 proteins, 69
beams, 52
behavior, 11, 15, 88, 92, 93, 94, 95, 103, 104, 106, 158, 159, 160, 161, 163, 164, 165, 166, 170, 176, 179, 185, 190, 191, 192, 194, 195, 203, 204, 205, 207, 208, 209, 210, 212, 214, 216, 217, 218, 222, 223, 225
behavioral change, 218
behavioral effects, 211
beneficial effect, 63, 69, 84
benzodiazepine, 203, 211
benzodiazepines, 174, 203, 211
beta, xii, 48, 49, 56, 221, 225, 226, 229, 231, 234, 238, 244
beta wave, xii, 221
bicarbonate, 77
bilateral, 122, 123, 131, 133, 134, 135
binding, 36, 40, 62, 73, 78, 169, 172, 196, 197, 223
biochemical, 34, 70, 166
biochemistry, 52
biological, vii, 52, 73, 160, 202, 203, 222, 226, 241, 244
biological systems, 222, 241, 244
biologically, 224
biology, 196
biomarker, 39
biomechanics, 85
biophysical, 17
biophysics, 16, 185
biotin, 62, 79
birth, 58, 59, 61, 65, 66, 67, 70, 71
black, 8, 9, 13, 228
blocks, 171, 193, 228
blood, 4, 5, 6, 17, 30, 60, 83
blood flow, 60
blood vessels, 17, 30
blurring, 144, 146, 154
body, viii, 33, 60, 67
body temperature, 60
Bohr, 51, 55
BOLD, vii, 1, 2, 3, 4, 5, 6, 7, 8, 9, 12, 13, 14, 15, 16, 17, 18, 19, 20, 21, 22, 23, 24, 27, 28, 29, 30, 31, 120
bonds, 37
bone, 60, 78
borate, 62
Boston, 188, 191, 193, 195
bovine, 59
brain activity, 92, 155, 160, 161, 165, 166, 171, 174, 177, 178, 190, 192, 241, 244
brain damage, 71, 115
brain development, 58
brain functioning, 163, 168, 191, 222
brain functions, xi, 114, 115, 138, 160, 167, 221, 222
brain injury, vii, ix, 57, 72, 75, 76, 77, 82, 84, 85
brain stem, 222
brain structure, xi, 65, 115, 123, 176, 199, 201, 202, 203, 214, 218, 222
brain tumor, 43
brainstem, xi, 199, 201, 203, 217
Brazil, 199
Brazilian, 216, 217
BRCA1, 37, 49, 55
BrdU, 46, 79, 81
breakdown, ix, 57, 58
Breast, viii, 33
breathing, 200, 201
Britain, 112
buffer, 61, 62, 78, 79
building blocks, 171, 193
Burma, 41, 48
burn, 239
bypass, 48

C

Ca^{2+}, 41, 70, 73
calcium, 82
calculus, 236
California, 74
cAMP, 41
Canada, 89
cancer, viii, 33, 35, 39, 41, 47, 50, 52, 53, 54, 55, 74
capacity, 44, 51, 76, 82, 83, 169, 170, 174, 202, 203, 218
capillary, 9
capital, 112
carbon, 44, 52
carboxymethylcellulose, 60
carcinogenesis, 35, 48

cardiovascular, 219
carrier, 170
case study, 129, 133
caspase, 46, 69, 71, 72
caspases, 36, 50, 69
castration, 73
catalytic, 40, 54
categorization, 124, 126
cats, 84
caudal, 217
causal model, 29, 237
causality, 24, 25, 26, 28, 29, 30, 31
causation, 25
CDK, 43
CDK4, 37
CDKs, 36, 55
CE, 218
ceiling effect, 211
cell, vii, viii, ix, 33, 34, 35, 36, 37, 38, 40, 41, 42, 43, 45, 46, 47, 48, 49, 50, 51, 52, 53, 56, 57, 58, 59, 60, 61, 62, 63, 65, 69, 70, 71, 72, 73, 74, 76, 78, 80, 82, 83, 84, 85, 86, 166, 167, 168, 169, 170, 171, 172, 188, 190, 192, 193, 194, 195, 222, 243
cell assembly, 167, 169, 190, 193
cell culture, 59, 63, 71, 72
cell cycle, viii, 34, 35, 36, 37, 41, 43, 45, 46, 47, 50, 51, 52, 53, 72, 73, 85
cell death, vii, viii, ix, 33, 34, 41, 42, 43, 48, 49, 50, 51, 56, 57, 58, 63, 69, 70, 71, 72, 73, 74, 76
cell fate, viii, 34
cell grafts, 84
cell growth, 73
cell line, 52, 85, 86
cell lines, 52, 86
cell signaling, 34
cells, 166, 168, 177
central nervous system (CNS), viii, 33, 34, 49, 50, 52, 55, 71, 74, 76, 82, 83, 84, 85, 86, 106
cerebellar granule cells, 46
cerebellum, 44
cerebral cortex, ix, 15, 42, 53, 61, 65, 66, 67, 69, 71, 75, 186, 187, 190, 194, 195
cerebral hypoxia, 74
cerebral ischemia, 51, 58, 73
cerebrospinal fluid, 52
c-fos, 206, 218
Chalmers, 164, 187
changing environment, 160
channels, x, 83, 87, 88, 96, 103, 104, 105, 106, 143, 181, 182, 183, 229
chaos, 162, 190, 191, 196, 243
chaotic, 162, 193, 196, 223, 242, 244
Checkpoints, 36, 54
chemical, 37, 39, 162, 165, 197, 206
chemical bonds, 37
chemical energy, 165
chemicals, 35
chemistry, 54
chemotherapeutic drugs, 74
Chicago, 185, 187
childhood, 120
children, 88, 89, 184
China, 75, 137
Chinese, 155, 156
chloral, 60, 78
chloride, 77
cholinergic, 86
chromatid, 38
chromatin, 34, 46, 58, 61, 63, 67, 68, 69, 70
chronic, 34, 42, 83, 84, 203, 217, 218, 227, 243
chronic diseases, 227
chronic pain, 243
classes, 89, 94, 96, 104, 162, 236
classical, x, 137, 163, 169, 177, 178, 207, 229
classical conditioning, 207
classification, x, 31, 39, 74, 88, 89, 90, 95, 96, 98, 100, 137
classified, 97
cleanup, 40
cleavage, 72, 73
clinical, x, 48, 88, 94, 105, 106, 111, 118, 121, 122, 125, 133, 137, 188, 203, 245
clustering, 95, 177
clusters, 95, 96, 231
Co, 186, 190
CO2, 58, 59
codes, 164, 195
coding, 163, 165, 166, 169, 187, 188, 190, 191, 193, 194, 196, 197
cognition, xi, 110, 117, 119, 121, 127, 157, 159, 161, 163, 166, 167, 169, 173, 175, 176, 185, 187, 188, 189, 191, 193, 195, 197, 201, 202, 243
cognitive, viii, x, 21, 33, 109, 113, 116, 117, 122, 125, 127, 128, 130, 137, 138, 158, 159, 160, 162, 163, 165, 166, 167, 169, 171, 172, 173, 174, 175, 176, 181, 182, 184, 186, 187, 190, 192, 193, 195, 196, 202, 223, 224, 236, 238, 242, 243
cognitive effort, 171

cognitive function, 116, 138, 175
cognitive impairment, viii, 33
cognitive load, 173, 192
cognitive process, 113, 128, 162, 167, 169, 186, 195, 202, 223, 238, 242
cognitive processing, 128, 167, 202
cognitive representations, 162
cognitive research, 193
cognitive science, 130, 162, 166, 186, 187, 196
cognitive set, 127
cognitive system, 162
cognitive tasks, 21, 158, 184, 242
coherence, 28, 92, 110, 113, 146, 158, 177, 181, 186, 195, 196, 225, 242, 243, 244, 245
cohort, 50
Columbia, 194
commercial, 227
commissure, 63
communication, 164, 166, 172, 200, 204
compensation, 25
complement, 4, 48
complementary, 4, 38
complex systems, 186
complexity, xii, 92, 93, 96, 97, 98, 99, 100, 101, 102, 103, 104, 106, 116, 130, 142, 159, 171, 176, 189, 195, 221, 225, 226, 228, 235, 236, 237, 238, 239, 241, 242, 243, 245
components, 3, 4, 10, 18, 22, 23, 24, 26, 44, 45, 77, 82, 91, 117, 127, 134, 162, 164, 169, 209, 214, 223, 224, 229
composite, 78, 169, 174, 184
composites, 164
composition, 3, 175
compounds, 40, 203
comprehension, 167
compression, 84
computation, 159, 163, 194, 197, 230
computer, 89, 107, 137, 155, 181, 184, 187
computers, 163, 188, 191
computing, 95, 140
concentration, 45
conceptualization, 159, 172, 174, 176
condensation, 34, 46, 58, 61, 67, 68, 70, 74
conditioned response, 203, 207, 208
conditioning, xi, 174, 199, 206, 207, 208, 209, 210, 211, 214, 218
conductance, 9
conductivity, 143
conductor, 138, 141, 143
cone photoreceptors, 31
confidence, 24, 182
confidence interval, 24
configuration, 37, 140, 142, 143
conformity, 210
confounding variables, 124
confusion, 97, 98, 99
Congress, iv, 192, 195
conjecture, 163
Connecticut, 188, 195
connectionist, 163
connectionist models, 163
connectivity, xi, 24, 28, 29, 31, 169, 171, 172, 175, 177, 181, 189, 190, 197, 221, 222, 237, 239
conscious awareness, x, 109, 113, 117, 126, 127, 128
consciousness, xi, 113, 126, 127, 129, 134, 157, 161, 163, 164, 165, 166, 175, 176, 185, 186, 187, 188, 190, 191, 194, 195, 196, 209
consensus, 49, 116, 166
consent, 227
consolidation, 117, 118, 119, 120, 132, 133
constraints, 16, 163, 172, 239
construction, 129, 169, 172, 175, 176, 181
consumption, 4
contamination, 229
context memory, 117, 126
continuity, 110
control, ix, 36, 42, 50, 57, 59, 60, 61, 62, 63, 64, 65, 66, 67, 68, 69, 75, 76, 78, 79, 82, 83, 116, 117, 124, 127, 155, 185, 192, 194, 201, 208, 211, 218
control condition, 208
control group, ix, 75, 76, 78, 82, 211
controlled, 17, 46, 85, 113, 124, 126, 143, 201
contusion, 84
convection, 162
convergence, 170, 236
conversion, 89
conversion rate, 89
convex, 138
coordination, 158, 159, 160, 164, 165, 172, 173, 174, 175, 187, 188, 191, 192, 194, 197
copyright, iv
corpus callosum, 121
correlation, x, 25, 26, 27, 29, 92, 93, 96, 97, 98, 104, 106, 137, 139, 140, 141, 142, 143, 145, 147, 148, 151, 153, 155, 162, 168, 169, 181, 196, 197, 201, 207, 223
correlation coefficient, 142, 143, 153
correlation function, 25, 27
correlations, 26, 30, 140, 141, 169, 177, 225, 235

cortex, viii, ix, xi, 1, 2, 3, 9, 11, 15, 22, 24, 27, 28, 30, 31, 42, 53, 57, 61, 65, 66, 67, 68, 69, 70, 71, 75, 81, 82, 83, 110, 115, 121, 122, 123, 124, 128, 129, 130, 131, 132, 133, 134, 135, 150, 151, 159, 167, 170, 175, 180, 186, 187, 188, 189, 190, 194, 195, 196, 197, 199, 202, 203, 204, 226, 238, 239, 242, 243
cortical, viii, x, xii, 1, 2, 3, 6, 8, 9, 13, 14, 16, 20, 21, 22, 23, 26, 27, 28, 29, 30, 31, 44, 45, 54, 67, 71, 72, 73, 83, 84, 85, 129, 133, 137, 138, 151, 154, 155, 158, 161, 165, 167, 170, 171, 172, 173, 174, 175, 177, 179, 181, 182, 186, 187, 188, 191, 194, 195, 196, 197, 217, 221, 222, 223, 225, 227, 231, 235, 236, 237, 238, 240, 241, 242, 244, 245
cortical neurons, 6, 9, 31, 44, 45, 54, 72, 170, 191
cortical processing, 3, 27, 196
corticosterone, 217
couples, 232, 233, 234, 235, 237
coupling, xii, 20, 29, 30, 181, 182, 190, 222, 223, 235, 236, 237, 241, 244
covalent, 38
covering, 121
CREB, 41, 55
crosslinking, 38
cross-validation, 96, 97, 98
C-terminal, 53
cues, 76, 83, 196, 207
cultural, 80, 126
cultural norms, 126
culture, 45, 59, 69, 72
curiosity, 213
currency, 171
Cybernetics, 189
cyclin D1, 83, 85
cyclin-dependent kinase inhibitor, 51
Cyclin-dependent kinases, 53, 54
cycling, viii, 34, 45, 46, 47
cyclins, 36
cycloheximide, 59, 63, 69
cystathionine, 44, 56
cysts, 128
cytoarchitecture, 82
cytokine, 82
cytokines, 34, 82, 83
cytology, 134
cytometry, 46
cytoplasm, 79
cytosine, 39
cytotoxic, 35, 39, 53, 74, 82

D

damage, viii, 33, 35, 36, 37, 38, 39, 40, 41, 42, 43, 45, 46, 47, 53, 55, 58, 60, 72, 76
danger, 202, 203, 204, 205, 208, 209, 213, 214, 215, 239, 245
Darwinism, 188
data analysis, 244
data base, 97
data collection, 229
data set, 29, 89, 93, 244
death, vii, viii, ix, 33, 34, 41, 42, 43, 48, 49, 50, 51, 52, 53, 54, 56, 57, 58, 63, 68, 69, 70, 71, 72, 73, 74, 76, 200, 203, 213, 228
debt, 185
decay, 10, 14, 25, 35
decision making, 106
declarative memory, 111, 117, 119, 131, 134
decomposition, 91, 153, 155, 165, 176
deconvolution, 2
decoupling, xii, 182, 222, 235, 236, 237, 238
deduction, 162
defecation, 212
defects, 41, 42
defense, viii, xi, 33, 35, 199, 200, 201, 204, 205, 206, 208, 209, 210, 212, 213, 215, 217
defense mechanisms, 35, 215
defensive strategies, 205
deficiency, 41, 44, 47
deficit, 115, 128, 129, 132, 210
deficits, viii, 1, 2, 27, 72, 86, 115, 120
definition, 172, 222, 223, 224, 242
degradation, 37, 39, 41, 55, 58, 63, 70, 163
degree, 35, 78, 92, 105, 116, 119, 121, 124, 125, 127, 158, 174, 175, 181, 201, 230, 231, 236
degrees of freedom, 160, 184, 225, 235, 237, 238, 239
delays, viii, 1, 2, 3, 5, 6, 15, 23, 24, 25, 26, 27, 145, 170
delivery, 3, 59
delta, xii, 54, 186, 221, 226, 229, 231, 236, 237, 238, 242
demand, viii, 1, 3, 4, 5, 8, 9, 16, 17, 18, 19, 23, 36
dementia, 122
dendrites, 159, 166
dendritic cell (DC), 216
density, 2, 7, 13, 59, 60, 61, 67, 77, 155, 231
dentate gyrus, 76
dephosphorylation, 41
depressed, 147, 211

depression, 207, 210, 211, 219
deprivation, vii, ix, 57, 58, 70
desire, 225
desires, 176
destruction, 35, 58, 128, 163
desynchronization, 226, 235, 238, 241, 243, 244
detection, 11, 12, 31, 38, 40, 47, 49, 50, 52, 54, 61, 70, 96, 100, 106, 107, 108, 126, 162, 174, 205, 223
deterministic, 24, 162, 222, 236, 243
developing brain, viii, 57, 58, 69, 72
developmental process, 34
deviation, 20, 92, 93, 95, 97, 230, 231
diagnosis, 192
diagnostic, 7, 17, 18, 19, 184
Diagnostic and Statistical Manual of Mental Disorders, 200, 216
diagnostic markers, 184
dichotomy, 191, 201, 203
differential equations, 161
differentiated cells, viii, 33, 43, 53, 76
differentiation, ix, 42, 75, 83, 85, 86, 115, 116, 122, 125, 127
diffusion, 162
digestion, 70, 74
dimer, 48
diodes, 11
dipole, x, 137, 138, 140, 142, 147, 148, 149, 151, 152, 153, 154, 155
directionality, 28
discharges, 88, 155
disclosure, 201
discomfort, 203
discrete emotions, 240, 241
discrimination, 188, 193
diseases, viii, 2, 27, 33, 34, 42, 47, 184
disorder, 41, 131, 162, 200, 204
displacement, 144, 187
dissociation, 48, 77, 83, 132, 188, 203, 208, 218, 240
distal, xi, 199, 202, 203, 205, 208, 214, 235
distilled water, 61
distraction, 179
distribution, 31, 140, 141, 142, 144, 145, 146, 148, 149, 151, 155, 172, 217, 222, 225, 227, 231, 232, 235
distribution function, 144
divergence, 236
diversification, 52
division, 82, 202
dizziness, 200
DNA, v, vii, viii, ix, 33, 34, 35, 36, 37, 38, 39, 40, 41, 42, 43, 45, 46, 47, 48, 49, 50, 51, 52, 53, 54, 55, 56, 57, 58, 61, 62, 63, 64, 65, 66, 67, 68, 69, 70, 71, 72, 73
DNA damage, v, vii, viii, 33, 35, 36, 37, 38, 39, 40, 41, 42, 43, 45, 46, 47, 48, 49, 50, 51, 52, 53, 54, 55, 56, 72, 73
DNA damaging agents, viii, 33
DNA lesions, viii, 33, 35, 37, 38, 42, 73
DNA ligase, 40, 48, 49, 51
DNA polymerase, 40, 46, 48, 49, 55
DNA repair, viii, 33, 35, 37, 38, 39, 42, 43, 45, 46, 47, 48, 50, 51, 53, 54, 55
DNA strand breaks, viii, 33, 40, 42, 49, 62
dopamine, 76, 217, 219
dopaminergic, 52, 84
dorsal, xi, 199, 203, 206, 209, 215, 216
double helix, 37, 40
drowning, 228
drugs, 74, 174
DSB, 39, 41, 42, 44, 51
DSM, 200
DSM-IV, 200
duration, 2, 8, 9, 11, 12, 13, 14, 15, 16, 17, 18, 19, 20, 21, 22, 89, 160, 170, 177, 178, 179, 188, 191, 224
dynamic systems, 162, 243
dynamical properties, 236
dynamical system, 29, 163, 164, 190, 196, 235, 242
dynamical systems, 29, 164, 190, 196, 235, 242

E

E2F, 36, 46, 48, 49, 50, 52, 53, 55
EA, 30, 31, 52, 85
EEG, v, vii, x, xi, 2, 24, 29, 87, 88, 89, 90, 91, 92, 93, 95, 96, 99, 100, 103, 104, 105, 106, 107, 108, 137, 138, 139, 144, 145, 153, 154, 155, 156, 157, 160, 161, 164, 167, 176, 177, 178, 179, 180, 181, 182, 183, 184, 186, 187, 188, 189, 191, 192, 193, 194, 195, 196, 221, 222, 223, 225, 226, 228, 229, 230, 231, 232, 235, 236, 237, 238, 239, 240, 241, 242, 243, 244, 245
EEG activity, 88, 188, 242
EEG patterns, 90
efficacy, ix, 76, 84
EGF, 77, 79, 84
eigenvalues, 140, 141, 145
elaboration, 128, 238, 239
election, 186, 209

electric current, 159
Electric Source Imaging, v, 137
electrical, 107, 138, 139, 144, 150, 151, 153, 154, 159, 175, 177, 186, 192, 193, 194, 206, 207, 209, 212, 218, 242
electrical fields, 177
electrochemical, 50
electrochemical detection, 50
electrodes, vii, x, xii, 87, 88, 89, 91, 93, 94, 95, 97, 98, 100, 101, 103, 104, 105, 106, 139, 177, 221, 229, 232, 233, 234, 235, 237
electroencephalogram, 138, 160, 178, 188, 244
electroencephalography, 155, 189
electromagnetic, 138, 154, 168, 183, 184
electromagnetic tomography, 154
electronic, iv
electrophoresis, ix, 57, 69, 70
electrophysiological, 21, 24, 28
electrophysiology, 72, 161
electrostatic, iv
embryo, 77
embryogenesis, 69
embryonic, 41, 48, 51, 54, 58, 59, 63, 64, 82, 83, 84
embryos, 59, 69
emergency response, 212
emission, 3, 62, 115, 131, 133, 134, 194
emotion, xii, 110, 117, 121, 122, 131, 188, 201, 222, 223, 224, 225, 226, 227, 228, 231, 232, 233, 234, 235, 236, 237, 238, 239, 240, 241, 242, 243
emotional, x, xi, xii, 109, 110, 113, 114, 117, 119, 120, 122, 123, 124, 125, 127, 131, 132, 133, 199, 201, 202, 211, 214, 215, 221, 223, 224, 225, 226, 227, 228, 230, 232, 234, 235, 236, 237, 238, 239, 240, 241, 242, 243
emotional experience, 202, 224, 226, 228
emotional memory, 117, 122
emotional state, xi, 199, 202, 215, 228
emotional stimuli, 202, 215, 226, 232, 236, 237
emotional valence, 225, 240, 241
emotions, xii, 163, 201, 217, 218, 221, 223, 224, 225, 226, 227, 228, 230, 231, 233, 235, 236, 237, 238, 239, 240, 241, 242, 243, 244, 245
empathy, 117
encoding, x, 46, 48, 109, 110, 111, 112, 113, 115, 116, 118, 119, 125, 126, 127, 128, 129, 131, 132, 134, 173
Encoding, 115
endocrine, 201
endocrine system, 201
endogenous, viii, 33, 35, 37, 40, 49, 56, 70, 74, 76
endogenous progenitors, 76
endonuclease, 40, 44, 56, 70, 71, 73, 74
energy, 4, 9, 11, 18, 19, 58, 70, 165
energy consumption, 4
engagement, 118, 119, 122, 126, 131, 134, 235
England, 242
English, 73, 185
engraftment, 81
Enhancement, 155, 189, 218
entorhinal cortex, 121, 130
entropy, 236, 241, 244
envelope, 177
environment, 38, 82, 122, 158, 166, 223
environmental, xi, 35, 40, 53, 139, 158, 159, 161, 199, 204
environmental factors, 53
environmental threats, 204
enzyme, 40, 44, 49, 54, 55
enzymes, 35, 36, 39, 45
epidermal, 59
epidermal growth factor, 59
epigenetic, 47, 76, 83
epilepsy, 72, 88, 105, 107
epileptogenesis, 106
episodic memory, x, 109, 110, 111, 112, 113, 114, 115, 116, 117, 118, 119, 120, 122, 123, 124, 125, 126, 127, 128, 129, 130, 131, 132, 133, 134
episodic memory tasks, 113, 114, 116, 117, 119, 123, 125, 126, 127
epithelial cell, 73
epithelial cells, 73
equipment, 89

F

factor analysis, 224
factorial, 123
failure, 83, 163, 171
false, 98, 100, 106, 148, 179
false negative, 98
false positive, 98, 106
family, 23, 36, 48, 49, 54, 69
fatigue, 9, 168
fear, xi, xii, 131, 199, 200, 201, 202, 203, 204, 205, 206, 207, 208, 209, 210, 211, 213, 214, 215, 216, 217, 218, 219, 221, 224, 225, 226, 227, 228, 230, 231, 232, 234, 235, 237, 238, 239, 240
fear response, xi, 199, 208, 210, 238, 239
February, 107
feedback, viii, 1, 3, 27, 186, 201, 202, 222

feeding, 18, 25
feelings, 200, 201
feet, 205
females, 227
fetal, ix, 56, 59, 71, 72, 75, 76, 83, 84, 85, 86
fetal tissue, 76
fetuses, 76
FGF-2, 79, 83
fibers, 83, 85
fibroblast, 59, 85
fibroblast growth factor, 59, 85
fibroblasts, 52
fidelity, 51
field theory, 191
figure-ground, 30, 196
filament, 83
film, xii, 221, 226, 228, 230, 231, 233, 235, 236, 239, 242, 243
films, 227
Finland, 157
fire, 158, 168
fires, 168
fixation, 78
flashbacks, 200
flexibility, 160, 163, 175
flight, 200, 212, 215
floating, 79
flow, 24, 46, 60, 164, 171, 187
fluctuations, 13, 106, 166, 177
fluid, 52, 85
fluorescence, 61, 62
fluoxetine, 203
fMRI, vii, viii, 1, 2, 3, 4, 5, 6, 15, 19, 20, 23, 24, 25, 28, 29, 30, 31, 110, 116, 119, 123, 124, 125, 129, 130, 131, 132, 133, 134, 138, 181, 187, 222, 243, 244
focusing, x, 87, 105, 202
food, 59
forebrain, 52, 58, 63, 64, 69, 72, 85, 170
forecasting, 225, 236, 241
fornix, 83, 128, 130
Fourier, 25, 225, 227, 231
Fox, 129
fractionation, 70
fractures, 77
fragility, 41
fragmentation, ix, 34, 42, 49, 57, 58, 61, 63, 65, 67, 68, 69, 70, 71, 72, 73, 74, 170
framing, 197
France, 57, 59, 60, 61, 62, 64
free radical, 40, 82, 84
free radicals, 40, 82
free recall, 112
freedom, 160, 184, 225, 231, 235, 237, 238, 239
free-radical, 34
freezing, 202, 203, 204, 205, 206, 207, 208, 209, 210, 211, 212, 214, 215, 217, 218
frontal cortex, 128, 203, 204, 239
frontal lobe, 130, 131, 133, 134, 240
frontal lobes, 130, 240
functional approach, 243
functional magnetic resonance imaging, 28, 30, 31, 130, 133, 135
functional MRI, 28, 30, 31
fusiform, 130

G

GABA, 189, 218
GABAergic, 218
Gamma, 7, 186, 196, 242
gamma rays, 35
gamma-ray, 52
gas, 60, 65
Gaussian, 143
gel, 62, 63, 64, 65, 66, 67, 68, 70
gels, ix, 57, 70, 71
gender, 115, 133
gene, 37, 46, 48, 52, 53, 56, 58, 71, 85
gene expression, 37
gene therapy, 85
general anesthesia, 77
general knowledge, 123
generalization, 163, 174
generalized anxiety disorder, 200
generation, 5, 13, 34, 37, 170, 188, 192, 211
generators, 144, 151, 154, 166
genes, 36, 38, 42, 54
genetic, 76, 205, 209
genetics, 49
genome, viii, 33, 35, 38, 40, 42, 55
genomic, viii, 33, 35, 36, 39, 43, 45, 51, 55, 68, 70
genomic instability, viii, 33, 35
genotoxic, 40, 43, 55, 56
genotoxins, 40
Germany, 79, 109
gestalt, 167
gestation, 59
GFAP, 80, 81, 83
glass, 60, 79

glia, 76, 158
glial, 3, 4, 5, 16, 30, 76, 83
glial cells, 3, 16
glial scar, 76
glucose, 17, 77, 216
glutamate, 9, 31
glutamic acid, 216
glutamine, 9, 77
glutathione, 35
glycerol, 61
glycolysis, 9
goal-directed behavior, 225
goals, 226
government, iv
grafting, 84
grafts, 76, 84, 86
grain, 25
grants, 106
granule cells, 46
gravity, 236
gray matter, 200, 219
Great Britain, 112
Greeks, 158
grids, 103, 106
grouping, 197
groups, ix, xi, 28, 75, 78, 93, 94, 95, 104, 106, 147, 167, 210, 211, 221, 222
growth, 14, 34, 41, 45, 46, 53, 59, 73, 83, 84, 85, 173, 179
growth factor, 34, 59, 83, 85
growth factors, 34, 59
guanine, 50
guidelines, 59
gut, 202
gyrus, 76, 124, 130, 131

H

H1, 66
handedness, 244
handling, 169
hanging, 96
happiness, xii, 221, 224, 226, 227, 228, 230, 231, 232, 234, 235, 237, 238, 239, 240
Harvard, 194
head, 77, 138, 139, 143, 151, 152, 205, 227
head injury, 77, 227
hearing, 223
heart, 44, 200, 201
heart rate, 200
hedonic, 176
height, 77, 212
helix, 37, 40
helplessness, 200
hemisphere, xii, 116, 221, 240
hemodynamic, 4, 5, 8, 9, 17, 20, 21, 29
hemodynamics, 2, 21
hemoglobin, 4
heterogeneity, 28, 76, 85
heterogeneous, 51
high resolution, 154
hippocampal, 76, 111, 117, 118, 119, 120, 121, 122, 123, 127, 128, 129, 131, 132, 133, 134, 166, 217, 226
hippocampus, xi, 44, 53, 60, 72, 77, 82, 110, 115, 117, 118, 119, 121, 122, 124, 127, 128, 130, 131, 132, 133, 134, 135, 187, 199, 203, 213, 218
histogram, 120
histological, 29
histone, 41, 52, 53
holistic, 163, 167
holistic approach, 167
Holland, 171, 191
holoenzyme, 40
homeostasis, 35, 69
homogeneity, 59
homogeneous, 3, 61
homogenized, 61
homology, 53, 239
horse, 62, 78
hospital, 89
host, 76, 82, 84, 86
hostile environment, 82
House, 197
hub, 50
human, vii, ix, 1, 2, 10, 12, 15, 20, 27, 28, 29, 30, 35, 42, 48, 49, 52, 53, 54, 59, 75, 76, 77, 84, 85, 96, 110, 111, 112, 115, 126, 131, 132, 133, 134, 135, 138, 154, 158, 159, 163, 164, 165, 186, 187, 189, 190, 191, 192, 193, 195, 227, 228, 239, 241, 242, 243, 244
human behavior, 159, 164
human brain, vii, 1, 2, 15, 27, 85, 111, 131, 138, 154, 163, 187, 189, 190, 191, 192, 244
human subjects, 49, 115, 135
humans, 29, 47, 111, 117, 119, 133, 190, 196, 224, 243, 245
hydrate, 60, 78
hydrodynamics, 162
hydrogen, 34, 62

hydrogen peroxide, 34, 62
hydrolysis, 35, 38
hydroxyl, 34
hyperhomocysteinemia, 44
hypersensitive, 41
hypertension, 212
hypnosis, 242
hypotensive, 214
hypothalamic, 44, 204, 213, 214, 216, 217, 218
hypothalamus, xi, 199, 200, 204, 212, 213, 215, 216, 217, 218
hypothesis, xi, 26, 129, 162, 165, 190, 196, 199, 209, 210, 211, 216, 236, 239, 240
hypoxia, vii, ix, 57, 58, 59, 60, 61, 63, 64, 65, 66, 67, 69, 70, 71, 72, 74
hypoxia-ischemia, 58, 70, 71, 74
hypoxic, viii, 57, 58, 61, 63, 64, 65, 66, 71, 72, 73
hypoxic-ischemic, viii, 57, 58, 71

I

ice, 44, 60, 78
id, 60, 95, 211, 238
identification, 24, 25, 125, 163
IgG, 62
illumination, 62
illusion, 174
imagery, 122, 161, 193, 236
images, 138, 158, 160, 162, 171, 174, 184, 224
imagination, 188
imaging, x, 3, 28, 29, 30, 31, 115, 130, 132, 133, 135, 137, 138, 140, 144, 145, 146, 149, 151, 153, 154, 155, 176, 181, 185, 191, 193, 195
imaging techniques, 138, 155
immune system, 216
immunodeficiency, 41
immunoglobulin, 52, 53, 78
immunoglobulin G, 78
immunohistochemical, 63, 79
immunohistochemistry, ix, 57, 62, 75
immunological, 211
immunoreactivity, 62, 68, 217, 218
immunosuppression, 216
impairments, ix, 57, 115, 118
implementation, 10, 25, 26, 92, 106, 195
in situ, ix, 55, 57, 62, 71, 82, 212
in vitro, viii, 33, 43, 46, 59, 70, 73, 76, 80, 83, 177, 193
in vivo, 43, 46, 61, 73, 83
inactive, 37, 53, 168
incidence, 42, 43, 47
inclusion, 54, 112
incubation, 59, 61, 79
indication, 48
indicators, 113, 157
indirect measure, 24
inducible protein, 72
induction, 36, 39, 41, 46, 71, 77, 235, 236
ineffectiveness, 211
infarction, 71
inferences, 25, 26
infinite, 171
inflammation, 34
inflammatory, 82
inflammatory cells, 82
information exchange, 237
information processing, x, 109, 110, 111, 113, 116, 117, 123, 124, 126, 158, 161, 165, 190, 191, 192, 237, 238, 239, 244
information retrieval, 126, 127
informed consent, 227
inhibition, 9, 16, 18, 19, 20, 53, 54, 83, 130, 161, 174, 189, 197, 238
inhibitor, 53, 63, 70
inhibitors, 49, 51, 54, 72, 73, 74, 203, 204
inhibitory, 8, 9, 17, 23, 26, 27, 83, 168, 177
initial state, 16
initiation, 35
injection, 60, 78, 83
injections, 81
injuries, 84
injury, iv, vii, viii, ix, 44, 52, 57, 58, 68, 70, 71, 72, 73, 75, 76, 77, 78, 80, 82, 83, 84, 85, 134, 227
innate capacity, 218
inspection, 89, 229
instability, viii, 33, 35
instruction, 126
insulin, 59, 77
insults, 34, 36, 58, 71
integration, xi, 5, 11, 12, 13, 14, 15, 18, 19, 28, 46, 83, 86, 106, 125, 126, 134, 154, 160, 164, 165, 170, 174, 188, 189, 194, 196, 197, 199, 212, 215, 222, 223, 225, 237, 239, 245
integrity, viii, 33, 35, 36, 42, 45, 55
intelligence, 163, 191
intensity, xi, 12, 62, 199, 206, 207, 208, 210, 212, 214, 215, 218, 224, 227, 228, 231
interaction, 35, 43, 47, 122, 137, 143, 164, 170, 222, 231, 232, 235, 240
interaction effect, 231, 232

interaction process, 240
interactions, viii, 1, 24, 27, 28, 29, 30, 54, 55, 84, 126, 127, 131, 154, 162, 164, 170, 172, 174, 180, 191, 193, 197, 226, 235, 237
interdependence, 175
interest, 76
interface, 76
interference, 31
interleukin (IL), 185
intermediaries, 4
intermolecular, 48
interpretation, vii, 8, 21, 48, 107, 158, 159, 174, 175, 176, 190, 196
interrelations, 181, 189
interrelationships, 181
interval, 13, 24, 114, 161, 172
intervention, vii, viii, 34
intraperitoneal, 60, 78
intravenous (IV), 200
intrinsic, 36, 43, 58, 159, 162
intuition, 185
invasive, 27
inversion, x, 9, 137
Investigations, 238
ionic, 83
ionizing radiation, viii, 33, 40, 49, 50
ions, 84
ipsilateral, 67, 68, 82
irradiation, viii, 33, 44, 50, 52
ischemia, 44, 49, 51, 52, 58, 60, 61, 67, 68, 69, 70, 71, 72, 73, 74
ischemic, viii, ix, 33, 42, 57, 58, 62, 68, 71
isolation, 61, 73, 163
isomorphism, 160, 187
Italy, 189, 195, 221
iteration, 137

J

jackknife, 24, 30
January, 107
Java, 112, 130
judges, 227
judgment, 113
Jun, 55
Jung, 60, 229, 243

K

kainic acid, 55
kernel, 2, 4, 5, 6, 8, 9, 13, 14, 17, 22
Ki-67, 45, 46
kinase, 36, 40, 43, 47, 49, 51, 52, 54, 55
kinase activity, 54
kinases, 36, 53, 54, 55, 72, 73
kinetics, 31
King, 37, 46, 51
knockout, 44, 45
Kolmogorov, 236, 241

L

L1, 140, 142, 236
L2, 140, 142
labeling, ix, 57, 61, 62, 65, 79
laminar, 29
language, 162, 186, 188, 192, 195
large-scale, xi, 28, 122, 128, 164, 172, 173, 175, 180, 187, 194, 197, 221, 222
latency, 28, 29, 30
lateral sclerosis, 35
laterality, 115, 116, 242
law, 29, 30
lead, vii, x, xi, 4, 16, 35, 36, 39, 42, 43, 45, 61, 72, 87, 88, 98, 100, 104, 105, 106, 167, 169, 199, 213, 216
leakage, 58
learning, 111, 112, 114, 119, 126, 127, 132, 134, 168, 169, 170, 186, 194, 210, 223, 244
learning task, 134
left hemisphere, 116
lesions, viii, 33, 35, 37, 38, 40, 42, 51, 73, 84, 86, 107, 115, 118, 119, 128, 133, 134, 206, 207, 216, 218
life experiences, 125
life span, 69, 123, 179, 194
lifetime, 114, 134
light-emitting diodes, 11
likelihood, 8, 105, 244
Likert scale, 227, 228
limitation, 2
limitations, 2, 3, 14, 27, 76, 138, 178, 181
linear, x, 3, 4, 5, 6, 9, 11, 12, 13, 16, 17, 18, 19, 22, 92, 94, 95, 97, 98, 107, 108, 116, 137, 138, 142, 191, 222, 225, 229, 235, 241, 242
linear function, 116

linear model, 229
links, 26, 51, 171
lipid, 34
lipid peroxides, 34
lipids, 35
literature, 163, 235
liver, 48
lobectomy, 128
localization, x, 87, 105, 113, 137, 138, 153, 154, 155, 225
location, x, 5, 12, 82, 87, 88, 94, 96, 118, 142, 152, 154, 155, 171, 179, 181
locomotion, 165
locus, 167
London, 74, 108, 112, 185, 188, 190, 196, 197
long-distance, 238, 244
long-term, 89, 96, 110, 111, 118, 127, 132, 133, 186
long-term memory, 110, 111, 133
lover, 28
low-level, 169
Lyapunov, 92, 162, 236, 241, 244
Lyapunov exponent, 92, 162, 236, 241, 244
lymphocytes, 53, 74
lysine, 59, 80
lysis, 61

M

M.O., 132
machinery, viii, 34, 36, 37, 38, 43, 46, 47, 51
magnetic, iv, 17, 28, 30, 31, 107, 115, 130, 131, 133, 135
magnetic resonance, 17, 28, 30, 31, 115, 130, 131, 133, 135
magnetic resonance imaging (MRI) , vii, 1, 2, 28, 30, 31, 88, 115, 130, 133, 135, 154, 138, 222
magnetoencephalogram, 160
magnetoencephalography (MEG), 138, 139, 154, 155, 157, 160, 164, 177, 178, 179, 180, 181, 182, 183, 184, 190, 192, 222, 244
maintenance, 46, 50, 51, 127, 245
maladaptive, xi, 199, 203, 212
males, 59, 227
Mammalian, 52
mammalian brain, 72, 76, 85, 222
mammalian cell, 35, 38, 49, 52, 53
mammalian cells, 38, 52, 53
mammals, 40, 53, 217
manipulation, 2, 20, 26, 127, 138, 207
manufacturer, 62
mapping, vii, viii, xi, 1, 2, 3, 6, 24, 29, 150, 154, 156, 157, 192, 195, 209
Massachusetts, 188, 195
mat, 163, 180
mathematical, 5, 88, 106, 139, 185, 222
mathematical methods, 222
mathematics, 94, 186
Matrices, 91
matrix, x, 91, 92, 98, 137, 138, 139, 140, 141, 142, 143, 145, 147, 148, 151, 153, 155, 232
maturation, 48
meanings, 236
measurement, 19, 24, 28, 124
measures, x, xi, 20, 87, 88, 92, 98, 108, 125, 162, 164, 207, 210, 221, 222, 225, 226, 230, 232, 235, 236, 241
mechanical, iv, 77, 165, 172
mechanical energy, 165
mechanics, 165
media, 170
medial prefrontal cortex, 124, 130, 135
median, 60, 155, 218
mediators, 127
medication, 227
medicine, 196
membranes, 166, 177
memory, x, 5, 86, 109, 110, 111, 112, 113, 114, 115, 116, 117, 118, 119, 120, 121, 122, 123, 124, 125, 126, 127, 128, 129, 130, 131, 132, 133, 134, 135, 164, 167, 170, 172, 173, 189, 190, 209, 223, 236, 243
memory deficits, 86, 115, 120
memory loss, 119, 120, 236
memory performance, 243
memory processes, 116, 127
memory retrieval, 115, 118, 124, 125, 126, 128, 131, 133
meninges, 59
mental activity, 167, 174
mental arithmetic, 236
mental disorder, 227
mental image, 122, 160, 171
mental imagery, 122
mental processes, 164, 167, 222, 241
mental representation, 158, 162, 164
mental state, 158, 160, 169, 171, 172
mental states, 158, 160, 171
meridian, 11
mesoscopic, 170, 171, 176, 185
messengers, 34

meta-analysis, 55, 122, 134, 244
metabolic, viii, 1, 3, 4, 5, 6, 8, 9, 14, 16, 17, 18, 19, 20, 21, 22, 23, 24, 30, 42
metabolic rate, 30, 42
metabolism, viii, 2, 17, 33, 34, 35, 41, 42, 44
metaphor, 159, 176, 187, 189
methanol, 62
methylation, 38
metric, 140, 141, 144, 146, 147, 148, 149, 151, 152, 236
Mg^{2+}, 70, 73
Miami, 87, 106
mice, 41, 42, 44, 45, 46, 47, 48, 49, 50, 51, 55
microenvironment, 83
microglia, 82
microphotographs, 62
microscope, 8, 12, 62, 79
microscopy, 61, 78, 80
micro-states, 193
microtome, 78
midbrain, 209, 216, 217
migration, 83, 85
MIT, 80, 129, 133, 134, 188, 189, 192, 193, 194, 195, 196, 197
mitochondria, 38, 51, 55
mitochondrial, 34, 42, 51, 53, 71
mitochondrial DNA, 42, 51
mitogenic, 37
mitosis, 43, 54
mitotic, 69
mobility, 92, 93, 96, 97, 98, 104, 106
modalities, 138, 174, 191
modality, 171, 174, 218
mode, 177, 190, 210
model system, 229
modeling, 14, 15, 16, 17, 19, 20, 21, 22, 23, 24, 29, 30, 114, 154, 155, 161, 179, 181, 202, 243
models, vii, ix, 16, 24, 25, 29, 56, 57, 58, 69, 70, 76, 140, 162, 163, 169, 177, 181, 192, 195, 201, 202, 215, 223, 225, 226, 233, 235, 239, 240
modulation, 2, 10, 28, 29, 131, 170, 190
modules, 158, 168, 184, 185
molecular weight, 70
molecules, 3, 9, 37, 38, 48, 50, 82, 83, 170
monkeys, 133, 194
mononuclear cells, 81
morbidity, 58
morphine, 218
morphogenesis, 162, 197
morphological, ix, x, 46, 57, 63, 65, 67, 69, 70, 73, 77, 80, 81, 83, 88
morphology, 63, 65, 67, 72, 80
mortality, 58, 60, 170
Moscow, 178, 181, 185, 186, 189
motion, 2, 197, 223, 227
motor activity, 209, 211
motor area, 175, 193, 238, 244
motor control, 185
motor coordination, 192
motor function, ix, 75, 78, 80, 83, 238
motor system, 208, 214
motor task, 227
Mountcastle, Vernon, 163, 165, 167, 193, 194
mouse, 42, 51, 52, 54, 85
mouse model, 42, 54
movement, 160, 176, 191, 206, 238, 244
mRNA, 44
mtDNA, 38
multidimensional, 142, 152, 161
multiple factors, 128
multiple sclerosis, 2, 30, 31
MUltiple SIgnal Classification (MUSIC), x, 137, 138, 139, 141, 145, 151, 153, 154, 155
multipotent, 82, 84, 85
multivariate, 153
muscle, 44, 60, 206
muscle cells, 44
muscles, 200, 205, 209
mutagenesis, 35, 49
mutagenic, 35, 39, 40
mutant, 42, 55
mutants, 51
mutation, 46, 51
mutations, 48
myoblasts, 50

N

NA, viii, 33, 35, 36, 39, 40, 42, 46, 49, 54, 58, 64, 68, 70, 178
NaCl, 61
naloxone, 218
national, 193
National Academy of Sciences, 185, 188, 190, 191
National Science Foundation, 106
natural, 24, 25, 124, 182, 213, 217
neck, 60, 202, 205
necrosis, 34, 58, 61, 62, 63, 64, 65, 67, 69, 70, 71, 74
needs, 58

negative emotions, xii, 221, 225, 227, 238, 239, 240
negative valence, 120
negativity, 22
neglect, 212
neocortex, 118, 120, 121, 166, 189, 193
neonatal, 71, 72, 73
neonate, 58, 71
neonates, 59
nerve, 50, 83, 85, 155
nerve growth factor, 83, 85
nervous system, vii, viii, 33, 34, 42, 44, 48, 49, 50, 53, 54, 56, 71, 73, 74, 76, 84, 85, 86, 201, 205, 209, 212
Netherlands, 192
network, 3, 14, 26, 28, 30, 55, 96, 97, 106, 108, 110, 131, 134, 158, 163, 164, 169, 173, 187, 193, 235, 238
neural development, 42
neural mechanisms, 15, 20, 126, 127, 133, 134, 201, 202, 204, 215
neural network, xii, 14, 95, 96, 106, 107, 108, 129, 134, 162, 163, 169, 172, 191, 192, 193, 197, 222, 226, 235, 236
neural networks, xii, 107, 108, 129, 162, 169, 172, 191, 192, 197, 222, 226, 235, 236
neural regeneration, 83
neural stem cell, 77, 85, 86
neural stem cells, 77, 85
neural systems, 187, 215, 223
neural tissue, 76, 77
neuritis, 30, 31
neuroanatomy, 130, 133, 242, 244
neurobehavioral, 83
neurobiological, 167, 203, 224, 225
neurobiology, 188, 190, 200, 201, 202, 243
neuroblastoma, 52
neuroblasts, 84
neurodegeneration, viii, 33, 34, 35, 42, 47, 48, 49, 50, 51, 54, 85
neurodegenerative, vii, viii, 34, 35, 41, 42, 43, 47, 50, 53, 83
neurodegenerative disease, vii, viii, 34, 42, 43, 50, 53
neurodegenerative diseases, vii, viii, 34, 42, 43, 50, 53
neurodegenerative disorders, 35, 42, 43, 47
neurodegenerative processes, 83
neurodynamics, 162, 190
neurofibrillary tangles, 50
neurogenesis, 71, 72
neuroimaging, vii, 110, 112, 115, 116, 117, 118, 119, 120, 121, 122, 123, 124, 125, 126, 129, 130, 131, 132, 164, 187, 224, 225, 236, 237, 239
neuroimaging techniques, 225
neurological disease, 27, 34
neurological disorder, 88
neuromotor, 41
neuron, 159, 160, 165, 166, 170, 190
neuron death, 50
neuronal apoptosis, viii, 33, 34, 43, 46, 48, 50, 51, 53, 73
neuronal cells, 59, 62
neuronal death, 34, 49, 72
neuronal degeneration, 41
neuronal loss, 34, 42, 71, 82
neuronal survival, viii, 34, 52
neuronal systems, 164
neurons, v, vii, viii, ix, 3, 6, 9, 22, 31, 33, 34, 41, 42, 43, 45, 46, 47, 49, 50, 51, 52, 53, 54, 55, 56, 58, 59, 60, 61, 62, 63, 64, 69, 70, 71, 72, 75, 76, 80, 82, 83, 84, 97, 158, 159, 163, 165, 166, 167, 168, 169, 170, 171, 172, 177, 179, 190, 191, 209, 213, 216, 219, 222
neurophysiology, 185, 191
neuroprotection, ix, 75
neuroprotective, vii, ix, 43, 49, 75, 76, 83, 84
neuroprotective agents, 49
neuropsychology, 188
neuroscience, vii, x, xi, 3, 107, 109, 137, 157, 163, 185, 187, 193, 194, 223, 224, 242, 244
neurotoxic, 34
neurotoxicity, 48
neurotransmitter, 3, 31, 217
neurotrophic, 48, 83
neurotrophic factors, 83
New Jersey, 107, 185
New York, iii, iv, 29, 31, 107, 134, 186, 187, 188, 191, 193, 197, 217, 243, 244
Newtonian, 197
Ni, 3, 5
Nielsen, 73, 156
nightmares, 200
nigrostriatal, 84
nitric oxide, 71
NMDA, 52, 72
NMDA receptors, 72
N-methyl-D-aspartate, 71
nociceptive, 209
nodes, 237, 240

noise, x, 2, 5, 24, 27, 31, 90, 91, 92, 137, 138, 139, 140, 141, 142, 143, 145, 146, 147, 148, 153, 162, 163, 170, 177, 187, 190, 200, 207, 209, 211
non-human, vii, 111
non-human primates, 111
non-invasive, 27
nonlinear, viii, xi, xii, 1, 3, 4, 5, 6, 13, 16, 19, 24, 25, 28, 92, 138, 152, 170, 190, 221, 222, 223, 225, 226, 227, 235, 236, 240, 241
non-linear, 3, 4, 28, 92, 107, 116, 138, 142, 191, 225, 229, 235
nonlinear dynamics, 19, 28
non-linear dynamics, 92
nonlinearities, 15, 16, 17, 31
non-linearity, 28
non-native, 37
nonparametric, 178, 187, 192
non-random, 177
nonverbal, 130
nonwhite, 138
norepinephrine (NE), 217, 219
normal, viii, 33, 34, 39, 40, 44, 47, 76, 78, 82, 83, 115, 122, 125, 150, 162, 167, 192, 200, 213, 215, 227
normal development, 34, 76
normalization, 25
norms, 126
North Atlantic, 218
NSC, ix, 76
NSCs, vii, ix, 75, 76, 77, 78, 79, 80, 81, 82, 83, 84
nuclear, 41, 42, 46, 61, 63, 65, 67, 70, 82
nuclease, ix, 39, 40, 58
nuclei, ix, 44, 51, 57, 61, 63, 65, 67, 69, 70, 79, 80, 184, 204, 213, 214, 216, 218
nucleic acid, 35
nucleoli, 80
nucleotide sequence, 36
nucleus, 58, 203, 204, 209, 213, 214, 218
nylon, 59

O

object recognition, 237
observations, 41, 42, 44, 46, 69, 70, 166
occipital, 173, 183
occipital regions, 227, 237
olive, 193
Oncogene, 48, 50, 52, 53, 54
Oncology, 33
online, 127
on-line, 96
open spaces, 212
opioid, 132
opposition, 224
optic neuritis, 30, 31
optimization, 14, 15, 23, 97, 107, 138, 142
organism, 83, 158, 163, 176, 213, 215, 225
organization, xi, 2, 30, 52, 92, 134, 159, 163, 166, 167, 169, 170, 175, 176, 179, 185, 186, 187, 189, 191, 192, 193, 199, 202, 205, 206, 212, 213, 214, 215, 216, 217, 226, 240
orientation, 129, 142, 200, 205, 210, 213, 215
oscillation, 187
oscillations, 28, 161, 171, 177, 186, 188, 190, 193, 222, 242, 243
ownership, 113
oxidation, 37, 49, 50
oxidative, viii, 33, 34, 38, 39, 40, 41, 42, 44, 46, 48, 49, 53, 55
oxidative damage, 35, 48, 53
oxidative stress, 34, 41, 45, 46, 48, 49
oxide, 71
oxygen, vii, ix, 3, 4, 5, 16, 17, 34, 38, 57, 58, 70, 86
oxygenation, 5
oxyradicals, viii, 33, 38

P

p53, 41, 42, 46, 47, 48, 52, 53, 55, 85
Pacific, 28
pain, 236, 243
pairing, 2, 211
palpitations, 200
panic attack, xi, 199, 203, 215
panic disorder, 204
paper, 2, 27, 84, 166
paradoxical, 201
paralysis, 202
parameter, 2, 7, 14, 23, 24, 92, 93, 94, 95, 97, 99, 100, 103, 104, 106, 145, 154, 162, 168
parameter estimation, 2, 24, 154
parasympathetic, 205, 206
parietal cortex, 61
Paris, 57, 59, 64, 190
Parkinson, viii, 33, 35, 51, 54, 76, 128
Parkinson's disease, 51, 76
parole, 187
PARP, 40, 42, 49
PARP-1, 40
partial seizure, 89

particles, 162
partition, 110
passenger, 200
passive, 158, 204
pathogenesis, 34, 47, 54
pathology, vii, viii, 33, 120, 122, 131, 134
pathophysiology, 201
pathways, viii, xi, 28, 30, 33, 34, 35, 38, 41, 42, 48, 51, 52, 54, 55, 71, 214, 221, 237, 239, 240
patients, viii, 33, 42, 43, 47, 48, 53, 76, 88, 89, 98, 100, 101, 103, 104, 105, 106, 115, 119, 120, 121, 134, 203, 243
PC12 cells, 70
peers, 138, 166
penumbra, ix, 57, 63, 67, 68, 71
peptide, 34, 48
perception, xi, 30, 130, 157, 158, 164, 166, 184, 185, 186, 188, 189, 196, 201, 202, 205, 223, 224, 242
perceptions, xi, 157, 169, 170, 176
performance, x, xi, 97, 98, 99, 101, 105, 110, 115, 137, 146, 147, 148, 153, 159, 199, 200, 210, 242, 243
periaqueductal gray matter, 200, 219
perinatal, viii, 57, 58, 71
permit, 83, 176, 180
peroxide, 34, 63
peroxynitrite, 34
personal, x, 109, 113, 117, 122, 123, 125, 130, 236, 243
perturbation, 161
PFC, 115, 116, 117, 127
pH, 61
phagocytosis, 34, 69
pharmacological, 184, 216
phase space, 92, 236
phenomenology, 164, 166, 174, 177, 191, 193
phenotype, 41, 50
phenotypes, 51
phenotypic, 76
Philadelphia, 74
philosophers, 158
philosophical, 113, 193
phosphate, 60, 61, 78
phosphorylates, 41, 45
phosphorylation, 41, 48, 49, 51
photoreceptor, 6
photoreceptors, 30, 31
phylogenetic, 209
physical activity, 209
physical environment, 163
physical sciences, 195
physicians, 88, 89
physics, 164, 165
physiological, ix, 5, 12, 37, 46, 57, 58, 60, 69, 74, 160, 163, 201, 203, 224
physiological arousal, 201
physiology, vii, viii, 33, 107, 185, 215, 243
piloerection, 201, 212
pilot study, 227
planning, 88, 116
plasma, 34
plasma membrane, 34
plastic, 60, 76, 77
plasticity, 70, 76, 85, 195, 196
Plato, 158
play, viii, 33, 36, 69, 117, 201, 213, 215, 222, 236
plus-maze, 209, 212, 217, 218
plus-maze test, 212, 218
Poincaré, 57
poisoning, 197
polarity, 6
polymerase, 40, 42, 46, 48, 49, 55
polypeptide, 83
poor, 163, 203
population, 3, 9, 16, 30, 76, 85, 165, 179, 195
population growth, 179
pore, 59
positive correlation, 207
positive emotions, 225, 238, 240
positron, 115, 131, 133, 194
positron emission tomography (PET), 29, 30, 115, 129, 131, 133, 138, 194, 244
post-hoc analysis, 230
postmitotic cells, 44
postsynaptic, 9, 34, 168, 177
post-translational, 34
post-traumatic stress, 200, 212
post-traumatic stress disorder (PTSD), 200, 201 , 200
posture, 207
power, 19, 20, 93, 95, 96, 97, 103, 169, 176, 195, 225, 226, 231, 232, 235, 243
powers, 195
pRb, 37
preclinical, 128
preconditioning, 72
precursor cells, 79, 80, 83, 84
predators, 205, 206
predictability, 225, 237, 238
prediction, 2, 9, 16, 22

predictors, 3, 105
prefrontal cortex (PFC), xi, 110, 115, 124, 129, 130, 131, 132, 133, 135, 199, 243
preparation, iv, 205, 209, 213
preparedness, 215
preprocessing, 92
pressure, 170
presynaptic, 168
prevention, 55
primary visual cortex, 28, 196
primate, 188, 196
primates, 111, 224
priming, 111
primitives, 163, 187
prior knowledge, 3, 24
probability, 7, 79, 92, 168, 177
probability density function, 7
procedural memory, 111
procedures, xi, 79, 199, 207, 210, 211, 214, 236
processing pathways, 239
processing stages, 4
production, xi, 83, 124, 199, 215
progenitor cells, 85
progenitors, 76, 83
progeny, 36, 82
progesterone, 59, 77
program, viii, ix, 33, 43, 45, 58, 69, 89, 128, 193, 195
programming, 95
progression, 175
progressive, viii, ix, 34, 42, 46, 47, 57, 65, 212, 218
proinflammatory, 83
proinflammatory effect, 83
proliferation, 43, 72, 82
promote, 54, 83, 86
propagation, 170
property, iv, 6, 8, 19, 24, 170, 174, 175, 176, 235
proportionality, 19, 20
proteases, 72
protection, 34, 35, 48, 53
protein, ix, 36, 37, 40, 46, 47, 49, 52, 53, 54, 55, 57, 62, 63, 64, 66, 67, 69, 70, 71, 72, 83
protein kinase C, 54
protein kinases, 55, 72
protein synthesis, 37, 63, 71
proteinase, 61, 79
proteins, ix, 35, 36, 37, 40, 43, 45, 46, 48, 57, 58, 62, 63, 66, 69, 72, 73, 85
proximal, xi, 47, 199, 202, 203, 205, 208, 212, 214
pseudo, 126
psychobiology, 197
psychological, 126, 185, 196, 223
psychological processes, 223
psychology, 113, 191, 196, 197
psychophysics, 12
psychophysiological, 223
psychophysiology, 242
psychotropic drug, 174
psychotropic drugs, 174
public, 75, 123
pulse, 5, 11, 12, 17, 19, 21, 22, 23, 70, 166
pulses, 16
Purkinje cells, 83, 85
putrescine, 59, 77
pyramidal, 82, 166
pyramidal cells, 82, 166
pyrimidine, 38

Q

quanta, 11, 12
quantum, 161, 165, 190
quantum mechanics, 165

R

race, 8, 9
radiation, viii, 33, 35, 40, 41, 49, 50
radical, 34, 52, 84
radiotherapy, viii, 33
radius, 141, 144
rain, 69, 71, 83, 115, 161, 175, 189, 193
random, x, 2, 7, 26, 58, 92, 103, 137, 139, 142, 146, 148, 177, 182, 228
randomness, 235
range, 5, 9, 11, 12, 13, 15, 16, 18, 20, 60, 91, 118, 158, 176, 178, 192, 196, 224
raphe, 218
rat, ix, 31, 44, 48, 49, 50, 55, 56, 57, 58, 59, 60, 61, 62, 63, 64, 65, 67, 68, 69, 70, 71, 72, 73, 74, 77, 78, 84, 85, 86, 205, 208, 217, 218, 219
rating scale, 228
ratings, 226, 230
rats, ix, 58, 59, 60, 65, 66, 67, 69, 74, 75, 77, 78, 80, 82, 84, 85, 119, 128, 133, 202, 206, 207, 208, 209, 210, 211, 214, 216, 217, 218
reaction time, 6
reactive oxygen species (ROS), 34, 35, 37, 38, 39, 40

reactivity, 211, 215
reading, 134, 202
real time, 164, 176
reality, 31, 125, 158
reasoning, 223
recall, x, 109, 110, 112, 113, 122, 123, 133
receptors, 3, 9, 72, 83, 132
reciprocity, 154
recognition, x, 107, 109, 110, 112, 113, 122, 124, 130, 131, 133, 166, 209, 237
recollection, x, 109, 110, 111, 112, 113, 114, 115, 116, 117, 119, 120, 122, 123, 124, 125, 126, 127, 128, 130, 133
recombination, 39, 40, 52, 53, 55, 171
reconstruction, x, 125, 137, 142, 146, 147, 154, 166
recovery, 4, 16, 20, 30, 38, 67, 68, 70, 77, 78, 86, 132, 219
recovery processes, 4, 20
recruiting, 175, 179
rectification, 16, 18, 19, 22
recycling, 9
reduction, 19, 43, 45, 209, 217, 218, 226, 235
reflection, 6
reflexes, 158, 209
refractory, 89
regeneration, 76, 83
regional, 30, 131, 155, 231, 242
regression, 25, 94, 95, 103, 104
regression line, 94, 95, 103, 104
regular, 37, 228
regulation, 37, 41, 44, 45, 48, 52, 55, 73, 168, 217, 218, 239
rehydration, 79
relationship, 3, 4, 6, 11, 44, 50, 125, 132, 164, 170, 219, 235, 243
relationships, 158
relevance, 11, 53, 126, 216
reliability, 31
remyelination, 83
reoxygenation, 59, 61, 62, 63, 64, 65, 71
repair, viii, 33, 35, 37, 38, 39, 40, 42, 43, 45, 46, 47, 48, 50, 51, 52, 53, 54, 55, 56, 70, 76, 83, 85, 86
repair system, 42, 43
reperfusion, viii, 33, 42, 58, 60, 67, 68, 73
repetitions, 117
replacement, 85
replication, 35, 36, 38, 43, 46, 51, 53, 54, 56
repression, 52
research, vii, x, 109, 127, 160, 161, 162, 163, 171, 193, 194, 195, 225, 226, 239, 240, 241
researchers, 163, 178
resection, 84
residual error, 15
resistance, 43, 71, 78, 177, 211
resolution, 2, 5, 6, 14, 15, 18, 24, 26, 27, 28, 138, 154, 156, 163, 176, 191, 225, 229
resources, 215, 239, 240
respiration, 39, 40
respiratory, 74
response, xi, 158, 163, 166, 167, 176, 199, 200, 201, 202, 203, 205, 207, 208, 209, 210, 212, 213, 214, 215, 217
response time, 4, 12, 15
restoration, 3, 60, 76
retardation, 50
retention, 114, 126, 173
retention interval, 114
retina, 3, 10, 31, 52, 193
retinoblastoma, 37, 46
retrograde amnesia, 118, 119, 121, 129, 131, 132
retrograde amnesia., 129
Reynolds, 82, 84, 85, 190
rhythm, 191, 195, 197, 226, 235, 238
rhythms, 195, 229, 232, 245
ribose, 40, 42, 49
ribosomes, 80
right hemisphere, 240
right visual field, 150, 152
risk, 55, 213
risks, 36
rodent, 76, 83
rodents, 69, 111, 112
rods, 31
room temperature, 61, 62, 79
Rössler, 162
Royal Society, 186, 190, 197
Russian, 168, 185, 186, 189, 192, 193, 197

S

S phase, 37, 43, 46
saccadic eye movement, 191
sadness, xii, 221, 224, 226, 227, 228, 230, 231, 232, 234, 235, 237, 238, 239, 240
safety, 209, 238
saline, 45, 60, 61, 77, 78, 211
salt, 60
sample, 26, 143
sampling, 13, 89, 161, 178
satisfaction, 225

saturation, 11
scaling, 7
scalp, x, 77, 106, 137, 138, 139, 143, 150, 155, 156, 164, 177
schema, 117
schizophrenic, 192
school, 168
science, 48, 130, 157, 160, 187, 189, 194
scientific, 158, 186, 195
scientific knowledge, 158
scientific theory, 186
sclerosis, 2, 30, 31, 34
scores, ix, 75, 78, 79, 80, 231
search, x, 76, 103, 106, 109, 110, 130, 138, 142, 151, 152, 162, 194, 204
searches, 138
searching, 142, 165
segmentation, 178, 180, 186, 187, 192, 193, 196
segregation, 110, 116, 117, 122, 123, 124, 126
seizure, vii, x, 87, 88, 96, 97, 98, 100, 101, 103, 104, 105, 106, 107
seizures, 88, 89, 105, 107, 108
selective attention, 223
selective serotonin reuptake inhibitor, 203
selenium, 77
self, 82, 83, 85, 155, 189, 196, 228, 242
self-organization, 166, 170, 186, 187, 192
self-organizing, 176
self-renewal, 82, 83
self-report, 226, 228, 231, 235, 236
semantic, 111, 117, 123, 126, 132, 134, 243
semantic categorization, 126
semantic memory, 111, 123, 132, 134
senescence, 35
sensation, 203, 213
sensations, 201, 202
sensing, 193
sensitivity, 24, 41, 58, 73, 100, 154, 211
sensitization, 210, 211, 216, 217
sensor proteins, 37
sensorimotor cortex, 194
sensory modality, 171
separation, 103, 104
sequelae, 58
series, 5, 13, 17, 18, 19, 20, 24, 26, 37, 76, 92, 105, 112, 159, 175, 176, 179, 187, 193, 196, 222, 228, 230, 234, 235, 236
serine, 36, 41
serotonergic, 212
serotonin, 203, 204, 219
serum, 59, 62, 70, 78
services, iv
shape, 7, 21, 31, 55, 79, 93
shares, 212
shock, 207, 208, 210, 211, 218
shocks, 208, 210
short period, 167
shortness of breath, 200
short-term, 170, 184, 195
short-term memory, 170
shoulders, 202
SI, xi, xii, 30, 155, 221, 226, 230, 232, 234, 235, 236, 237, 238, 239, 240, 241
sign, 5, 12, 105
signal transduction, 37, 38
signaling, 34, 35, 36, 38, 41, 43, 45, 47
signaling pathway, 34, 35, 41
signaling pathways, 34, 35
signalling, 48, 52, 189
signals, vii, viii, x, xi, 1, 2, 3, 5, 6, 7, 10, 12, 13, 14, 15, 17, 18, 19, 20, 22, 23, 24, 25, 26, 27, 29, 31, 36, 53, 83, 84, 87, 94, 104, 106, 107, 151, 153, 165, 174, 176, 199, 203, 205, 206, 207, 215, 222, 223, 224, 229, 231, 236, 237, 245
significance level, 233
signs, 101
similarity, 22, 92, 240
simulation, xi, 7, 26, 137, 142, 143, 144, 145, 153, 154, 155, 181
sine, 143
Singapore, 185, 190
singular, 91, 92, 142, 144, 145, 146, 147, 148, 150, 151, 169
sites, 37, 41, 62, 78, 117, 174, 228, 231, 235, 236, 237, 238
skin, 60
skull fracture, 77
sleep, 166, 192
social, 117, 126, 130, 200
social cognition, 117
social perception, 130
social performance, 200
society, 187
sodium, 61, 77, 83
sodium dodecyl sulfate (SDS), 61
software, 6, 21, 62, 65, 153, 185
solution, 166, 169
somatic, 202, 203
somatosensory, 196
sounds, 188, 208, 210, 211

South Carolina, 194
space-time, 172, 173
spatial, vii, x, 2, 3, 15, 21, 27, 28, 29, 30, 37, 92, 109, 110, 112, 113, 119, 124, 125, 129, 132, 137, 138, 139, 142, 143, 145, 146, 147, 148, 153, 154, 158, 170, 171, 173, 175, 176, 189, 222, 225
spatial learning, 132
spatial memory, 124
spatial representations, vii
spatiotemporal, 160, 161, 174, 190
specialization, 116, 135, 224
species, 34, 38, 224, 239
specificity, vii, viii, 1, 25, 29, 57, 100, 114, 196, 202
spectral analysis, 3, 225
spectrophotometric, 60
spectrophotometric method, 60
spectrum, 3, 6
speech, 174, 189
speed, 178, 179
S-phase, 36, 46, 51, 56
spheres, 79, 143
spinal cord, 76, 84, 86
spinal cord injury, 76
stability, 40, 51, 55, 158, 179
stabilization, 48, 118, 158, 190
stages, 4, 5, 16, 71, 83, 120, 121, 167, 173, 178, 202
stainless steel, 77
standard deviation (STD), 92, 93, 95, 96, 97, 100, 103, 230, 231
Standards, 49
stars, 3
statistical analysis, 105, 232
statistics, 25, 100, 101, 166, 172, 229
steel, 77
Stem cell, 82
stem cell lines, 86
stem cells, 76, 77, 82, 83, 85
sterile, 77
Stimuli, vi, 20, 221, 227, 228
stimulus, 2, 3, 5, 6, 8, 9, 10, 12, 13, 14, 15, 16, 17, 19, 20, 21, 22, 23, 24, 30, 31, 116, 122, 123, 125, 150, 158, 159, 165, 170, 177, 188, 189, 201, 202, 205, 206, 207, 209, 210, 214, 215, 228, 237, 238, 239
stochastic, 181, 182, 183, 190, 222
storage, 31, 117, 118
strategic, 116, 127
strategic planning, 116
strategies, x, 77, 85, 109, 110, 117, 134, 187, 205, 208, 213
strategy use, 206
stream of consciousness, 185
strength, 13, 25, 168, 207, 210
stress, 34, 42, 44, 46, 48, 49, 51, 54, 55, 56, 164, 171, 176, 200, 203, 209, 210, 211, 212, 216, 217, 218
stress level, 210
stressful events, xi, 199
stressors, xi, 199, 215, 216
striatum, 82, 86, 132
stroke, 34, 49, 53
structural equation model, 24, 28, 181
structural equation modeling, 24
students, 153
subcortical structures, 209, 224, 239
subcutaneous (SC), 182, 183
subjective, x, 96, 109, 110, 117, 125, 126, 153, 159, 163, 174, 176, 200, 201, 203, 224, 226, 228
subjective experience, 176, 224
substantia nigra, 48
substrates, xi, 41, 127, 161, 199, 202, 204, 212, 213, 214, 215, 216, 218, 224, 239, 245
subtraction, 179, 186
subventricular zone, 76, 83
sucrose, 78
suicide, 34
sulfate, 61
Sun, 6, 33, 50, 72, 191
superoxide, 34, 37, 71
superposition, 2, 169
supply, 17, 58
supply chain, 17
suppression, 43, 47, 174, 211
suppressor, 41, 46
surgery, 60, 88, 105
surgical, 88, 89
survival, viii, 34, 52, 54, 56, 58, 60, 63, 76, 83, 84, 213, 224, 239
surviving, ix, 60, 67, 69, 75, 80, 82
suspensions, 83
suture, 60
swallowing, 171
sweat, 201
swelling, 58
switching, 215
symbolic, 161, 162, 164, 191, 239
symbols, 12, 162, 176, 192
symmetry, 159
sympathetic, 54, 56, 202
symptoms, 200

synapse, 72
synapses, 16, 158, 163, 187, 217
synaptic plasticity, 195
synaptic vesicles, 31
synchronization, xi, xii, 159, 164, 166, 174, 179, 181, 182, 183, 190, 193, 197, 221, 222, 223, 225, 226, 227, 229, 230, 232, 233, 235, 236, 237, 238, 239, 240, 241, 242, 243, 244
Synchronization Index, xi, 221, 240
synchronous, 138, 139, 140, 141, 145, 148, 151, 152, 166, 172, 177, 181, 191, 229
syndrome, 42
synergetics, 162, 191
synthesis, 37, 38, 40, 63, 71, 133, 174, 188, 209, 242
systematic, 173
systems, xi, xii, 20, 26, 28, 29, 35, 39, 40, 43, 110, 111, 125, 131, 132, 133, 134, 160, 161, 162, 164, 177, 185, 186, 187, 190, 196, 199, 204, 208, 213, 215, 216, 217, 221, 222, 223, 224, 225, 226, 227, 229, 235, 241, 242, 243, 244

T

T lymphocyte, 74
T lymphocytes, 74
tachycardia, 212
tactile, 209, 212
tangles, 50
targets, 43, 53, 97
task conditions, 160
task demands, 116
task performance, 242
technicians, 96
technological, 27
technology, 178, 181
telangiectasia, 36, 41, 42, 44, 48, 49, 51, 52
temperature, 60, 61, 62, 79
temporal, vii, viii, ix, x, 1, 2, 3, 5, 8, 10, 11, 12, 13, 14, 15, 18, 19, 21, 24, 25, 26, 27, 57, 60, 69, 108, 109, 110, 112, 115, 116, 119, 121, 123, 124, 125, 126, 127, 128, 130, 131, 132, 133, 134, 135, 137, 138, 141, 154, 155, 158, 159, 161, 164, 169, 170, 171, 174, 175, 177, 182, 187, 190, 191, 196, 209, 222, 229, 231, 236, 238
temporal lobe, 108, 119, 121, 128, 130, 131, 132, 133, 134, 209
territory, 205
Tesla, 2
testis, 56
thalamus, 209
theoretical, 7, 17, 154, 155, 159, 179, 195, 223, 227, 236, 240
theory, xi, 29, 92, 107, 117, 118, 119, 120, 130, 134, 140, 142, 157, 159, 160, 163, 164, 166, 167, 168, 169, 185, 186, 188, 191, 193, 194, 196, 197, 201, 209, 224, 226, 242, 243, 244
therapeutic, vii, viii, 34, 76, 203
therapy, 82, 85, 243
thermal, 35, 166
thermodynamics, 162
theta, xii, 186, 221, 225, 226, 229, 231, 235, 236, 237, 238, 242, 243
theta band, 238
theta waves, xii, 221
thinking, 161, 189, 193, 195
threat, 131, 202, 204, 205, 216
threatened, 202
threatening, xi, 199, 202, 203, 207, 209, 214, 216
threats, 203, 204
three-dimensional, 28, 138
threonine, 36
threshold, 12, 92, 229
thresholds, 11, 12, 181, 182, 207, 209
throat, 202
thymocytes, 74
Ti, 167
tiger, 218
time, vii, x, 1, 2, 3, 4, 5, 6, 7, 9, 10, 12, 13, 14, 15, 16, 17, 18, 19, 20, 21, 23, 24, 25, 26, 29, 31, 45, 52, 54, 58, 59, 60, 61, 62, 63, 65, 66, 67, 69, 87, 91, 92, 93, 94, 95, 96, 97, 99, 103, 104, 105, 109, 110, 112, 113, 117, 118, 119, 120, 121, 125, 127, 132, 138, 140, 141, 143, 145, 146, 147, 148, 153, 155, 158, 159, 161, 163, 164, 165, 167, 169, 170, 171, 172, 173, 175, 176, 178, 179, 180, 181, 182, 183, 187, 190, 191, 195, 196, 197, 200, 205, 206, 207, 211, 215, 216, 222, 223, 227, 228, 230, 235, 236, 242
time lags, 25
time resolution, 5, 14
time series, 24, 26, 92, 105, 187, 222, 235, 236
timing, 27, 169, 188
tissue, x, 42, 45, 51, 60, 61, 67, 76, 77, 79, 81, 83, 84, 86, 87, 121
tolerance, 212, 217
tonic, 9, 28, 83, 205, 212, 214
topographic, 132, 154, 164
Topoisomerase, 74
topological, 172, 184
topology, 97

toxic, 34
toxicity, viii, 33, 53, 72
toxins, 35
tracking, 178
trade, 27
trade-off, 27
training, 96, 97, 98, 99, 210, 217
transactions, 190
transcription, 35, 36, 39, 41, 42, 49, 53, 55, 58, 72
transcription factor, 36, 41, 49, 72
transcription factors, 36, 49, 72
transcriptional, 34, 36, 55
transducer, 5, 41
transduction, 3, 30, 37, 38
transection, 130
transfer, 83, 138, 139, 140, 141, 142, 147, 148
transferrin, 59, 77
transformation, 36, 43, 50, 231
transgenic, 42
transgenic mice, 42
transition, 12, 36, 46, 164, 168, 172, 177, 178, 183, 192
transition period, 168, 178, 183
transitions, 160, 161, 171, 177, 190
translation, 55, 58
translational, 34
transmission, 25, 36, 175, 186
transmits, 159
transparency, 6
transparent, 174, 209, 216
transplant, 83
transplantation, 76, 77, 78, 82, 83, 85, 86
transport, 86
trauma, 34, 58, 77, 86, 200, 216, 218
traumatic brain injury (TBI) , vii, ix, 75, 76, 77, 78, 80, 82, 83, 84, 85
traumatic events, 213
travel, 110, 113, 119, 127
treatment, 210
trend, 95, 104, 106, 242
trial, 141, 142, 148, 182, 212, 217, 228
trial and error, 141, 142, 148
triggers, 50, 63, 72, 200, 209
tumor, 41, 46
tumors, 43
tumour, 130
turbulence, 162
two-dimensional, 224
two-way, 212

U

ubiquitin, 41
ubiquitous, 58
UK, 130, 132
ultraviolet, 35
unconditioned, xi, 199, 201, 203, 204, 206, 207, 208, 212, 213, 214, 215
unconditioned response, 208
undifferentiated, 82
undifferentiated cells, 82
uniform, 7, 21, 22, 83, 144, 181, 222
uniformity, 170
unilateral, 30, 58, 73, 128, 134
United States, 185, 188, 190, 191, 193
unpredictability, 235, 237
upper alpha band, 242
URL, 187, 189
UV, 35, 37, 62
UV light, 37

V

vaginal, 59
valence, xii, 120, 130, 221, 224, 225, 226, 227, 230, 235, 236, 239, 240, 241, 242
validation, 96, 97, 98, 216
validity, 98, 115, 231
values, 12, 19, 20, 22, 45, 63, 65, 67, 69, 91, 92, 95, 97, 103, 104, 105, 142, 145, 147, 148, 151, 174, 178, 179, 181, 182, 183, 208, 224, 226, 230, 231, 232
variability, 20, 31, 179, 189
variable, 8, 25, 38, 160, 218
variables, 7, 124, 162, 172, 229
variance, 23, 24, 31, 79, 93, 230
variation, 3, 19, 22, 54, 115, 238, 241
vascular, 21
vasculature, 4
vector, 24, 25, 29, 92, 97, 142
vehicles, 84
vein, 60, 161
ventricle, 128
ventricular, 52, 82
ventricular zone, 82
versatility, 95
vertical integration, 237
vessels, 17, 28, 30
victims, 239

video, 239
virtual reality, 125
virtual reality (VR), 125
viscera, 205, 209
viscosity, 162
visible, 14, 81, 95, 206
vision, 12, 28, 30, 185, 200, 227, 228, 231
visual, viii, 1, 2, 10, 12, 20, 21, 22, 28, 30, 31, 89, 103, 124, 128, 150, 151, 154, 161, 171, 174, 189, 190, 191, 196, 223, 229, 237, 238, 242, 243
visual acuity, 150
visual area, 22, 28, 31, 124
visual attention, 190
visual field, 150, 152, 171
visual images, 174
visual perception, 11, 30, 223
visual processing, viii, 1, 10, 12
visual stimuli, 2, 21, 174, 196
visual stimulus, 237
visualization, vii, 63, 95, 166
voiding, 206
vulnerability, 49

W

waking, 171, 242
walking, 171
Washington, 33, 194
water, 59, 60, 61, 112, 170
water maze, 112
Watson, 40, 130, 134
wavelet, 24, 31, 187, 230
wavelets, 107
wealth, 113
web, 35
wells, 79
white matter, 82
William James, 161, 190, 201
windows, 93, 97, 103, 178, 181, 182
Wistar rats, 77
withdrawal, 223, 225, 226, 239, 240, 241
work, 41, 44
workers, 224, 236
working memory, 116, 127, 129, 131, 133, 134
workspace, 186
worry, 200
writing, 187

X

X-axis, 183
X-irradiation, 50
X-linked, 46
x-ray, 52, 54
X-rays, 52

Y

Y-axis, 183
yield, 78, 120, 162

Z

zygomatic, 60
zygomatic arch, 60